Aging is a Group-Selected Adaptation

Theory, Evidence, and Medical Implications

T0074640

Aging is a Group-Selected Adaptation

Theory, Evidence, and Medical Implications

Josh Mitteldorf, PhD.

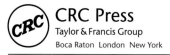

CRC Press
Taylor & Francis Group
Boca Raton London New York

CRC Press is an imprint of the
Taylor & Francis Group, an **informa** business

A SCIENCE PUBLISHERS BOOK

Cover Acknowledgement: Cover art by Doris Lane Grey "Old Darwin and Young Darwin, Tortoise and Hare".

CRC Press
Taylor & Francis Group
6000 Broken Sound Parkway NW, Suite 300
Boca Raton, FL 33487-2742

First issued in paperback 2020

© 2017 by Taylor & Francis Group, LLC
CRC Press is an imprint of Taylor & Francis Group, an Informa business

No claim to original U.S. Government works

ISBN-13: 978-1-4987-1528-7 (hbk)
ISBN-13: 978-0-367-78273-3 (pbk)

Library of Congress Cataloging-in-Publication Data

Names: Mitteldorf, Josh, author.
Title: Aging is a group-selected adaptation : theory, evidence, and medical implications / Josh Mitteldorf.
Description: Boca Raton, FL : CRC Press/Taylor & Francis Group, [2016] | "A Science Publishers book." | Includes bibliographical references and index.
Identifiers: LCCN 2016029598| ISBN 9781498715287 (hardback : alk. paper) | ISBN 9781498715300 (e-book)
Subjects: | MESH: Aging--genetics | Adaptation, Physiological | Biological Evolution | Population Dynamics
Classification: LCC QP86 | NLM WT 104 | DDC 571.8/78--dc23
LC record available at https://lccn.loc.gov/2016029598

Visit the Taylor & Francis Web site at
http://www.taylorandfrancis.com

and the CRC Press Web site at
http://www.crcpress.com

Preface

During Orientation Week for Harvard freshmen, I learned this: The chapter is there for people who didn't read the chapter summary at the end. Later, in grad school, I learned that the journal article was written for people who didn't read the Abstract; and as a theorist, I extrapolated to deduce that the book is for people who didn't read the Preface.

We might stress-test this procedure by exploring limits to its domain of validity. Maybe the title is all we need to know. *Aging is a group-selected adaptation.* That thesis is indeed the core of this volume. It is preposterous, provocative, and pregnant with far-reaching implications.

The lion's share of my work has been devoted to substantiating the statement. First, evidence is adduced from every corner of biology, diverse lines of reasoning, all pointing to the same conclusion. Then, prevailing evolutionary theories of aging are examined and found wanting.

Why is adaptive aging excluded by evolutionary theory? The theoretical foundations of population genetics are deconstructed, until we arrive at the source of the belief that group selection is vanishingly weak (and at any rate far too weak to overcome individual selection against senescence).

Only when the fact of adaptive aging is firmly established and the theoretical landscape is thoroughly depopulated do I venture to speculate about a replacement theory that might suggest an evolutionary history for what we see and provide a plausible selective mechanism.

In the final two chapters, I propose a beginning toward a long process of re-evaluation, following the consequences of a new idea out into the larger realms of evolutionary theory, medical paradigms, the place of humanity in the global ecosystem, and the future of the planet.

What is the Evidence Pointing to an Adaptive Origin for Aging?

Most of the interventions currently known to extend lifespan in lab animals are based on *hormesis*. That is to say, the body overreacts to stress by activating a response mechanism that not only abate the insult but, surprisingly, make the body healthier and better-defended for a longer lifespan in the presence of stressors than it was without stressors. Familiar examples of stressors that extend lifespan include caloric restriction and exercise. Less familiar but also well-documented are heat shock, physical trauma, radiation, and powerful oxidants in small doses. Extension of life in the presence of insults is only possible because the body is holding some of the protective response in reserve, undeployed when the body is fully fed and unstressed. It follows that the body is not evolved to live as long as possible. This suggests a picture in which the death rate is being modulated for homeostasis, with senescence functioning as a complement to environmental hardships.

"Aging genes" have been discovered in every model organism in which they have been sought. By "aging genes" I mean that when the gene is mutated so as to be ineffective, or excised with gene editing chemistry, or silenced with RNAi, the animal lives longer. Some of these genes have pleiotropic benefits that might explain their presence within the framework of classical evolutionary theory. Some do not.

What is more, some of these genes have an ancient origin. They have homologs in organisms across the tree of life, going back to the simplest eukaryotes. Of course, there are very many genes that have been conserved since the origin of eukaryotic life, but they all have core metabolic functions that are essential to life. Natural selection has treated aging with the same conservatism as these other essential biological functions.

At the heart of classical evolutionary theory is Fisher's Fundamental Theorem. The theorem offers a test for determining whether a trait has been subject to affirmative selection pressure or whether it is a happenstance of genetic drift. The criterion is called *additive genetic variance*. The additive genetic variance of senescent mortality is low, and becomes ever lower at advanced age. This implies that aging is no accident, but the result of selection. Death has not been left to chance.

In semelparous organisms, there is also clear biochemical evidence of programmed death, and circumstantial evidence that death is not a necessary cost of a burst of fertility. Some mechanisms of death in semelparous organisms have homologs in iteroparous species.

Single-cell protists are subject to two modes of programmed death. This was not predicted by classical evolutionary theory; in fact, biologists quite broadly believed (until recently) that senescence in one-celled organisms was a logical impossibility. But we now know that

- When starved, yeast cells are subject to apoptosis. The majority will fall on their swords, turning themselves into food so that the remaining minority might have a better chance of survival.
- Ciliates are subject to cellular senescence through telomere shortening. They withhold telomerase during replication, allowing telomeres to shorten with each cell division. The effect of this is to enforce an imperative to share genes, because it is only during sex (conjugation) that telomere length is restored.

Both apoptosis and cellular senescence appear in multi-celled eukaryotes, including you and me, and both mechanisms play a role in the dynamics of human senescence.

What is Wrong with the Current Theories?

Many biologists continue to believe that aging is dictated by physical law, traceable ultimately to the increase of entropy demanded by the Second Law of Thermodynamics. But the Second Law applies only to closed systems, not interacting with the outside world. Living organisms are open systems; their essence is to extract free energy from the environment and to excrete entropy with their waste. If living things were subject to the Second Law, then life would be impossible, because there would be no growth or evolution of increased complexity or accumulation of information. This reasoning has been appreciated at least since the mid nineteenth century, and today's evolutionary biologists generally understand that aging must command an evolutionary explanation; but among gerontologists and other scientists, the misconception continues.

All prevailing evolutionary theories are based on a low (or vanishing) cost of aging in the wild. But field studies have consistently revealed that senescence takes a substantial bite out of fitness, typically 20 to 30% – far too large to be explained by genetic load or, for that matter, many of the tradeoff theories.

Most prevailing theories are based on explicit assumptions about constraints that force natural selection to accept shorter lifespans when longer ones would support higher individual fitness. However, when we consider the broad variety of aging phenotypes in nature, each one of these constraints is violated in turn. There are a few animals and many plants that do not age at all; there are organisms that experience mortality acceleration and mortality deceleration; there are species that can revert from mature to larval form, aging backwards; many more species are characterized by long periods of "negative senescence", in which mortality decreases steadily while fertility increases. The diversity of aging schedules in nature tells us that there are no absolute constraints, and casts doubts on particular constraints that are postulated in support of particular theories.

"Antagonistic pleiotropy" underlies a number of popular theories based on tradeoffs, and while there is evidence for tradeoffs in some cases, there are many other cases where aging seems gratuitous, in the sense that no tradeoff has yet been identified.

The most clearly formulated of all theories of aging hypothesizes specifically that aging derives from the necessity of rationing a limited supply of caloric energy. The body must choose between expending energy on fertility in the present or diverting the same energy for the molecular repair functions that are necessary to maintain the body's integrity for the future. This theory is the one most clearly falsified by experiment. In particular, animals that are starved take in much less total caloric energy, and yet they live longer than animals that have plenty to eat. The theory also predicts a cost of reproduction in the form of decreased life expectancy; but multiple studies in humans and zoo animals have failed to detect a negative association between realized fertility and longevity.

Programmed Aging Runs Afoul of Theory, but that Theory was Already Tottering

For aging to evolve as an adaptation in its own right requires violation of fundamental notions of population genetic theory which have been taken as solid for about 80 years. But the body of classical evolutionary theory is not without its critics. Some scientific luminaries have written that evolutionary theory is overdue for a workover if not an overhaul. Some great phenomena of nature that classical population genetics cannot explain include

- the evolution of sex (especially the maintenance of dioecious sex at a fitness cost of a full factor of two)
- the maintenance of diversity
- the hierarchical structure of the genome, with hox genes turning on whole suites of downstream genes
- other evolvability adaptations
- epigenetic inheritance
- horizontal gene transfer

How big a scandal would it be, then, to add the evolution of senescence to such a list?

What is the Least Radical Theory that Might Account for Aging as an Adaptation?

I propose a Demographic Theory of Aging. Population dynamics can provide a swift and efficient mode of natural selection at the group level, handily able to compete with individual selection for higher fertility, and often pushing in the opposite direction. If all deaths were circumstantial, then populations would grow exponentially until overcrowding becomes fatal to all. During famines and epidemics, everyone dies at once. Aging contributes to the stability of ecosystems by providing a steady, predictable death rate. Without aging, deaths would be tightly clustered and populations would rise and fall chaotically, risking extinction. This is selection not just at the level of the deme or community, but ecosystem-level selection. Natural selection on the level of ecosystems is classically implausible– many would say absolutely proscribed by theory. But I demonstrate with simulation (for simple cases) that population dynamics can be quite as strong a selective force as the most direct individual selection for survival and reproduction.

There are other communal benefits of aging that accrue to the population, and the best recognized of these are based on evolvability. Populations with senescence have greater diversity and shorter generation times, other things being equal. I agree that evolvability is important, but quantitative numerical models confirm what population geneticists have long told us: the benefit for evolvability is too weak and too slow to compete with individual selection against senescence. However, once the population dynamic mechanisms (from the Demographic Theory) have dulled the sharp edge of individual selection, then selection for evolvability can take its place as an important evolutionary force.

Maintenance of diversity was the greatest question that continued to mystify Darwin throughout his career. We now have some answers that were unavailable to Darwin, though I daresay a full solution to the mystery remains elusive to this day. Aging may be catalogued as contributing to the maintenance of diversity that is essential for persistence of life in the long-term, taking its place alongside phenotypic plasticity, co-evolution, assortative mating, and sex itself.

Some Implications of Adaptive Aging

Here is where I invite you to imagine along with me. The implications of this new paradigm for aging extend widely into biological and medical sciences, and beyond into sociology, politics and philosophy. I can only begin to sample the directions that creative thought might pursue.

Having made great inroads in the 20th Century against infectious disease and traumatic injury, medical research is now focused on the Big Three diseases of old age: cardiovascular disease, cancer, and dementia. The paradigm and methodology of the field continues to be: first diagnose what has gone wrong with the body, then guide the metabolism back on track. But this approach has been less effective for the Big Three. Now we can begin to see the reason: When people at advanced age fall prey to disease, they are precisely on track, performing as they were evolved to perform the deadly business of metabolic dismemberment. We seek in vain for what has "gone wrong" in the body, because the body is performing exactly as intended*. Eating organic vegetables, taking statin drugs and irradiating tumors all have this in common: none of them addresses the underlying, programmed failures that make the body exponentially more vulnerable to disease with each passing year.

The aging program is accomplished through signals in the blood and transcription factors that control gene expression. When we understand aging on this level, we will be able to turn it off, and revert the Big Three diseases to the modest risk levels encountered by a twenty-year-old.

In just the last few hundred years, humans have come to dominate the planet's ecology, and we have done this via pursuit of our individual self-interests. But tragedies of the commons loom in plain sight, the predictable result of an imbalance between individual and communal adaptations. We see the consequences in the form of depleted fisheries, global climate change, collapse of biodiversity, and the absurd mundanity of traffic congestion.

On my computer screen, entire ecosystems flash in and out of existence. One of the quickest ways to destroy an ecosystem is for its top predator to lapse into unrestrained growth, supported by unsustainable exploitation of the trophic base. In agent-based simulations, populations explode and crash within the space of just a few generations. The possibility that these models may offer glimpses of our human future may be too horrific to contemplate, but we neglect it at our peril.

Got it? Is there Still a Reason to Read the Book?

It has been 50 years since I was a Harvard freshman, and what have I learned in the interim? That the Preface and the Abstract and the Chapter Summary are fine ways to add twigs and whole branches to the tree of knowledge. But to be a scientist

---

* See note on teleologic language, p 3.

means to be open to the possibility that, from time to time, the tree must be uprooted and replanted. If the operation is successful, almost all the leaves and branches survive intact, and maintain the same relationship to one another...but they are part of a different tree, growing in a different place.

The latter is a process that requires thoughtful re-evaluation. For me, it has meant allowing time to test new ideas against many other things I know, going for long walks in the woods, talking to colleagues, asking myself what I really believe and why I believe it.

In this spirit, I invite you to savor the chapters that follow. Let's start digging.

Josh Mitteldorf
Philadelphia, PA
July, 2016

Acknowledgments

This book is the culmination of my nineteen years' journey into evolutionary research. I came as a carpetbagger in 1996 and was immediately welcomed by an online community, precursor to the *list serve*, in a time entirely innocent of spam. But my ideas were too radical and my credentials too foreign to be accepted for publication. It was David Sloan Wilson who mentored me in my early forays into the field, co-authored my first paper, and shepherded it through peer review. He introduced me to Charles Goodnight and John Pepper, who have become long-term colleagues and allies in our quest to make the world safe for group selection. Michael Rosenzweig was another early mentor and had the courage and vision to accept my Demographic Theory for publication in his journal, *Evolutionary Ecology Research*. In a similar vein, it was Aubrey de Grey who welcomed me into the world of radical gerontology, taught me a great deal, and offered me a venue for two of my early publications (though he did not and does not to this day support my primary thesis that aging is a group-selected adaptation).

My teachers over the years included Warren Ewens and Paul Sniegowski, who patiently trained me in population genetics. Vladimir Skulachev reached out to offer me encouragement and advice early in my biology career. Uri Wilensky has been a lifelong friend and colleague, since long before our career paths centered on agent-based modeling. Nick Fisher has been my friend since pre-school, has encouraged my better angels at key points in my career, and introduced me to the most prominent aging theorist of the previous generation. Justin Travis, Calvin Dytham, and Peter Taylor all contributed to my development as a modeler. Greg Fahy has offered me connections, publication opportunities, and a trove of medical knowledge that is off the beaten path. Jeff Bowles contributed creative insights into the aging metabolism. Gustavo Barja, Ted Goldsmith, and Giacinto Libertini paved the way for me with early publications on programmed aging. Dario Valenzano, Cynthia Kenyon, Dale Bredesen, and Len Guarente all welcomed me to their labs and offered invaluable feedback on my thinking.

Among people who critiqued and corrected this volume, highest honors go to Meng-Qiu Dong and George Martin, who offered references, perspectives, and even sound advice. I received feedback on style from Enid Kassner and Dorion Sagan and on content from Alexei Sharov, Bill Andrews, Michael Fossel, Daniel Promislow, Steve Austad, João Pedro de Magalhães, Russell Bonduriansky, Bruce Ames, and Rhonda Patrick.

Thanks to all the above and nameless others from who have helped shape my thinking and encourage me on.

Foreword by Michael Rosenzweig

If you were to say that Natural Selection changes life for the good of the species, almost any biologist who specializes in evolution would make a fuss. "No, no, no!" you'd hear, "Natural Selection increases the fitness of individuals."

But what's the difference? If individuals are improving, isn't the species also improving? Not always. Consider the individuals of a predator species. If its individuals improve, they might entirely destroy their prey! What is good for the individual might exterminate the group. And so a paradox emerges.

Can it be resolved? Can Natural Selection improve the chances that our predator will behave prudently? Or like Samson, does Natural Selection doom it to topple the pillars of its temple and bring destruction down upon its head?

Getting evolution to produce individuals that age, and getting it to produce a prudent predator, turn out to be closely related problems. Both improve the likelihood that the group of individuals survives. That may sound like a wonderful idea but generations of evolutionists have resisted all the evidence that it exists because they could not come up with a mechanism to counteract the selfishness of natural selection. After all (p 167), "the impact of senescence on the individual is wholly detrimental, depleting its ability to survive and to reproduce."

But, dear biologists, hold onto your hats! "Evidence [suggests] that aging is chosen not despite its fatal consequences for the individual, but because of them" (p79). Ouch! This book will make your head explode. And the more you think you know about evolution, the greater the shrapnel field.

In science, eventually, facts rule. And during the past quarter century those facts have been piling up. Mitteldorf reviews them and treats them with dignity. They range from computer simulations — that pit prudence against selfishness — to the genetics and biochemistry of aging. And they amount to a body of evidence that declares (see p75), "Aging is an adaptation. Aging evolves."

Make no mistake. If you have come here to collect evidence and arguments against evolution, you are wasting your time. Mitteldorf does not argue against evolution and natural selection. Not at all. Instead he strengthens immeasurably the case for an alternative mechanism of evolution, i.e., group selection. Having a robust case for group selection means that evolutionists will be able to explain more of life's features. Some puzzles that have resisted even the cleverest wielders of natural selection will fall to the strokes of group selection. Foremost among them is surely the evolution of sex itself, which Mitteldorf discusses briefly.

Evolutionists have known about group selection for generations but have rejected it. They rejected it because individuals die faster than groups become extinct. So anything that led to a reduction in death rate would overwhelm any opposing gene that led to a smaller extinction rate. Case closed! Mind, too.

As if to make matters worse, the only accepted paper in favor of group selection (Lewontin & Dunn, 1960) modeled a system of semi-isolated mouse families and a somewhat weird allele-family called tailless. Most male mice homozygous for this allele have a fitness of zero; either they die before birth or are merely sterile. Heterozygotes do reproduce and the tailless allele they carry occurs in their offspring with a frequency of about 95% (instead of 50%). In other words, compared to wild types, tailless alleles enjoy a competitive advantage in fertilizing ova. Otherwise tailless would be eliminated by natural selection.

Tailless alleles are selfish in the extreme. Lewontin & Dunn noted that if the population of a typical mouse semi-isolate is small, tailless can destroy that population in one unlucky generation. With group extinction rates that high, group selection can assert itself. Tailless and the wild type both remain in the gene pool because group selection and natural selection are similarly influential.

As a graduate student, I remember reading Lewontin & Dunn in a study seminar. It was viewed as a special case, a case so difficult to achieve that it demonstrated the implausibility of group selection. We'd be just fine if we paid no further attention to group selection as long as we lived.

At about the same time, V. C. Wynne-Edwards published his massive tome mustering empirical case after empirical case of apparent prudence in wild animals. It had no mechanism and no math. So it inspired only our hoots and vilification. We students took an unspoken oath to ignore it.

In 1962 we were faced with the ultimate test. Richard Levins published his seminal paper on fitness in heterogeneous environments (Amer. Natur. 96: 361-373). We read it and discussed it and we agreed: Brilliant, yes, but his models of extended fitness sets relied on a tacit, unproven mechanism, namely, group selection. We swept that under the rug and carried on with the rest of the paper's glories.

Once, I challenged Levins face-to-face about his assumption of group selection and he brushed it aside. He was a Marxist even before he was scientist. So belief in group selection was integral to his mindset because, without group selection, Marxism would fail. Since that was unthinkable, group selection had to be real.

You get the picture: Two parties, one of true believers in group selection who had never subjected it to a scientific test; and the rest of us who believed just as strongly that it must not be taken seriously.

Now, half a century later and in my mid-seventies, I find myself writing a highly laudatory foreword for a book that culminates in the demonstration that group selection matters. When I was twenty-five, I might have used such a book to start a campfire. What happened?

Well, Josh Mitteldorf happened. And Greg Pollock, too. And a great deal of biochemistry that laid out the nuts and bolts of the aging process. Yet I confess that all the brilliant biochemistry in the world would not have helped me personally. First, I am biochemically illiterate; I leave that material entirely to others. But even if I did read biochemistry, it would not have changed my mind; I would have lumped all the biochemical advances as submicroscopic empirical examples to add to the unsatisfying Wynne-Edwards pile. I needed mechanism and even Richard Levins had not supplied it.

On 20 March 2000, I received an ms as editor-in-chief of *Evolutionary Ecology Research*. It was from Josh Mitteldorf, and it set me up for a personal intellectual revolution. It discussed the phenomenon of life span increase when calories are restricted, an important topic Josh reviews fully in the book. Then on 5 November 2002, I took the body blow that sent me reeling, i.e., the ms of "Ageing selected for its own sake". Heresy, pure heresy!

Thank heaven I always keep my science brain far away from my editor brain. As an evolutionist, I wanted to suppress this ms, but as an editor, I saw that it was courageous and I owed it a chance. And that's a good thing. Mitteldorf was working toward the missing part of group selection, its mechanism. It took me over a year to shed my prejudices but the paper made it through the usual gauntlet of academic review and was published (*Evol Ecol Res* 6: 937-953. 2004). It was followed by a daring theory that seals the deal: Chaotic population dynamics and the evolution of ageing (*Evol Ecol Res* 8: 561-574. 2006). Its full throated form emerges as the very thesis of this book (p4): "Aging and the regulated timing of death evolved for the purpose of stabilizing ecosystems."

Let me put it this way. Do you believe in population dynamics? Fine. Then you ought to realize that senescence is an adaptive consequence of 'variation in population size that is not wholly deterministic.' But we know of no species with wholly deterministic population sizes. Q.E.D.

You see why I warned you that this book will make your head explode?

While intransigence was being attacked from one side by Mitteldorf, it was also being pummeled on its other side by the independent studies of Gregory Pollock whose mss. I began to see on 11 June 2003 (On suicidal punishment among *Acromyrmex versicolor* cofoundresses: the disadvantage in personal advantage, *Evol Ecol Res* 6: 891-917 (2004) & 14: 951-971 (2012)). And then it was made to look foolish by the theoretical simulations of Simon and Nielsen (Numerical solutions and animations of group selection dynamics (*Evol Ecol Res* 14: 757-768 (2012)). My intransigence became acceptance, albeit with the emotional reluctance that follows when facts force one to discard a cherished belief.

What has happened here? Evolutionists are not being asked to relinquish their opinion that life span evolves. The evidence for that is overwhelming. They are, however, being shown that they must discard their belief that life span is an adaptation selected for by natural selection. Instead they must accept the likelihood that group selection does the job. Unwillingly and unwittingly, to keep our species alive we must all self-destruct by following a program that brings us to death on a schedule. Mouse or man; moth or mollusc; the schedule may be different but the end is the same, and it exists for the same reason, the good of the species.

Michael L. Rosenzweig
Ecology & Evolutionary Biology
University of Arizona
26 August 2016

Contents

Introduction

A Divergence of Theory and Evidence

"Aging as an adaptation" is not simply a new idea, a scientific revolution waiting to happen. It is an idea that has been considered and decisively rejected by generations of evolutionary scientists. You might say that in the evolutionary competition of ideas, selection (by scientists) has driven this species to the brink of extinction.

The reasons for this are sound. Aging is the opposite of fitness. Aging destroys first fertility, then viability. Genes that cause aging impose a selective cost on the bearer without conferring any benefit. So for the majority of evolutionary scientists who believe that individual selection is the only kind of selection there is, "aging as an adaptation" is an oxymoron.

From the perspective of the individual, affirmative selection for aging is a non-starter. In recent decades, there has been a growing, if controversial, movement to reconsider group selection as an evolutionary force. Can the idea of affirmative selection for aging be framed in the language of group selection? Not in an easy or obvious way.

Those who believe there is some merit in the idea of group selection usually ground their theory in the equation of Price [1, 2] which, in turn, is generalized from Hamilton's Rule [3, 4]. It was Hamilton (following Haldane [5]) who gave us the theoretical foundation for kin selection. Altruism can evolve to the extent that the benefit provided by a gene to other copies of that same gene in close relatives outweighs the fitness cost to the native copy of the gene at home. It is easy to understand, for example, why a mother bird might risk her life in defense of her hatchlings.

Price's contribution was to realize that external copies of the gene need not be in close relatives. A warrior might sacrifice himself for a tribe in which the gene for courage which he bears is shared sporadically through a larger group of indeterminate genetic relationship. The critical thing is that the total benefit to all of the copies of the gene for this trait outweighs the cost to the bearer of the gene for this trait. This is the substance of the Price Equation.

With Price as a foundation, Wilson developed a theory of Multilevel Selection that has become the standard alternative to purely individual selection [6]. Wilson formulated the useful but subtle notion of a "trait group," defined neither by kinship nor by locality but by Price's criterion exactly: *for a given altruistic behavior*, it is the set of individuals that stand to benefit from that behavior. It is the prevalence of the trait (and its genetic basis) within the trait group that is critically important.

The relevant "group" in group selection is not a geographic cluster nor a familial collective, but it is defined as the set of beneficiaries of the particular altruistic behavior in question.

In this model, an altruistic trait (which imposes fitness cost on its bearer) can be positively selected if its benefit is focused sufficiently on other bearers of the altruistic trait. But in the case of aging, the only benefit is to get out of the way, vacating a place in the niche which is no more likely to be filled by an altruist than by anyone else. In other words, the trait group for the trait of aging is far too large and the prevalence of aging in that group is not necessarily high. And worse: even if it could be guaranteed that the slot vacated by aging unto death is always filled by another individual that carries the aging gene, the result is only break-even, with no net benefit for prevalence of the aging gene. This reasoning constitutes a rigorous proof that aging (without pleiotropic benefit) cannot evolve as an adaptation on its own, within the framework of standard population genetic thinking, even as extended by Price.

Thus, even within the wing of the evolutionary community which embraces MLS, affirmative selection for aging is not easy to understand.

So why does the idea of "adaptive aging" refuse to die? The answer is that empirical science is shouting at us: aging has all the hallmarks of an adaptive trait, programmed into the genes. Laboratory manipulation of individual genes in model animals has been available since the 1980s, and the scientific community was not as stunned as it should have been to discover how easily lifespan of worms and flies can be extended, often by deletion of a single gene. Sometimes these genes were found to have countervailing (pleiotropic) benefits, but half of such genes had no identifiable benefit [7, 29]. What could we call these, but "aging genes"?

The genetic basis of aging is deeply conserved, with families of homologous genes that can be traced to the earliest eukaryotes. Of course, there are many other genes that have been conserved by evolution, but all of them serve a core purpose. All of them are essential for life. Evidently, natural selection has treated aging as an essential life function.

There are two mechanisms of programmed cell death in protists, both well-accepted to be adaptations shaped by natural selection. These are apoptosis and telomere attrition. Both these mechanisms have been preserved and modified over evolutionary time and both contribute to senescence in humans [30-36].

A great diversity of aging schedules has been found in nature, varying widely both in shape and duration. This attests to a feature under genetic control [37].

An accelerating cascade of experimental findings has affirmed the perspective that aging is "voluntary," in the sense that the body knows how to keep itself in a pristine state of repair, but chooses not to. Epigenetic programming changes with aging, and if we expected that protective signaling should be enhanced and repair ramped up with age, we would be in for a surprise. In fact, pro-inflammatory signaling (e.g., NFκB, TNF-α) increases with age, while protective enzymes like glutathione and SOD are dialed down with age. Epigenetic changes with age are exactly what we might expect a suicide program to look like.

After marginalizing the issue for decades, the community of biological scientists seems ready to embrace a debate on the gulf that now separates evolutionary theory from the genetics and biodemography of aging.

There are prominent biochemists and bench scientists who have been convinced by what they see in the laboratory that aging is an adaptation. Cynthia Kenyon made some of the earliest discoveries of single genes in lab worms that dramatically shorten lifespan; that is to say, when one of these genes is knocked out, the animal lives longer [7, 8]. Valter Longo is a microbiologist at USC who has demonstrated programmed death in yeast cells [9]. Vladimir Skulachev [10] is a senior biochemist of the University of Moscow who has written extensively on mechanisms of aging and programmed death. Dale Bredesen [11] is former director of the Buck Institute for Aging Research in California. Rafael de Cabo [12] heads a prominent research group at the National Institute on Aging. Maria Blasco and her colleagues at Spanish National Cancer Research Center have demonstrated that simple telomere erosion is a substantial factor in aging and that activating telomerase is a viable anti-aging strategy [13-15]. Greg Fahy is a biochemist at Twenty-First Century Medicine, long-time board member and former president of the American Aging Association, and author/editor of an encyclopedic book on The Future of Aging [16]. Kerry Kornfeld and his research group at Washington University in St Louis have elucidated pathways by which lifespan is regulated in *C. elegans* and identified pharmacological agents that extend lifespan [17, 18]. Tom Rando's lab at Stanford has pioneered the study of blood factors that control aging and has characterized an epigenetic "aging clock" [19]. Gustavo Barja and his research group at Complutense University in Madrid elucidated the reasons why free radicals have a double-edged relationship to aging [20, 21]. Bill Andrews identified the human telomerase gene while working at Geron Corp and has developed the most efficient cellular assays for telomerase [22, 23]. Dario Valenzano documented the first evidence for life extension from resveratrol supplementation in a vertebrate, while still a graduate student [24], and presently studies genetics of aging at the Max Planck Institute in Rostock. Justin Travis is a rising star in evolutionary ecology at University of Aberdeen [25]. Yaneer Bar-Yam is director of New England Complex Systems Institute [26]. John Pepper has written seminal papers demonstrating the profound impact of ecology on evolution and now studies cancer from an evolutionary perspective at National Institutes of Health [27]. Charles Goodnight (University of Vermont) developed some of the fundamental theory establishing the viability of multilevel selection [28]. These researchers and others have found evidence in their own research to convince them that aging has the genetic features of an evolutionary adaptation. Some of them have told me privately that they have been ignored, patronized, ridiculed, and censored when they write about aging as an adaptation.

A Crisis for Evolutionary Theory

If we collect all this evidence in one place and face it squarely, we must acknowledge a crisis for evolutionary theory. There is a deep disconnect between predictions and experiment. Aging is one of Michael Brooks's *13 Things that Don't Make Sense* [38]. "Why Do We Age?" is one of Sherratt and Wilkinson's "Big Questions in

Ecology" [39]. This is not an artifact that can be accommodated with a tweak of the theory or a footnote in the textbook. To reconcile the phenomenology of aging within evolutionary theory will require new foundations, new mechanisms, a fundamentally different model.

Not incidentally, standard population genetic theory is vulnerable in other respects and ripe for overhaul. The theory has been validated in many thousands of artificial selection experiments, but its validity in the wild has never been established. Large features of the biosphere that appear incompatible with classical evolutionary theory include dioecious sex, the maintenance of diversity, and the structure of the genome, manifestly optimized for evolvability. Prominent scientists who have called for an overhaul of evolutionary theory include Carl Woese [40], Lynn Margulis [41], Massimo Pigliucci [42], Eva Jablonka [43], James Shapiro [44], and Marc Kirchner [45].

The emphasis of the present volume is on the importance of population dynamics as a driver of selective local extinctions, the basis of a neglected evolutionary force. By itself, consideration of population dynamics will not resolve any of the above issues, nor even fully explain aging; however, consideration of population dynamics undermines the notion that natural selection is concerned exclusively with maximizing reproductive potential. Individual selection in animal species for higher and higher fertility with longer and longer lifespans inevitably leads to population overshoot, to chaotic population dynamics, and quickly to local extinction [46]. At the population level, selection for ecological homeostasis is an efficient and powerful force, counterbalancing selection for ever higher individual reproductive fitness. Thus the one and only selective force recognized by standard population genetics is effectively neutered, and a door is open that may lead to a diversity of selective forces. Only in this context can we understand the evolution of aging.

References

1. Price, G.R., *Selection and covariance.* Nature, 1970. **227**(5257): p. 520-1.
2. Price, G.R., *Extension of covariance selection mathematics.* Ann. Hum. Genet., 1972. **35**(4): p. 485-90.
3. Hamilton, W.D., *The genetical evolution of social behaviour. I.* J. Theor. Biol., 1964. **7**(1): p. 1-16.
4. Hamilton, W.D., *The genetical evolution of social behaviour. II.* J. Theor. Biol., 1964. **7**(1): p. 17-52.
5. McElreath, R. and R. Boyd, *Mathematical Models of Social Evolution: A Guide for the Perplexed.* 2008, University of Chicago Press.
6. Wilson, D.S., *A theory of group selection.* Proc. Natl. Acad. Sci. U.S.A., 1975. **72**(1): p. 143-6.
7. Arantes-Oliveira, N., J.R. Berman and C. Kenyon, *Healthy animals with extreme longevity.* Science, 2003. **302**(5645): p. 611.
8. Guarente, L. and C. Kenyon, *Genetic pathways that regulate aging in model organisms.* Nature, 2000. **408**(6809): p. 255-62.

9. Fabrizio, P., et al., *Superoxide is a mediator of an altruistic aging program in Saccharomyces cerevisiae.* J. Cell Biol., 2004. **166**(7): p. 1055-67.

10. Skulachev, I.V., *Phenoptosis: programmed death of an organism.* Biochemistry (Mosc), 1999. **64**(12): p. 1418-1426.

11. Bredesen, D.E., *The non-existent aging program: how does it work?* Aging Cell, 2004. **3**(5): p. 255-9.

12. de Cabo, R., et al., *The search for antiaging interventions: from elixirs to fasting regimens.* Cell, 2014. **157**(7): p. 1515-1526.

13. Tomás-Loba, A., et al., *Telomerase reverse transcriptase delays aging in cancer-resistant mice.* Cell 2008. **135**(4): p. 609-622.

14. Bernardes de Jesus, B., et al., *Telomerase gene therapy in adult and old mice delays aging and increases longevity without increasing cancer.* EMBO Molecular Medicine, 2012: p. n/a-n/a.

15. Vera, E., et al., *The rate of decrease of short telomeres predicts longevity in mammals.* Cell Reports, 2012. **2**(4): p. 732-737.

16. Fahy, G., *Precedents for the biological control of aging: postponement, prevention and reversal of aging processes*, In: *Approaches to the Control of Aging: Building a Pathway to Human Life Extension*, G.M. Fahy, et al., Editors. 2010, Springer: New York.

17. Hughes, S.E., et al., *Genetic and pharmacological factors that influence reproductive aging in nematodes.* PLoS Genet, 2007. **3**(2): p. e25.

18. Huang, C. and K. Kornfeld. *A Screen for Mutations that Affect Caenorhabditis elegans Aging, In:* Mid-west Worm Meeting. 2002.

19. Rando, T.A. and H.Y. Chang, *Aging, rejuvenation and epigenetic reprogramming: resetting the aging clock.* Cell, 2012. **148**(1): p. 46-57.

20. Barja, G., *Mitochondrial free radical production and aging in mammals and birds.* Ann. N.Y. Acad. Sci., 1998. **854**: p. 224-38.

21. Sanz, A., R. Pamplona and G. Barja, *Is the mitochondrial free radical theory of aging intact?* Antioxid. Redox Signal, 2006. **8**(3-4): p. 582-99.

22. Andrews, W.H., et al., *Assays for TERT promoter modulatory agents using telomerase structural RNA component*, U.P. Office, Editor. 2007: USA.

23. Harley, C.B., et al., *A natural product telomerase activator as part of a health maintenance program.* Rejuvenation Res., 2011. **14**(1): p. 45-56.

24. Terzibasi, E., et al., *Large differences in aging phenotype between strains of the short-lived annual fish Nothobranchius furzeri.* PLoS One, 2008. **3**(12): p. e3866.

25. Travis, J.M., *The evolution of programmed death in a spatially structured population.* J. Gerontol. A Biol. Sci. Med. Sci., 2004. **59**(4): p. 301-5.

26. Werfel, J., D.E. Ingber and Y. Bar-Yam, *Programed death is favored by natural selection in spatial systems.* Phys. Rev. Lett., 2015. **114**(23): p. 238103.

27. Mitteldorf, J. and J. Pepper, *Senescence as an adaptation to limit the spread of disease.* J. Theor. Biol., 2009. **260**(2): p. 186-195.

28. Mitteldorf, J. and C. Goodnight, *Post-reproductive life span and demographic stability.* Oikos, 2012. **121**(9): p. 1370-1378.

29. Stearns, S.C., *The Evolution of Life Histories.* 1992, Oxford; New York: Oxford University Press. xii, 249 p.

30. Cawthon, R.M., et al., *Association between telomere length in blood and mortality in people aged 60 years or older.* Lancet, 2003. **361**(9355): p. 393-5.

31. Rode, L., B.G. Nordestgaard and S.E. Bojesen, *Peripheral blood leukocyte telomere length and mortality among 64 637 individuals from the general population.* Journal of the National Cancer Institute, 2015. **107**(6).

32. Kimura, M., et al., *Telomere length and mortality: a study of leukocytes in elderly Danish twins.* Am. J. Epidemiol., 2008. **167**(7): p. 799-806.

33. Beirne, C., et al., *Age-related declines and disease-associated variation in immune cell telomere length in a wild mammal.* PloS one, 2014. **9**(9): p. e108964.

34. Bredesen, D., *Neural apoptosis.* Annals of Neurology, 1995. **38**: p. 839-851.

35. Warner, H.R., *Aging and regulation of apoptosis.* Curr. Top Cell Regul., 1997. **35**: p. 107-21.

36. Dirks, A. and C. Leeuwenburgh, *Apoptosis in skeletal muscle with aging.* Am. J. Physiol. Regul. Integr. Comp. Physiol., 2002. **282**: p. R519-27.

37. Jones, O.R., et al., *Diversity of aging across the tree of life.* Nature, 2014. **505**(7482): p. 169-173.

38. Brooks, M., *13 Things That Don't Make Sense: The Most Baffling Scientific Mysteries of Our Time.* 2008, Knopf Doubleday Publishing Group.

39. Sherratt, T.N. and D.M. Wilkinson, *Big Questions in Ecology and Evolution.* 2009, Oxford University Press.

40. Woese, C.R., *A new biology for a new century.* Microbiology and Molecular Biology Reviews, 2004. **68**(2): p. 173-186.

41. Margulis, L. and D. Sagan, *Acquiring Genomes.* 2002, Basic Books. 240p.

42. Pigliucci, M., *Evolution and its major transitions.* Evolution, 2011. **65**(12): p. 3642-3644.

43. Jablonka, E. and G. Raz, *Transgenerational epigenetic inheritance: prevalence, mechanisms and implications for the study of heredity and evolution.* The Quarterly Review of Biology, 2009. **84**(2): p. 131-176.

44. Shapiro, J.A., *Evolution: A View from the 21st Century.* 2011, FT Press.

45. Kirschner, M. and J. Gerhart, *The Plausibility of Life.* 2006, New Haven, CT: Yale University Press. 336.

46. Mitteldorf, J., *Chaotic population dynamics and the evolution of aging: proposing a demographic theory of senescence.* Evol. Ecol. Res., 2006. **8**: p. 561-574.

1
CHAPTER

Hormesis

Hormesis is where it began for me, though I did not yet know the word. In 1996, I learned for the first time [1] that many animals live longer when they are underfed and their lifespans continue to increase right up to the threshold of starvation.

Lifespan of Calorie-Restricted Mice (data from Weindruch et al., 1986)

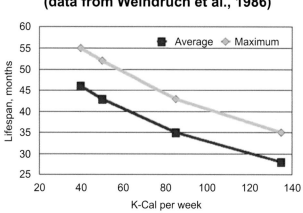

Lifespan plotted against percent CR, based on data from Weindruch and Walford.

This alone is sufficient to imply that aging is an adaptive evolutionary program. Since the Caloric Restriction (CR) phenomenon is reproducible robustly across widely-separated taxa, it must have a general evolutionary basis, a benefit that applies as well to spiders and flies, to dogs and mice, to crustaceans, yeast cells, and worms. But how are they able to extend their lives under the duress of starvation? From what reserve of strength do they pull this ability when starved? And why do they not perform the same trick when they are not starved? All these animals cannot be lengthening their lives when starving unless they hold some capacity in reserve, shortening their lives when they have plenty to eat. Even when they are slightly underfed, they must be holding something back, to be applied only when they are severely underfed. And of course, the feat of maximum life extension is performed under circumstances when the resources available are barely enough for survival.

This behavior contradicts expectations from the "damage" theories that dominate gerontology [2] and the tradeoff theories that dominate evolutionary theory of aging. Most popular and most inconsistent with CR [3] is the Disposable Soma theory [4], based on the idea that the underlying cause of aging is that the body short-changes the calorie budget for repair and maintenance in order to goose the budget for survival and reproduction. If longevity were a function of sufficient caloric energy, then lifespan would not be maximized when consumption is minimized.

When they have enough to eat, animal metabolisms are not trying to live as long as possible. They have evolved to have a shorter lifespan than the maximum of which they are capable. Lifespan is an evolutionary program.

The adaptive benefit of this program is demographic, as articulated by Harrison and Archer [5-7]. The ability to toughen up and to extend lifespan when starved helps the population to survive a famine and delivers the survivors into a world with plentiful resources and thinned competition, in which their progeny may prosper.

When the comparison is made in this way—as extended life during a famine—it appears that there is a benefit for the community and also for the individual. The community resists extinction from famine; the individual delivers its genes into a world where much of the competition has been eliminated, with the opportunity to found a new community. But suppose we frame the same statement conversely: what is the advantage to shortening lifespan when fully fed? This makes it clear that the benefit is only to the community and not to the individual. The individual that dies early just because it has enough to eat does not secure thereby a selective advantage—quite the contrary; dying early carries a cost*. But there is a communal benefit from death on a schedule. If lifespan were indeterminate and open-ended, awaiting a cause of death sufficient to knock out a robust individual in the prime of life, then deaths would be dangerously clumped in time. When conditions were good, almost no one would die; when there was a famine or an epidemic, everyone would die at once. Aging puts death on an individual schedule, so deaths can be spread out through time. Without aging, common sources of death are tightly correlated within a local community, so population swings wildly up and down. Ecosystems are routinely stretched to their demographic extremes and each boom and subsequent population crash poses a risk of extinction.

The evolutionary meaning of fixed individual lifespan is to promote population homeostasis, to make possible stable ecosystems, to avoid population overshoot that risks extinction. In order to have some extra slack to extend lifespan when food is scarce, it is logically necessary to keep lifespan shorter when food is plentiful. You could say that nature invented aging so she would have some room to relent and extend life in times of famine.

This is the thesis on which the remainder of this volume is an elaboration.

---

* If fertility has already declined to zero before death, then there may be no fitness cost, but in this case we only kick the can down the road, for we must explain why evolution has permitted the loss of fertility.

A Note on the Use of Teleological Language

"Nature invented aging so she would have some room to relent and extend life in times of famine."

By convention, biologists avoid this kind of sentence construction. There are no purposes in evolution, just blind mutation and differences between what survives and what does not. To write in terms of purposes encourages a kind of sloppy thinking, with which we may fool ourselves about what may evolve by natural selection and what may not. To be really accurate, what we ought to write instead is:

"Plasticity of mortality under genetic control is an adaptation that aids in the prevention of population overshoot. Populations in which the death rate is left to fluctuate widely with seasonal and stochastic changes in the environment have suffered extinctions, effectively selecting those groups in which there was an adaptive death rate. Plasticity of aging implies higher death rates in the absence of stress, and although this imposes a cost against individual fitness, it delivers a much larger communal benefit through avoidance of extinctions."

The plausibility of the hypothesis, stated in this way, can only be established by quantitative models, using explicit assumptions about the selective mechanism. This I have done [8-11] and these models will be fully described in Chapter 7.

However, elsewhere in this book, I will honor convention in the breach, freely deploying teleological language and anthropomorphizing nature. I think that the language of purpose helps us to gain intuitive understanding. In practice, every working biologist thinks in terms of purpose and function. The leaf grows toward the light. The sperm swims upstream, seeking the egg. The human metabolism is regulated by a network of chemical signals that makes decisions and transmits message to each cell in the body, to carry them out. Coded in those messages are meanings. It would be absurd to describe biology without this level of understanding.

I was trained in another discipline, physics, in which there is no such proscription. We frequently deploy language such as the following:

"The electron wants to live as near the nucleus as it can get."

"The photon searches the entire space of pathways from A to B and chooses the one for which the integrated action is a minimum."

"The crystal seeks its lowest energy state as the temperature is gradually lowered, but may become trapped in an elevated valley, separated from the ground state by a hill."

Physicists understand that such statements are powerful aids to intuitive understanding, though of course they are no substitute for a quantitative, predictive theory. No one makes the mistake of imagining there is a little man who lives inside the electron and tells it where to go.

In this book, as an experiment, I will defy the convention unapologetically, with a promiscuous use of teleologic language. I will write about evolution with the language of purpose, using metaphors of human intent. I ask the reader to accept this as a shorthand for quantitative, predictive models that will be described in appropriate detail in due course.

The thesis of this book is that:

"Aging and the regulated timing of death evolved for the purpose of stabilizing ecosystems."

What is Hormesis?

Many homeostatic systems (living and non-living) respond to a disturbance in such a way as to lessen its impact. This is the chemical principle of Le Chatelier [12]. It is a basic property of equilibrium dynamics. When a system is in equilibrium and you push it left, it comes back part-way to the right. It settles in a position further left than originally, but not as far left as you had pushed it. In a homeostatic chemical or physical system that includes a component C, when some of C is removed, the equilibrium shifts in such a way that C is partially restored. The amount of C will still be less than the system had originally, but more than there was after the system was disturbed by removing some C. Conversely, if some C is added, the equilibrium shifts the other way, so that some of the additional C is used up. For example, a buffered solution may have a pH of 7. If you add acid with a pH of 2, it will become only slightly more acidic, perhaps 6.5.

We expect that if there is a shortage of resource X in the environment, an animal or plant, evolved for a plastic adaptive response, adjusts its metabolism so as to mitigate its loss. It adapts by shifting strategies or by substitution, so that it uses less of X. Thus, despite the condition of scarcity, it does almost as well with less X than with sufficient X.

Hormesis is far stranger than this. Animals (and sometimes plants) over-compensate to a stressor, such that they actually do better with stress than without. They live longer when stressed compared to the unstressed lifespan. When X is scare, the animal overcompensates and lives *longer* than when X was plentiful. When poisoned with toxin Y, the animal overcompensates and actually lives longer than if it were not poisoned.

Hormesis is a property of biological systems, with no analog in physical systems. Compensation is a natural result of homeostasis, but over-compensation is an active process. Hormesis is an evolved system for actively maintaining homeostasis.

Without aging, death would only be from external causes. These tend to be tightly clustered in time. When there is sufficient food in the environment, no one is dying of starvation; in a famine, everyone dies at once. Aging evolved as a way to take control of the death rate from within the genome. We die one by one on an individual schedule to avoid the eventuality that we might all die at once in a famine. When food is scarce, there is plenty of death from starvation and no need for additional deaths from aging. But when food is plentiful, there is no death from starvation and the death toll from aging rises to take up the slack. Hormesis is an adaptation for leveling the death rate in good times and bad.

Implicit in this logic is that the organism is evolved explicitly to shorten lifespan in the absence of stress.

Examples of Hormesis

An Overview of Caloric Restriction

The connection between less food and longer life predates modern scientific study. Hippocrates hints at it [13]. In 15th-century Venice, Luigi Cornaro wrote a volume titled *Discorsi della vita sobria* (Discourses on the Temperate Life) about his personal experiments with caloric restriction, supplemented by half a litre of wine daily. Cornaro lived to 102. Benjamin Franklin wrote in Poor Richard's Almanac (1737, while he was still a skinny youth), "To lengthen thy life, lessen thy meals." (Franklin grew portly and died of pleurisy, an inflammatory disease, at age 84).

In the depression of the 1930s, the issue of widespread malnutrition was discussed in America. How would it affect people's health and longevity if they did not have enough to eat? Would children's growth be stunted permanently? Clive McCay was a young researcher at Cornell when he received a grant to study the relationship between delayed growth and lifespan in rats.

McCay framed his experiment in terms of growth rather than nutrition. He knew that he could slow the rats' development and maturation by limiting their food intake. How would that affect their health? Would they be able to resume growth at a later time if they were provided with *ad libitum* daily rations? Would delayed maturation lead to delayed aging?

McCay was working before Dobzhansky counseled us that "Nothing in biology makes sense except in the light of evolution" [14]. His logic was physiological and nowhere did he give evidence of having thought about aging in an evolutionary context or the adaptive value of life extension under CR.

In modern CR experiments, restricted animals are supplied with a constant amount of food daily, a percentage of what *ad libitum* control animals are observed to eat. But McCay was working from a different premise and carefully monitored the animals' weight, feeding them just enough to keep them alive, but not growing. When he discovered he could not do this without killing them, he modified his protocol minimally. His protocol was to alternate between keeping the animals from growing until the first signs of adverse effect on their health appeared, then increasing their rations until they gained 10 g of body mass, then holding their weight constant again for as long as possible. These step functions are apparent in the growth curves of restricted rats published in McCay's second paper on CR [15].

McCay saw his challenge as keeping the animals alive and healthy while delaying their growth as long as possible. To this end, he decided to provide them with a diet rich in nutrients. He did not add required micronutrients in measured amounts, as a modern researcher might, but he offered his CR rats a diet based on casein for proteins, yeast and cod liver oil for vitamins. He emphasized that his results contrasted with previous studies, which had reported shortened lifespans from restricted feeding, and surmised that their results were due to inadequate micronutrients rather than restricted calories.

The theme of optimizing nutrition while restricting calories set a precedent for experimental designs through the 20th century, and it was not until the 1970s that McCay's protocol was varied substantially. It was discovered that life extension could be achieved even if CR were begun after animals had achieved full body size [16] and that restricting protein or even a single amino acid could have benefits for life extension almost as great as CR [17].

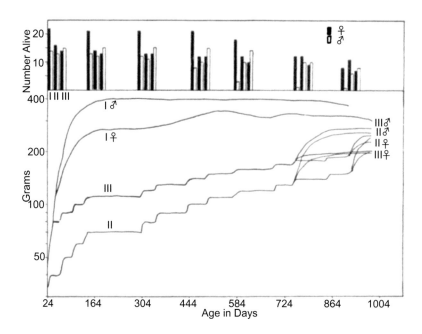

Growth curves for rats allowed to grow rapidly, no I and for those retarded in growth by limiting the calories, nos. II and III. The columns at the top show the numbers alive by sex and group at various periods of the experiment. The top of these columns provides a mortality curve.

CR works with many animals. Experiments have been done with yeast cells, worms, fruit flies and other inspect species, arachnids [18], crustaceans, fish, various rodents, dogs, horses, and rhesus monkeys. A project at Washington University has followed the health histories of people who practice CR [19], though mortality comparisons may not be available for a long while. Shorter-lived animals tend to show greater proportional life extension, but health and (arguably) longevity benefits were discerned even in the monkeys, with a lifespan of 25 years [20, 21].

CR works when begun in adulthood. Life extension is not as great as when begun earlier, but qualitatively the effect is the same. The life extension phenomenon has been thoroughly distinguished from McCay's original hypothesis about delayed maturation.

CR increases both mean and maximum lifespan. It is often useful to distinguish between, on the one hand, interventions that protect health and avoid premature death and on the other, those that actually slow or delay the aging process. Both kinds of interventions increase life expectancy (mean lifespan); but only the latter increases maximum lifespan. Sometimes the former is referred to as "squaring the mortality curve" and we can see why in the example below, which is a qualitative representation, valid for no animal in particular.

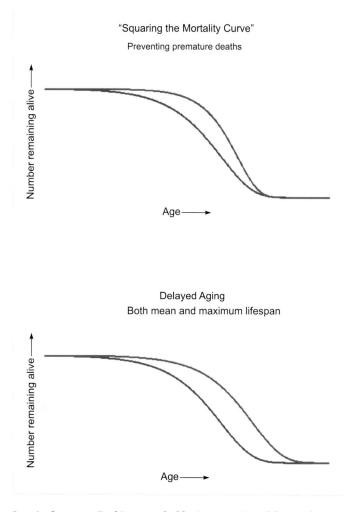

"Squaring the Mortality Curve"
Preventing premature deaths

Delayed Aging
Both mean and maximum lifespan

Survival curves: Red is extended by intervention, blue without.
Top: Early mortality is reduced, but late life mortality is increased so that the two curves converge at late ages.
Bottom: Aging is delayed. The red mortality schedule is the same as the blue, but with a time delay.
These curves are illustrative only, and represent no experiment in particular.

In the first case, mortality begins to increase later in life, but then increases faster, so that the curve drops more steeply. Only the early stages of aging are softened. In the second case the curve is actually shifted over to the right, indicating delayed aging.

The top curve is typical of what happens when dangers can be avoided or infectious diseases treated.

It is the second curve that is typical of CR experiments in rodents. And indeed, in one dramatic experiment with fruit flies, the mortality schedule was observed to jump from the curve on the left to the curve on the right within two days, when caloric restriction was initiated in mid-life [22]. Such results cast doubts on theories that aging can be characterized as a self-reinforcing, irreversible accumulation of damage.

Signaling a Famine

McCay's framing of the issue still dominated discussion of the issue of caloric restriction half a century later, when, at last, the usefulness of CR as a powerful probe to understand aging was finally appreciated and research was renewed. Emphasis was on full nutrition, and it was thought that caloric intake was the irreducible bottom line that determines lifespan. In McCay's classic view, the macronutritional content of foods and the schedule on which food is consumed are unimportant variables.

But during the renaissance of caloric restriction research, it became clear that the classic view was in error. Macronutrient proportions are important, micronutrient supplementation is not always helpful, and feeding schedule can have a large effect. As details of the landscape have been filled in, it has become increasingly clear that life extension is not a direct physiological effect of a low-food environment (or of shutting off reproduction, another popular hypothesis [3, 23]); rather, lifespan extension is initiated by a change in the signaling environment. It follows that shortening the lifespan in the presence of abundant food is not an unavoidable side-effect of enhanced fertility, but an independent choice that the body makes. A major research effort is now underway in universities and pharmaceutical laboratories to find "caloric restriction mimetics" that induce longevity signals even in the presence of plentiful food.

Macronutrient proportions have a major effect on the longevity response to diet. The response to CR is mediated through insulin [24], thus foods with high glycemic index may induce greater shortening of life, calorie for calorie. This has led to strategies that minimize carbohydrates in the diet [25]. An opposite approach has also proved effective. Low protein above a threshold does not increase lifespan, but when protein is sufficiently restricted, substantial increases in lifespan are observed, comparable to those obtainable with CR [26, 27]. Furthermore, restriction of a single essential amino acid, methionine, also extends mouse lifespan remarkably [28]. To see this effect, methionine intake must be restricted at a level lower than any natural protein source would permit, so the experiment is done with synthetic chows, containing refined and re-mixed amino acids.

Timing of food intake is also important in a way that escaped the notice of CR researchers for many years. Intermittent fasting can lead to substantial life extension, even if total caloric intake is unaffected. Mice that are fed every other day tend to double-up when food is available, so that their total caloric intake is barely diminished from *ad libitum* fed mice. But their lifespans are substantially extended nonetheless [29-31]. Sketchy but promising results from blood analysis of human volunteers suggest that intermittent fasting can promote a younger metabolism [32-34]. Some field clinicians report promising health results with diets for seniors based on periods of severely restricted food, alternating with *ad libitum* access [35].

McCay's original studies emphasized an abundance of micronutrients in the context of a low-calorie diet. The wisdom of this approach was not questioned for fifty years, and indeed micronutrients have long been considered an unmitigated boon to good health. But since 1990, this premise has been qualified, if not falsified outright. The ATBC study enlisted 29,000 male smokers from Finland to study the effects of the antioxidant vitamins C, E and beta carotene on cancer rates. The study was halted early when it was discovered that those men receiving placebo had significantly lower rates of cancer and lower overall mortality than those taking the vitamins [36]. As early as 1971, it was reported that vitamin E could worsen the performance of competitive swimmers [37]. Ubiquinone in the mitochondria declines with age and supplementing with ubiquinone (CoQ10) has become common in recent years, especially for heart patients taking statin drugs. But CoQ10 has also been reported to reduce running speed for trained sprinters and cross-country skiers [38-40]. One theory is that the longevity benefits of exercise are mediated through ROS signaling and that neutralizing ROS with antioxidant supplements can diminish the benefits of exercise [41-43].

Though it was long assumed that the lifespan benefits of low calories and high exercise were metabolic effects, there is now abundant evidence that lifespan is increased via signaling. In fact, it has been shown in flies and worms that chemically sensing food can interfere with life extension from CR, even when no calories are consumed. *C. elegans* worms live longer when their capacity to sense food chemically is impaired; conversely, their lifespan is shortened even on CR if they are allowed to sense but not ingest food [44]. Calorically restricted fruit flies exposed to food-derived odors don't live as long as the same CR flies without food odors [45].

The central role of signaling implies that there is latent capacity for extending lifespan that the body does not always deploy, but must be instructed to do so with signals that can be triggered by environmental cues.

Smart Worms

C. elegans worms have an opportunistic lifestyle. They are exquisitely adapted for population growth when conditions are favorable, and for hunkering down and surviving when conditions are harsh. What is more, their simple nervous system is honed for the purpose of sensing and deciding whether current conditions favor their growth and reproduction. The biggest decision that every worm is called upon to make is whether to hibernate as a *dauer*. At the first or second larval stage (the first day of life), the worm smells the concentration of food in the water it is constantly filtering and also the pheromones [46] of other worms in the vicinity. If food is high and competition is low, it chooses "now" over "later". It completes its growth cycle, eats what it can find, and if all goes well, goes on to lay about 300 eggs, self-fertilized. (Fewer than one worm in a thousand is a male, but if a hermaphrodite can find a male to fertilize its eggs, it may lay 1,000 or more.)

Fertility ends for the vast majority of worms (hermaphrodites) when they run out of sperm [47]. Sperm are small and metabolically "cheap". It is hard to imagine an energetic reason that sperm should be the bottleneck in fertility. This is a plain indication that the worms are not evolved to maximize their individual reproduction. I suggest that this is because intraspecific competition is the worms' worst enemy. The best strategy is to leave enough eggs but not too many; if too many offspring all grow up in the same place at the same time, they compete with one another for food and the entire cohort can starve before each worm can find enough food to mature. Math modeling suggests, and the worms' own adaptation confirms, that the ideal number of offspring is not "as many as possible" and that laying fewer eggs can lead to a better probability that some will survive to continue the lineage.

Another surprise in the worms' life history is that they continue to live and to eat after their fertility is finished. Why have they evolved a post-reproductive phase? Simulations show that the existence of a weak, non-productive age class can help stabilize population cycles [9]. In the worms' case in particular, it may be that post-reproductive elders contribute to a pheromone pool that signals to the next generation about how crowded the environment is and helps them to decide whether to mature now or to dauer. (This is my own speculation. Dauer pheromone is known [46], but its source has not been well characterized.)

A dauer is like a spore, hard and well-protected, resistant to predation, needing no food and hardly any water. Dauers can survive up to six months, waiting for more propitious conditions. Even though most life systems are shut down, the dauer still monitors the environment, sensing and evaluating whether now might be the right time to make its move. And they are not entirely passive. Dauers also exhibit the "get me out of here" behavior known as *nictation*. A dauer's dream is to deposit its eggs in a better world.

As a life history strategy, the dauer phase is just a more extreme form of the near-universal Caloric Restriction adaptation. Similar to the dauer, the CR response is a decision to forgo immediate reproduction, to lengthen lifespan, to bet on survival and an opportunity to reproduce later. CR and the dauer adaptation have a common genetic basis.*

In addition to the extremes of dauering, the worms also have a CR adaptation, and they decide how long to live and how rapidly to reproduce based on chemical signals they pick up about how much food is around and how many other worms are competing for that food.

All this is done with 302 nerve cells. We know that the nerves are making the decision, rather than some purely chemical signaling, through elegant experiments at Ruvkun's Harvard lab [48] and Guarante's lab at MIT [49]. In the first, mosaic worms were engineered, in which an insulin-receptor gene (*daf-2*) that causes lifespan to be shortened in the presence of food was disabled selectively in different tissues of the same worm. When the genes were disabled in the digestive system or the muscles, the worms were still able to modify their life history in response to environmental cues. But when the genes were disabled in the nerve cells, the worms had the long lifespan (typical of *daf-2* mutants) always. In the second, control of the CR response was traced to the transcription factor *skn-1* acting in two neurons in

---

* The best known of these genes is called *daf16* in the worm and its homolog in mammals is called *foxoA3*. (Yes, daf stands for **da**uer **f**ormation, but no, foxo has nothing to do with foxes.)

the brain. This is a clear example of a "deliberate" adaptation to shorten the length of life for the sake of population regulation, and it is not arranged automatically through chemical signals, but actually "calculated" by the nerve cells, based on sensory input.

Caloric Restriction and Population Regulation

The Caloric Restriction adaptation is very general across the animal kingdom. The fact that it is controlled by the same genes that cause the *C. elegans* worm to die early when there is danger of overpopulation is a powerful hint. The purpose of the CR adaptation is to adjust lifespan to complement the death rate from starvation. When starvation deaths are high, aging deaths are low and vice versa.

In starving animals, it is also true that stress resistance is enhanced. In fact, the genes that signal life extension have very generally been found to be the same genes that fortify stress resistance. The mechanisms are one and the same. Animals respond to caloric restriction with better resistance to disease [50], enhanced agility and speed [51], and quicker, more reliable neuronal responses [52]. Conversely, this means that when there is plenty of food, nature has arranged for animals to age more rapidly and also to be more vulnerable to death from every kind of stress. Individuals are giving up a portion of their fitness in good times, just so they can get it back when times are tough. Thus it has been arranged for the death rates in good times and hard times to be somewhat more equal, more level than they might have been if everyone were at their peak of fitness all the time.

Even without the CR effect, aging would serve to help level the death rate. The effect of aging is very different from just adding extra mortality. Aging is able to complement the death rate from starvation or disease, because it only adds to the death rate when the other threats to the population are low enough that individuals are living long enough that aging can kick in. In other words, when everyone is dying of starvation (or of an epidemic, earthquake, or forest fire), they are not dying of old age. Aging has little effect on the death rate at such times, but only when these other threats to life have backed off sufficiently that some animals can live into old age.

What is the Mechanism by which Caloric Restriction Extends Lifespan?

No one theory has explained the physiology or the signaling that mediates life extension from CR. Genes are involved that have been conserved since the dawn of eukaryotic life, but there is also evidence that the mechanism may be different in different animals. For yeast, worms, flies, and mammals, life extension is mediated through insulin/IGF-1 signaling and also TOR. But the response of flies in particular has unique characteristics that suggest that the CR effect has been both a conserved adaptation and also the target of convergent evolution [53].

Commonly, life extension entails, in addition to preserved insulin sensitivity, a lower level of inflammation, higher available NO, enhanced autophagy, and not lower oxidative stress, but enhanced response to oxidative stress [54].

Can Life Extension from CR be Reconciled with Accepted Evolutionary Theories?

There are ideas in the literature that would purport to explain CR within the context of traditional evolutionary theory, but none has been fully explored or set forth in detail.

Harrison and Archer [5] were the first out of the starting gate, with a theory that extension of lifespan was an artifact of the breeding of laboratory rodents. (Harrison and Archer have worked many years at the Jackson Laboratories, which not only sponsor first-rate research, but also breed mice commercially for most lab studies the world over.) They focus appropriately on the huge advantage available to an animal that can survive through a famine and reproduce in the period of thin competition that follows. To their credit, they recognize, at least obliquely, that it is mysterious why, if their physiology permits, mice don't *always* extend their lifespans, even when food is plentiful. In their attempt to account for this, they hypothesize a linkage between extended fertility and extended longevity that has been incidentally magnified in the recent breeding of laboratory mice.

Phelan and Austad [55] responded to Harrison and Archer by noting that the CR adaptation is not restricted to lab animals, and they fell back on McCay's original reasoning that the response derives from slowing the developmental clock with delayed early growth. In a rejoinder [55], Harrison and Archer correctly point out that mice that begin CR at six weeks and at six months have about the same lifespan and that CR increases lifespan even when begun later in life.

In a fuller exposition a few years later, co-authored with Edward Masoro [6], Austad seems to come around to Harrison's view that brief periods of famine in nature were the origin of the adaptive advantage of the CR response. They frame their theory in terms of compromises in the allocation of unnamed "resources". The bottleneck resource cannot be caloric energy for obvious reasons, and the nature of the resources and reason for the compromise is left unspecified. Times of food scarcity are an unpromising time to invest in reproduction, hence "resources" are diverted from reproduction to protection and repair. One point on which Masoro and Austad are convincing is that life extension is achieved in conjunction with an enhanced stress response, which is evidenced as greater resistance to toxins and carcinogens. The points on which they are less convincing are why enhanced stress response is inconsistent with fertility and how the enhanced state is achieved under stress of food shortage, but not otherwise.

This hypothesis depends crucially on the link between life extension and curtailment of fertility. Genetic extension of lifespan must be tightly associated with fertility depression; in fact, it is predicted that the fertility effect must be primary and that extension of lifespan must be a downstream effect:

Hormonal signal → Effect on reproduction → Effect on aging

But the experiments imply that reproduction and aging are separately regulated:

Effect on reproduction

Hormonal signals

Effect on aging

Two worm experiments have clarified this separation of pathways. In the first [56], the timing of *daf-2* signals was manipulated via RNA interference to separate effects on lifespan from effects on fertility. Animals in which *daf-2* expression was curtailed only after maturation experienced full lifespan extension without incurring the fertility cost. In the second experiment, destruction of the germ line (via laser ablation) was found to lengthen lifespan [57]. If the surrounding gonads were removed with the worm's germ cells, the effect was negated and no life extension was observed. This observation rules out a simple explanation in terms of conserved resources (Disposable Soma theory). Rather, two signals must have been involved: a life-lengthening signal from the gonads and a life-shortening signal from the germ line (as Kenyon has emphasized).

There are general observations as well that cast doubt on the hypothesis that life extension in CR is mediated by fertility loss. All lab experiments in caloric restriction are performed with animals housed without mates, so they cannot breed. Yet the theory is based on the idea that starved animals that do not breed are spending much less "resource" on reproduction than well-fed animals that do not breed. So we must assume that the "resource" is invested in some potentiator of fertility and not fertility itself. Males lose a portion of their fertility, sometimes none, while female mammals typically lose all their fertility under caloric restriction, yet the increases in lifespan afforded to males and females are typically the same [58]. Fertility is reduced but not completely curtailed in male mice, even under severe calorie restriction [59]. The male control, fed *ad libitum*, was consuming only half as much energy as a pregnant female to begin with. This male mouse on 50% caloric restriction still has most of his fertility and weighs 60% as much as the control, yet he is more active [60], supports a stronger immune system [61], and lives 1/3 longer than the control [1].

Even for females, the schedules of fertility loss and life expectancy gain are not commensurate. In mice exposed to progressively lower feeding levels, fertility vanishes completely by about 30% restriction, and yet lifespan continues to increase with further restriction, down to 60%. In the range between 30% and 60% CR, there is nothing left to tradeoff in exchange for the gains in longevity.

More Theories with Less Credibility

A more general theory is that starvation is the default condition of nature and it is to be expected that animals are better adapted to the environment of their evolutionary past than to an artificial environment of plenty [13]. It is difficult to support or refute such broad claims about the condition of nature generally in the deep past. I prefer to think that natural environments include both periods of food scarcity and also periods of food abundance, which provide opportunities for populations that can expand quickly to fill a niche. But in any case, the observation that protected, domestic environments with unlimited food are unnatural fails to explain why an organism would do so much better in a difficult environment than in an easy one. A marathon runner may train under conditions of steep mountain slopes with reduced atmospheric oxygen, but when he runs his race on a flat course at sea level, we don't expect him to run a slower pace because he is maladapted to the easier conditions.

Sinclair [62] reviewed theories of the CR adaptation and found explanation in terms of hormesis most promising. He appropriately puts CR in the context of other over-compensations to stress, but he does not confront the essential paradox of over-compensation. In times of stress, where does the latent capacity for increased lifespan come from and why is this potential not realized in the absence of stress?

One thing all these papers have in common is the explicit assumption that the cost of aging in the wild is low, because nature is a tough environment in which almost everyone dies of something else before death from old age can take place. This idea was first set forth in Medawar's seminal lecture of 1952 [63], and has been accepted without question by too many researchers for too many years. In fact, broad surveys of animals in the wild have consistently confirmed a high fitness cost of aging [64-67] as predicted much earlier by Williams [68]. The high cost of aging in the wild underscores the paradox that so many species have failed to avail themselves of the latent metabolic capacity to extend lifespan, of which the CR adaptation is a clear indication.

The phenomenon of CR is utterly incompatible with all classical (non-programmed) theories of aging. When we re-frame the question as life shortening from food sufficiency, rather than life extension from scarcity, the paradox is sharpened. There is no escaping the conclusion that animals un-stressed by caloric deprivation are leaving a major portion of their fitness on the table by not extending their lives, at a time when there is plenty of energy available both for repair and reproduction and plenty of room in the environment to expand the population.

The only way to understand the fact that life is shortened just when resources are most abundant is to invoke dangers to the population if numbers are expanded too rapidly under these conditions. This is the Demographic theory, which will be fully expounded upon in Chapter 7.

How Much Reproduction is Enough?

Some biologists who do not specialize in evolution succumb to fuzzy thinking about the strength of selection for longer lifespan. They imagine that natural selection is an on/off switch that accepts those individuals that are able to reproduce their numbers and rejects those whose net reproduction falls below unity.

But in the standard paradigm of individual selection, relatively more reproduction implies a competitive advantage regardless of any notion of absolute sufficiency of offspring. In the standard paradigm, population is held steady from one generation to the next by intense competition for resources. More offspring means more tickets in the lottery for a fixed number of places in the niche. There is no notion of "enough offspring" within standard thinking about individual competition; there can be no such thing as "enough tickets" for you so long as your neighbor has more. If an individual dies early, it is forgoing the opportunity to continue procreation and it must be at a competitive disadvantage to a similar individual that continues to live and to reproduce.

Explaining the Caloric Restriction Effect within the Disposable Soma Theory

One of the most popular and frequently-cited evolutionary theories of aging is based on the body's energy budget. In the Disposable Soma theory [4], reproduction, repair, and current metabolic needs all use food energy. With limited caloric resources, the body is evolved to compromise in allocation of energy and the portion for repair/ maintenance functions is subordinated to uses that offer a more immediate payoff. On its face, this theory would seem to predict that decreased caloric energy would lead to a harsher compromise, with less energy available for repair. Thus the Caloric Restriction response predicted by the Disposable Soma (DS) theory is opposite to the one observed. Such a basic predictive failing should be considered a fatal flaw for the DS theory. This point has been ignored in a great body of literature based on DS reasoning. The first attempt to reconcile DS with CR came from Holliday [69], who proposed that caloric restriction extends lifespan via curtailment of reproduction as an essential intermediary. Energy savings from shutting down reproduction are so great as to more than compensate for the lower calorie intake and thus *more* net calories are available for repair when fewer calories are consumed. This theme was picked up by Kirkwood himself, in a strained attempt to make it work quantitatively [23, 70]. But, in contradiction to the positive spin provided in the discussion and abstract, the Shanley/Kirkwood model demonstrates clearly what our intuition tells us is true: fewer total calories consumed translates to fewer calories for repair. The severely limited scope of this model was demonstrated in a rejoinder article [3]. I offer more details of this and other failings of the DS theory in Chapter 4.

Exercise

The fact that exercise increases mean lifespan in animal models and lowers mortality in humans is widely appreciated, though it is seldom described in terms of hormesis. The familiarity of this phenomenon makes it difficult to appreciate how unexpected it is. Exercise burns calories that might otherwise be used for repair and maintenance. Exercise generates macroscopic damage to bones and muscles that require extra repair and generates copious free radicals that cause chemical damage [71]. Cells must proliferate to repair this damage, and cell proliferation leads to DNA copying errors and telomere attrition, and yet people who exercise are observed to have longer age-adjusted telomeres and lower age-adjusted DNA damage than sedentary people [72]. They also enjoy 30-40% lower mortality rates [73]. In CR experiments with rodents, the longest-lived mice are both eating least and exercising most [17, 74]. This phenomenon demands an explanation in terms of overcompensation to stress, i.e., hormesis. If the body is shortening its lifespan when un-stressed by exercise, this is not because of any metabolic necessity, but simply that it is choosing a shorter lifespan. Exercise hormesis, like the CR effect, is impossible to reconcile with any of the non-programmed theories of aging. But it poses particular difficulty for theories of aging from oxidative damage, since exercise increases oxidative stress and increases lifespan. Exercise is most demanding on mitochondria. It induces mitochondrial oxidative damage and promotes mitochondrial autophagy. According to the popular mitochondrial free radical theory [75], exercise ought to accelerate aging and antioxidants should offer some mitigation, but the truth is the opposite. It has been common knowledge for at least many decades that exercise benefits almost every aspect of health and lowers mortality, especially for diseases of old age. And since the turn of the millennium, evidence is accumulating that antioxidants lessen the benefit of exercise [42, 43] and may lead to higher mortality [76, 77], especially from cancer [36, 78].

Life Extended with Toxins and Other Stressors

Many animal experiments have been done demonstrating the phenomenon of hormesis for a broad variety of chemical and physical challenges [79]. Chloroform is a neurotoxin (used in the 19th century as a surgical anesthetic in low doses until too many people died on the operating table). In the 1970s, tiny amounts of chloroform were discovered to appear in toothpaste as a contaminant, and regulatory agencies demanded that the toothpaste companies study the long-term effects on health with animal experiments. The surprising result was that dogs, mice, and rats could be fed small quantities of chloroform for their entire lives and they actually lived longer on average than control animals that were not poisoned [80, 81].

Paraquat is a defoliant, a "pro-oxidant" so strong that it burns leaves on contact. It was sprayed by American planes on Mexican marijuana fields, before it came out that too many of the local people were dying from groundwater pollution. Paraquat can poison *C. elegans* lab worms, but it can also increase their lifespan. Tiny doses of paraquat have little effect and high doses kill the worms, but if the dose is adjusted just right, the worms live 70% longer [82].

Rats have been forced to slog through cold water for hours every day and the result is that they live longer [83]. And shocking worms with short-term exposure to heat that is not quite sufficient to kill them actually makes them live longer [84]. Exposure to pathogens enhanced both lifespan and fertility in fruit flies, compared to flies maintained in a sterile environment [85]. Mice exposed to 25 or 50 times the normal background level of gamma radiation lived 20% longer than mice that received only the ordinary background [86].

(Radiation hormesis has been embraced by the nuclear power industry and their apologists to support the fiction that nuclear power is safe. Routine, low-level releases of radiation from power plants operating under optimal conditions are not a danger to public health. However, there are much better reasons to oppose nuclear power, with Fukushima, Chernobyl, and Three Mile Island at the top of the list. There is also the question of building secure waste storage facilities and burdening our grandchildren's grandchildren with guarding them for the next 20,000 years, and ultimately there is the economic reality that without legislated immunity from liability, the industry would be uninsurable and bankrupt.)

Chemical hormetic phenomena are reviewed by Calabrese [79] and by Forbes [87]. Radiation hormesis has been reviewed by Luckey [88-90] and by Neafsey [91], updated by Jolly [92].

What all hormetic phenomena have in common is that the animal is treated in some way that we have good reason to believe ought to be harmful. Not surprisingly, the animal's strength and resistance rise in response. But what is completely unexpected: the body overcompensates, so that over the long haul, the animal does better and lives longer. This cannot be reconciled with the picture we may have of a metabolism bravely fighting off challenges, but being worn down in the end by accumulated stresses. Whatever mechanisms the body is using to resist stress and maintain itself against aging are not being deployed effectively in the absence of stress. This evidence forces us to see aging as "voluntary," in the sense that the body knows how to live longer, but normally it does not do so.

Is there an Alternative Account of Hormesis that does not Imply Programmed Aging?

For many years, the biological community marginalized reports of hormesis [93]. We may presume that the instinctive skepticism of hormesis came from a general view of how evolution works and an unarticulated appreciation that hormesis is difficult to reconcile with individual-based evolutionary theory. There has been little attempt to square hormesis with evolutionary theory, but rather a passive refusal to acknowledge hormesis as a general phenomenon.

More recently, the reality of hormesis has become accepted in the mainstream of biological literature, but there remains an uncomfortable dissonance between the phenomena and traditional perspectives on evolution. Forbes [87] undertook one of the few efforts to confront the contradictions head-on. Forbes roots his analysis firmly in the classical theory of independent genes competing for growth in frequency within a static or slowly-varying environment. And yet, he concludes that "the occurrence of hormesis of individual life-history traits can be explained as an evolutionary adaptation that acts to maintain fitness in a changing environment." He arrives at this place by asking the question whether fitness is increased in a stressful environment (of course, it is), but never confronting the converse question, whether fitness is *decreased* in a stress-free environment (also affirmative).

Blagosklonny has his own theory of aging, and it is not a communal adaptive function. Nevertheless, he is the only theorist to have confronted the essential challenge to evolutionary theory in the fact that animals shorten their lifespans in the absence of stress [2]. "If aging were caused by damage, then damaging stresses would accelerate aging. However, mild stresses (including oxidative stress) can extend lifespan in different species... If hormesis induces damage and slows down aging, then aging is not driven by damage." He is not shy about exposing the absurdity of the conventional view: "No one will advocate 'mild and repeated' smoking to prevent lung cancer." Blagosklonny goes on to conclude that aging must be driven by signaling and goes on to describe some of the signal molecules that are known to trigger self-destruction, especially *mTOR*. How to reconcile this with natural selection? Blagosklonny invokes a kind of hormonal inertia, such that the expression of *mTOR* is favored while it is useful for growth and development, and later in life it is not properly turned off. Why then is it not turned off? At this point, he invokes the standard fiction, that there has been insufficient selection against it, because "in the wild, organisms do not live long enough to experience aging. Therefore, forces of natural selection against aging are weak." So this is the point at which I part company with Blagosklonny. I have stated above that there is a high fitness cost of aging in the wild and I shall return to describe this evidence in more detail in Chapter 4.

The hormonal signals that cause aging are not an inertial holdover from youth, but a re-purposing of existing, useful mechanisms like inflammation and apoptosis, co-opted in old age to accomplish self-destruction. This is the natural conclusion of Blagosklonny's reasoning, and he escapes this conclusion only because (a) he accepts the discredited hypothesis that natural selection against aging is weak and (b) he does not recognize that there are plausible mechanisms of group selection that can explain how aging evolved (to be fully described in Chapter 7).

Conclusions

Hormesis is a general evolutionary phenomenon. Animals lengthen their lifespans under duress. This attests to the fact that, under most conditions, the metabolism is evolved *not* to live as long as possible.

A more provocative and enlightening definition of hormesis is the converse: animals are evolved to shorten their lifespans in the absence of stress. This can only have a communal adaptive function, because the impact of shortened lifespan on individual fitness is always negative. The benefit is to promote demographic stability, to help maintain the homeostasis of ecosystems by leveling the death rate. Evolution has arranged matters such that the death rate from aging is at its minimum just when the death rate from starvation and other environmental challenges is at its maximum.

In common forms of hormesis, there is a general benefit from upregulating stress hormones and shifting gene expression in a direction that offers greater protection. Often there is no tradeoff, no down side. From the individual's perspective, this shift should be on all the time, not just under stress. The fact that it is turned off in the absence of stress harms the individual, though it benefits the community.

Hormesis is a profound and very general ecosystem-level adaptation.

References

1. Weindruch, R., *Caloric restriction and aging.* Sci. Am., 1996. **274**(1): p. 46-52.
2. Blagosklonny, M.V., *Hormesis does not make sense except in the light of TOR-driven aging.* Aging (Albany NY), 2011. **3**(11): p. 1051.
3. Mitteldorf, J., *Can experiments on caloric restriction be reconciled with the disposable soma theory for the evolution of senescence?* Evolution Int. J. Org. Evolution, 2001. **55**(9): p. 1902-5; discussion 1906.
4. Kirkwood, T., *Evolution of aging.* Nature, 1977. **270**: p. 301-304.
5. Harrison, D.E. and J.R. Archer, *Natural selection for extended longevity from food restriction.* Growth Dev. Aging, 1989. **53**(1-2): p. 3.

6. Masoro, E.J. and S.N. Austad, *The evolution of the antiaging action of dietary restriction: a hypothesis.* The Journals of Gerontology Series A: Biological Sciences and Medical Sciences, 1996. **51A**(6): p. B387-B391.

7. Walford, R.L. and S.R. Spindler, *The response to calorie restriction in mammals shows features also common to hibernation: a cross-adaptation hypothesis.* The Journals of Gerontology Series A: Biological Sciences and Medical Sciences, 1997. **52A**(4): p. B179-B183.

8. Mitteldorf, J., *Chaotic population dynamics and the evolution of aging: proposing a demographic theory of senescence.* Evol. Ecol. Res., 2006. **8**: p. 561-574.

9. Mitteldorf, J. and C. Goodnight, *Post-reproductive life span and demographic stability.* Oikos, 2012. **121**(9): p. 1370-1378.

10. Mitteldorf, J. and J. Pepper, *Senescence as an adaptation to limit the spread of disease.* J. Theor. Biol., 2009. **260**(2): p. 186-195.

11. Mitteldorf, J. and A.C. Martins, *Programmed life span in the context of evolvability.* The American Naturalist, 2014. **184**(3): p. 289-302.

12. Le Chatelier, H. and O. Boudouard, *Limits of flammability of gaseous mixtures.* Bull. Soc. Chim. (Paris), 1898. **19**: p. 483-488.

13. Dehmelt, H., *Re-adaptation hypothesis: explaining health benefits of caloric restriction.* Med. Hypotheses, 2004. **62**(4): p. 620-624.

14. Dobzhansky, T., *Nothing in biology makes sense except in the light of evolution.* 1973.

15. McCay, C., M. Crowell and L. Maynard, *The effect of retarded growth upon the length of life span and upon the ultimate body size. 1935.* Nutrition (Burbank, Los Angeles County, Calif.), 1935. **5**(3): p. 155.

16. Barrows, C., Jr. and G. Kokkonen, *Diet and life extension in animal model systems.* AGE, 1978. **1**(4): p. 131-143.

17. Masoro, E.J., *Minireview: food restriction in rodents: an evaluation of its role in the study of aging.* J. Gerontol., 1988. **43**(3): p. B59-B64.

18. Austad, S.N., *Life extension by dietary restriction in the bowl and doily spider, < i> Frontinella pyramitela </i>.* Exp. Gerontol., 1989. **24**(1): p. 83-92.

19. Holloszy, J.O. and L. Fontana, *Caloric restriction in humans.* Exp. Gerontol., 2007. **42**(8): p. 709-712.

20. Mattison, J.A., et al., *Impact of caloric restriction on health and survival in rhesus monkeys from the NIA study.* Nature, 2012.

21. Colman, R.J., et al., *Caloric restriction reduces age-related and all-cause mortality in rhesus monkeys.* Nature communications, 2014. **5**.

22. Mair, W., et al., *Demography of dietary restriction and death in Drosophila.* Science, 2003. **301**(5640): p. 1731-1733.

23. Shanley, D.P. and T.B. Kirkwood, *Calorie restriction and aging: a life-history analysis.* Evolution Int. J. Org. Evolution, 2000. **54**(3): p. 740-50.

24. Masoro, E.J., *Overview of caloric restriction and aging.* Mech. Ageing Dev., 2005. **126**(9): p. 913-22.

25. Bell, S.J. and B. Sears, *Low-glycemic-load diets: impact on obesity and chronic diseases.* Crit. Rev. Food Sci. Nutr., 2003. **43**(4): p. 357-377.

26. Youngman, L.D., *Protein restriction (PR) and caloric restriction (CR) compared: effects on DNA damage, carcinogenesis and oxidative damage.* Mutation Research/DNAging, 1993. **295**(4): p. 165-179.

27. Fontana, L., et al., *Long-term effects of calorie or protein restriction on serum IGF-1 and IGFBP-3 concentration in humans.* Aging Cell, 2008. **7**(5): p. 681-7.

28. Orentreich, N., et al., *Low methionine ingestion by rats extends life span.* J. Nutr., 1993. **123**(2): p. 269-274.

29. Goodrick, C.L., et al., *Effects of intermittent feeding upon growth and life span in rats.* Gerontology, 1982. **28**(4): p. 233-241.

30. Goodrick, C.L., et al., *Effects of intermittent feeding upon body weight and life span in inbred mice: interaction of genotype and age.* Mech. Ageing Dev., 1990. **55**(1): p. 69-87.

31. Anson, R.M., et al., *Intermittent fasting dissociates beneficial effects of dietary restriction on glucose metabolism and neuronal resistance to injury from calorie intake.* Proc. Natl. Acad. Sci., 2003. **100**(10): p. 6216-6220.

32. Johnson, J.B., D.R. Laub and S. John, *The effect on health of alternate day calorie restriction: eating less and more than needed on alternate days prolongs life.* Med. Hypotheses, 2006. **67**(2): p. 209-211.

33. Anson, M., B. Jones and R. de Cabod, *The diet restriction paradigm: a brief review of the effects of every-other-day feeding.* AGE, 2005. **27**(1): p. 17-25.

34. Longo, V.D. and M.P. Mattson, *Fasting: molecular mechanisms and clinical applications.* Cell metabolism, 2014. **19**(2): p. 181-192.

35. Varady, K.A. and M.K. Hellerstein, *Alternate-day fasting and chronic disease prevention: a review of human and animal trials.* Am. J. Clin. Nutr., 2007. **86**(1): p. 7-13.

36. Heinonen, O.P. and D. Albanes, *The effect of vitamin E and beta carotene on the incidence of lung cancer and other cancers in male smokers. The Alpha-Tocopherol, Beta Carotene Cancer Prevention Study Group.* N. Engl. J. Med., 1994. **330**(15): p. 1029-35.

37. Sharman, I., M. Down, and R. Sen, *The effects of vitamin E and training on physiological function and athletic performance in adolescent swimmers.* Br. J. Nutr., 1971. **26**(02): p. 265-276.

38. Malm, C., et al., *Effects of ubiquinone-10 supplementation and high intensity training on physical performance in humans.* Acta Physiol. Scand., 1997. **161**(3): p. 379-384.

39. Ylikoski, T., et al., *The effect of coenzyme Q 10 on the exercise performance of cross-country skiers.* Mol. Aspects Med., 1997. **18**: p. 283-290.

40. Östman, B., et al., *Coenzyme Q10 supplementation and exercise-induced oxidative stress in humans.* Nutrition, 2012. **28**(4): p. 403-417.

41. Powers, S.K. and M.J. Jackson, *Exercise-induced oxidative stress: cellular mechanisms and impact on muscle force production.* Physiol. Rev., 2008. **88**(4): p. 1243-1276.

42. Ristow, M., et al., *Antioxidants prevent health-promoting effects of physical exercise in humans.* Proc. Natl. Acad. Sci. U.S.A., 2009. **106**(21): p. 8665-70.

43. Yfanti, C., et al., *Effect of antioxidant supplementation on insulin sensitivity in response to endurance exercise training.* Am. J. Physiol. Endocrinol. Metab., 2011. **300**(5): p. E761-70.

44. Apfeld, J. and C. Kenyon, *Regulation of life span by sensory perception in Caenorhabditis elegans.* Nature, 1999. **402**(6763): p. 804-9.

45. Libert, S., et al., *Regulation of Drosophila life span by olfaction and food-derived odors.* Science, 2007. **315**(5815): p. 1133-7.

46. Butcher, R.A., et al., *A potent dauer pheromone component in Caenorhabditis elegans that acts synergistically with other components.* Proc. Natl. Acad. Sci., 2008. **105**(38): p. 14288-14292.

47. Goranson, N., J. Ebersole and S. Brault, *Resolving an adaptive conundrum: reproduction in Caenorhabditis elegans is not sperm-limited when food is scarce.* Evol. Ecol. Res., 2005. **7**(2): p. 325-333.

48. Wolkow, C.A., et al., *Regulation of C. elegans life span by insulinlike signaling in the nervous system.* Science, 2000. **290**(5489): p. 147-50.

49. Bishop, N.A. and L. Guarente, *Two neurons mediate diet-restriction-induced longevity in C. [thinsp] elegans.* Nature, 2007. **447**(7144): p. 545-549.

50. Good, R.A., et al., *Nutritional deficiency, immunologic function and disease.* Am. J. Pathol., 1976. **84**(3): p. 599-614.

51. Yu, B.P., *Modulation of Aging Processes by Caloric Restriction.* 1994, Boca Raton, FL: CRC Press. 281.

52. Martin, C.K., et al., *Examination of cognitive function during six months of calorie restriction: results of a randomized controlled trial.* Rejuvenation Res., 2007. **10**(2): p. 179-90.

53. Mair, W., M.D. Piper and L. Partridge, *Calories do not explain extension of life span by dietary restriction in Drosophila.* PLoS Biol., 2005. **3**(7): p. e223.

54. Ungvari, Z., et al., *Mechanisms underlying caloric restriction and life span regulation: implications for vascular aging.* Circul. Res., 2008. **102**(5): p. 519-528.

55. Phelan, J. and S. Austad, *Natural selection, dietary restriction and extended longevity.* Growth, Development and Aging: GDA, 1988. **53**(1-2): p. 4-6.

56. Dillin, A., D.K. Crawford and C. Kenyon, *Timing requirements for insulin/IGF-1 signaling in C. elegans.* Science, 2002. **298**(5594): p. 830-4.

57. Hsin, H. and C. Kenyon, *Signals from the reproductive system regulate the life span of C. elegans.* Nature, 1999. **399**(6734): p. 362-366.

58. Weindruch, R., et al., *The retardation of aging in mice by dietary restriction: longevity, cancer, immunity and lifetime energy intake.* J. Nutr., 1986. **116**(4): p. 641-54.

59. de Paolo, L., *Dietary modulation of reproductive function, In: Modulation of Aging Processes by Dietary Restriction,* B. Yu, Editor. 1994, CRC Press: Cleveland, OH. p. 221-246.

60. McCarter, J., *Effects of exercise and dietary restriction on energy metabolism and longevity, In: Modulation of Aging Processes by Dietary Restriction,* B. Yu, Editor. 1994, CRC Press: Cleveland, OH. p. 157-174.

61. Fernandes, G. and J.T. Venkatraman, *Role of omega-3 fatty acids in health and disease.* Nutrition Research, 1993. **13**: p. S19-S45.

62. Sinclair, D.A., *Toward a unified theory of caloric restriction and longevity regulation.* Mech. Ageing Dev., 2005. **126**(9): p. 987-1002.

63. Medawar, P.B., *An unsolved problem of biology.* 1952, London,: Published for the college by H. K. Lewis. 24 p.

64. Promislow, D.E., *Senescence in natural populations of mammals: a comparative study.* Evolution, 1991. **45**(8): p. 1869-1887.

65. Ricklefs, R., *Evolutionary theories of aging: confirmation of a fundamental prediction, with implications for the genetic basis and evolution of life span.* Am. Nat., 1998. **152**: p. 24-44.

66. Bonduriansky, R. and C.E. Brassil, *Senescence: rapid and costly aging in wild male flies.* Nature, 2002. **420**(6914): p. 377.

67. Jones, O.R., et al., *Diversity of aging across the tree of life.* Nature, 2014. **505**(7482): p. 169-173.

68. Williams, G., *Pleiotropy, natural selection and the evolution of senescence.* Evolution, 1957. **11**: p. 398-411.

69. Holliday, R., *Food, reproduction and longevity: is the extended life span of calorie-restricted animals an evolutionary adaptation?* Bioessays, 1989. **10**(4): p. 125-7.

70. Kirkwood, T.B. and D.P. Shanley, *Food restriction, evolution and aging.* Mech. Ageing Dev., 2005. **126**(9): p. 1011-1016.

71. Cooper, C., et al., *Exercise, free radicals and oxidative stress.* Biochem. Soc. Trans., 2002. **30**(2): p. 280-284.

72. Puterman, E., et al., *The power of exercise: buffering the effect of chronic stress on telomere length.* PLoS One, 2010. **5**(5): p. e10837.

73. Nocon, M., et al., *Association of physical activity with all-cause and cardiovascular mortality: a systematic review and meta-analysis.* Eur. J. Cardiovasc. Prev. Rehabil., 2008. **15**(3): p. 239-246.

74. Holloszy, J.O., *Mortality rate and longevity of food-restricted exercising male rats: a reevaluation.* J. Appl. Physiol., 1997. **82**(2): p. 399-403.

75. De Grey, A.D., *The Mitochondrial Free Radical Theory of Aging.* 1999, Austin, TX: Springer/Landes. 212 pp.

76. Hollar, D. and C.H. Hennekens, *Antioxidant vitamins and cardiovascular disease: randomized trials fail to fulfill the promises of observational epidemiology, In: Antioxidants and Cardiovascular Disease.* 2006, Springer. p. 305-325.

77. Bjelakovic, G., et al., *Mortality in randomized trials of antioxidant supplements for primary and secondary prevention: systematic review and meta-analysis.* JAMA, 2007. **297**(8): p. 842-57.

78. Sayin, V.I., et al., *Antioxidants accelerate lung cancer progression in mice.* Sci. Transl. Med., 2014. **6**(221): p. 221ra15-221ra15.

79. Calabrese, E.J. and L.A. Baldwin, *Hormesis as a biological hypothesis.* Environ. Health Perspect., 1998. **106 Supp 1**(Supplement 1): p. 357-362.

80. Heywood, R., et al., *Safety evaluation of toothpaste containing chloroform. III. Long-term study in beagle dogs.* J. Environ. Pathol. Toxicol., 1979. **2**(3): p. 835-51.

81. Palmer, A.K., et al., *Safety evaluation of toothpaste containing chloroform. II. Long-term studies in rats.* J. Environ. Pathol. Toxicol., 1979. **2**(3): p. 821-33.

82. Yang, W. and S. Hekimi, *A mitochondrial superoxide signal triggers increased longevity in Caenorhabditis elegans.* PLoS Biol., 2010. **8**(12): p. e1000556.

83. Holloszy, J.O. and E.K. Smith, *Longevity of cold-exposed rats: a reevaluation of the "rate-of-living theory".* J. Appl. Physiol., 1986. **61**(5): p. 1656-60.

84. Yashin, A.I., et al., *Aging and survival after different doses of heat shock: the results of analysis of data from stress experiments with the nematode worm Caenorhabditis elegans.* Mech. Aging Dev., 2001. **122**(13): p. 1477-1495.

85. McClure, C.D., et al., *Hormesis results in tradeoffs with immunity.* Evolution, 2014. **68**(8): p. 2225-2233.

86. Caratero, A., et al., *Effect of a continuous gamma irradiation at a very low dose on the life span of mice.* Gerontology, 1997. **44**(5): p. 272-276.

87. Forbes, V., *Is hormesis an evolutionary expectation?* Funct. Ecol., 2000. **14**: p. 12-24.

88. Luckey, T.D., *Hormesis with Ionizing Radiation.* 1980, CRC Press, Boca Raton, FL.

89. Luckey, T.D., *Radiation hormesis.* 1991, CRC Press.

90. Luckey, T.D., *Nurture with ionizing radiation: a provocative hypothesis.* Nutr. Cancer, 1999. **34**(1): p. 1-11.

91. Neafsey, P.J., *Longevity hormesis. A review.* Mech. Ageing Dev., 1990. **51**(1): p. 1-31.

92. Jolly, D. and J. Meyer, *A brief review of radiation hormesis.* Australas. Phys. Eng. Sci. Med., 2009. **32**(4): p. 180-187.

93. Calabrese, E.J., *Toxicological awakenings: the rebirth of hormesis as a central pillar of toxicology.* Toxicol. Appl. Pharmacol., 2005. **204**(1): p. 1-8.

2
CHAPTER

The Diverse Demography
of Aging

Synopsis

This chapter is just for fun and is not logically necessary for the theme of the book. In another sense, this chapter is the core of the book, a broad survey of what theorists have before them to explain. The message is that aging (and non-aging) in nature is about as diverse as it can be. Every attempt to reconcile aging with orthodox evolutionary theory has invoked one constraint or another that has stayed the hand of biological evolution. My purpose in this chapter is, then, to show you that exceptions abound to every one of these hypothesized constraints and that nature gives no evidence of having been constrained. Every conceivable schedule of actuarial and fertility senescence, forward, backward and sideways, has handily evolved somewhere, in some species. We can only conclude that the life history of each species has been selected as optimal for that species in its particular niche.

Classical theories have attempted to account for aging as we know it in the human species. Some theorists have even attempted to prove that gradual aging is inevitable [1, 2] or that mortality rates must increase exponentially (the Gompertz law) [3, 4]. Theorists might have saved themselves a deal of trouble if they had surveyed before hand the diversity of life history patterns found in nature [5]. Life histories observed in nature span time scales from hours to millennia. And within each time frame, there are examples of gradual aging, sudden aging, no aging and reverse aging. There is reproductive senescence without mortality acceleration and there is mortality acceleration with no reproductive senescence. To call any mode of aging "normal" can only be a product of anthropocentric myopia.

Semelparity is one extreme of sudden aging. By definition, *semelparous* animals reproduce just once and it is striking how quickly and consistently they die once their eggs are laid. We might be tempted to draw a causal connection and infer that it is the reproduction that kills them; except that their modes of death are wildly different: male praying mantises are consumed by their mates, while octopuses starve themselves to death and Pacific salmon poison themselves with steroids. For separating death and reproduction, the pansies in the backyard are an even better example: How can it be that they will grow layer upon layer of new flowers, so long as we remember to snip off the dead ones; but the week that we let the pods go to seed, the entire plant shrivels and dies?

Other animals have lifespans that extend long beyond the end of their fertility. Post-reproductive lifespan is not limited to humans or even to social mammals—guppies and round worms are more extreme examples. Lifespan that considerably exceeds the span of fertility explicitly violates a core prediction of pleiotropy theory [2]. At the other end of the spectrum, there are animals that seem not to age at all or to age so slowly that it cannot be detected, demonstrating that there is nothing inevitable about aging and that attempts to cast aging as necessary consequence of physical or evolutionary law are misguided. Sharks grow larger, more powerful and more fertile with each passing year. Whales have been captured with 130-year-old harpoon tips stuck in their flesh. Hydra, sea urchins and some sea mollusks have periods in their life cycles where they seem to be getting younger. And many researchers claim to detect "mortality plateaus", a phenomenon in which the relentless exponential increase in mortality slows or stops altogether late in life.

Diverse Modes of Aging

In America, humans begin aging around puberty, when mortality is at its minimum [6]. Aging proceeds very slowly in children and young adults, accelerating exponentially, until shortly past age 100, humans have a life expectancy less than one year.

We know that other animals and plants in nature don't follow the human model. Modes of aging are surprisingly diverse for anyone considering this field for the first time. At one extreme, there are animals that experience sudden death. The mayfly may live several years in the water, feeding on algae, going through several larval stages. Then she grows wings, lays eggs and dies, all in a single day. At the other extreme, there are whales and sharks, perhaps lobsters and clams that just get larger, stronger and more fertile as they grow older. Eventually, they will succumb to an accident (nature knows no "immortality") but when they die, age will not be a factor. It is considered normal for the risk of dying to increase gradually, starting with sexual maturity. But there are many plants and some animals whose death rates go steadily down with age through most of their lives. This demography has been characterized as "negative senescence" [7].

Protists get old in a few hours, while quaking aspen may live ten thousand years. The breathtaking scope of these modes of aging and their time scales attests nature's full control over the process. Natural selection has crafted aging, in all its varieties and all its vagaries, its slow and its rapid forms, its inevitability and its remarkable plasticity.

Actuarial Definitions of Aging

A common way of thinking about aging is a general weakening and loss of function. But markers of aging vary widely from one species to the next, so there is no universal metabolic definition. The two most standard definitions come from increasing mortality and declining fertility, respectively. To a demographer, aging means that an individual loses resilience over time, so that the same hazard has a greater probability of killing it this year as it did last year.

In a meadow in Sweden, the *Sanicula* shrub has been studied continually since the middle of the last century. It is a common plant and not particularly impressive to look at and perhaps the only remarkable thing about it is that it has been studied intensively. About one shrub in 70 dies each year, apparently from environmental factors, so that the plants have an average lifespan of 70 years. But the curious thing is that a 70-year-old plant does not seem to have a different mortality risk than a 10-year-old plant. Humans have a comparable lifespan to *Sanicula*, but because we age, very few humans reach 100 years old and none reach 150 years. Aging means that death is biologically determined and this limits our lifespan. But in *Sanicula*, death is merely a matter of constant chance. With one plant in 70 dying each year, there will be about half left at the end of 48 years (because $e^{-48/70} = \frac{1}{2}$); but that half will be untouched by age. So at the end of another 50 years, one quarter still remain and an eighth are still alive after 150 years. At this rate, about one in a million would live a thousand years. If human lifespans followed the same distribution as *Sanicula*, there would be a few people still alive who could give firsthand accounts of Leonardo da Vinci (1452-1519) and perhaps one or two who were in England at the time of the Norman Conquest (1066).

Demographically, *Sanicula* does not age and humans do age. This is true even though both *Sanicula* and humans are mortal and have similar lifespans. All will eventually die and in fact the *average* human may live longer than the average *Sanicula* shrub; but the last human of our generation will be long gone while *Sanicula* that came into the world at the same time are still hanging on.

Semelparity Equals Sudden Death

A *semelparous* plant or animal is defined by the fact that it reproduces just once in a lifetime; but as it happens, almost all semelparous animals and plants die promptly after reproduction. There is no aging, no weakening or loss of function, no increase in mortality for the entire time before the reproductive burst. But once reproduction is done, death follows promptly.

How and why do semelparous organisms die? The "how" varies widely, but the "why" has an evolutionary answer. Natural selection does not want a parent to be competing with its offspring. Evolution has programmed a death schedule into the genes, gratuitously and with no concomitant benefit to the individual. Theory proclaims that there is no such thing as genetically programmed death; it is an evolutionary oxymoron. But in the case of semelparity, some of the most orthodox evolutionary theorists will admit an exception [8].

Pansies and other annuals familiar from domestic gardens will flower once for the year, then the buds "go to seed" and the plant dies. Does death result from the effort of making the flower? No! In fact, snipping off the flower gives the plant a new lease on life. Pansies can be made to bloom continuously through the summer, if their flowers are snipped before they go to seed. Evidently, the plant can create a lot more flowers, had it in mind to do so. Evolutionary theory asserts that the plant is maximizing its reproductive output, because maximizing reproductive output is the very direction of natural selection. That would mean that the plant which dies after flowering is incapable of producing a second crop of flowers. But in defiance of theory, the pansy seems perfectly capable of going on to flower multiple times in the proper circumstances*.

Are there animals like the pansy, capable of resurrecting their fertility in a pinch? The female velvet spider limits herself to a single clutch of eggs—but only if she is successful. She stays with her eggs until they hatch and if she should lose her brood, she'll lay another clutch of eggs and another; but if her eggs hatch, she'll die a happy mother. Clearly, it is not producing eggs that kills her. Just like your pansies, the spiders belie the notion that death derives from an all-out effort at reproduction [9].

Evolutionary theorists continue to imagine a causal link between "reproductive effort" and death, because they believe programmed death to be an impossibility. It has been assumed that natural selection has pushed for an ever stronger burst of reproduction, usurping all the body's resources, so that the body is thoroughly wasted when reproduction is complete. "Semelparity may arise because the amount that must be allocated to reproduction so drains the organism's resources that its death is certain". This is a quote from a 1992 textbook by Derek Roff that is still a much-referenced standard of the field [10 p 247]. Roff's chapter on semelparity is dominated by theoretical analysis of the tradeoffs in fitness when energy is allocated for survival or for reproduction. The implicit assumptions that fitness is entirely a matter of individual reproductive output and that this measure of fitness is optimized by natural selection—these assumptions are so standard that they are not questioned or even mentioned. Tom Kirkwood, author of the Disposable Soma theory for the evolution of aging [11] wrote: "An important source of misunderstanding of the evolutionary theory of aging has been to regard post reproductive death in semelparous species as an instance of programmed aging, when in fact its evolutionary explanation appears likely to be very different" [12]. "[T]here is little evidence that semelparous organisms are actively destroyed once reproduction is complete; they tend simply to fall apart" [8].

Other neo-Darwinian theorists have published elaborate mathematical demonstrations that semelparity pays for some animals but not others. All of them are based on a major assumption: that investing less in offspring would allow an animal or plant to invest more in longevity [10]. That is, they assume it would only be possible to live longer by reducing fertility. No one knows if this is true in general or even in individual cases. It is easy enough to assume a numerical value for the tradeoff and crank the equations through to make a prediction about semelparity. But how can we know if this value is reasonable? What experiment could be done that would measure this tradeoff, even in theory? The only thing we can say with assurance about these equations is that if they apply at all, there must be some

---

* A partisan of the theory might argue that it was the seed, not the flower, that required extraordinary "reproductive effort" and it was this effort that finally kills the plant.

loopholes, because pansies and velvet spiders constitute clear exceptions. Are there others?

Salmon and Century Plants

The Century Plant (maguey) is a desert succulent, familiar to health food aficionados as the source of agave nectar. Maguey deploys the same reproductive strategy as annual plants, but on an augmented time scale. From a central root, it spreads spiny, fat leaves which collect water over a period of decades. The roots spread close to the surface and sprout other century plants in the local area. But to spread its seed further afield (and to share its genetic material), the plant creates a flowering spectacle. A stalk develops over a few weeks' time in the spring, rising at up to an inch per hour, until it reaches a height of more than 20 feet. Several pounds of purple flowers appear and scatter their seeds to the wind. Then the plant dies, roots and all (but not the runners, which live on to sprout a circle of clones around the dead parent). The nickname "Century" may be a stretch for Maguey, but Mediterranean cousins of the Century Plant actually have better claim to the name [13] and Peruvian Puyas live up to 150 years before flowering. We may wonder how a plant that flowers so infrequently can coordinate with neighbors for pollination. Flowers are pollinated by a particular species of bat (*Leptonycteris nivalis*) with a range of several kilometers so that it can locate and cross-pollinate distant magueys.

Semelparity does not work for birds and mammals, because their life cycle requires substantial investment in nourishing and protecting the young. This task can best be performed over an extended time period, so there is an advantage in spreading reproduction over a lifetime, not reproducing in one burst. Mammals bear their young a few at a time, so mothers will be able to supply enough milk. You might suppose that, since this argument applies only to females, there is nothing to stop male mammals from indulging in semelparity. And in fact, there are a few marsupials in which the males die after mating. They are western opossums and quolls, squirrel-sized marsupials of tropical Australia. They mate in the spring, after which the females carry their young and often live to see another season. But the male metabolisms pump out a lethal dose of steroid hormones (glucocorticoids) and die promptly. Selective death of the males presents a difficulty for theories that rely on reproductive effort and in fact the evolutionary paradox has been acknowledged by ecologists [14, 15]. We might imagine that males disappear so there is more food available for the females and their young; or we might note that the male die-off after a single mating promotes genetic diversity. But both these explanations require strong group selection, so they are eliminated from consideration in the mainstream of evolutionary theory.

Birds, too, invest care in their offspring and they spread their reproduction over time so they can sit on their eggs and forage for their hatchlings. Frequently the males participate in feeding the young. There are no semelparous birds, but there are a few semelparous reptiles and amphibians, many fish and mollusks and insects.

The Pacific salmon is probably our best-known example of semelparity in animals. The adults spawn in fresh water, sometimes hundreds of miles upstream from the ocean. Male and female both migrate inland and the male spreads sperm over the eggs after the female deposits them in a nest, a dimple (a 'redd') that she digs in the streambed or river pool. In some species, the hatchlings remain there just a few weeks and return to the ocean when they are only an inch or two in length. Others stay up to two years, becoming fully mature before migrating downstream. The majority of the salmon's life is spent in the sea, where, presumably, the hunt is richer and more reliable. All salmon return to breed in the very same pool in which they hatched. Most impressive are the Chinook salmon, which stay in the ocean up to seven years and range up to 2500 miles from the mouth of the stream where they first entered the sea. (How do they navigate? How do they distinguish their own stream or river from hundreds of others on the same coast? Science has yet to answer this question. There are theories involving taste and magnetic fields and polarized light, but there is nothing like a full hypothesis about their mechanism, let alone a demonstration or definitive experiment.)

By the time the adult salmon reach their spawning ground, their metabolisms are in terminal collapse. Their adrenal glands are pumping out steroids (glucocorticoids) that cause accelerated aging (perhaps "instant" would be a better word). They have stopped eating. The steroids have caused their immune systems to collapse, so their bodies are covered with fungal infections. Kidneys atrophy, while the adjacent interregnal cells (associated with those glucocorticoids) become greatly enlarged. Their arteries develop lesions that appear akin to those responsible for heart disease in aging humans. The swim upstream is arduous, but it is not the mechanical beating of the rocks (and dams) that does the body in. Rather it is the biochemical change that is genetically programmed to accompany spawning. These symptoms occur in both males and females, despite the fact that it is the females who carry the metabolic ball, in the form of eggs that may constitute a third of their body mass on the trip upstream. The sperm burden of the male is trivial—yet they die just as surely.

During their last weeks, metabolisms of these fish are in terminal collapse. How much of the damage is due to a flood of sex hormones that serve to up the egg harvest and how much is programmed death, with no other purpose? In nature it is hard to tell, but controlled experiments suggest the hypothesis of programmed death. First, the adrenal tissue—source of the glucocorticoids—can be removed from the salmon *after she spawns* and the result: she lives. Second, salmon in captivity go through all the sexual development leading to egg-laying, but they don't have to fight their way upstream and they don't lay eggs. Nevertheless, they die and die from the same glucocorticoid malady. One further reason to believe that death is separable from reproduction: The Pacific salmon have cousins in the Atlantic that routinely 'double dip'. They have milder versions of the same bodily symptoms and they can recover, returning to the ocean for another round trip. They even swim upstream to lay their eggs, but they survive to tell the tale; and the tale they tell is that death is not an inherent metabolic price that the salmon must pay for their fertility.

Semelparity as Programmed Death

To the field biologists who study the details of their life history, the Pacific salmon are a clear example of programmed death. The people most intimately familiar with the salmon's metabolism accept programmed death as a starting point, taking off from there to debate the anatomic details. It is only orthodox evolutionary theorists who insist without need of evidence that genetically programmed death is not logically possible. If the target of natural selection is deemed to be individual reproductive success, then they are correct.

But if we follow observations rather than theory, we might accept the evidence that these salmon are killing themselves with glucocorticoids; then we wonder why. A venerable theory states that the fish are fertilizing the streams where their young ones will grow up, adding nutrients to the ecosystem [16]. Although ecologists have been able to show that salmon carcasses are an important source of nitrogen and phosphorous in streams and pools where they die, it is still difficult to imagine how programmed death could evolve on that basis. The problem is that these chemical resources are widely shared. The benefit of a salmon's death is not limited to its own offspring. If some salmon die while others go back to the sea for another round, then all their offspring benefit, so there is no advantage to separate the offspring of the salmon that die from the offspring of the salmon that don't die. There is no kin selection for the trait, no force driving programmed death to evolve.

This is an instance of a common problem, perhaps the central problem that has led the neo-Darwinists to conclude that 'cooperation cannot evolve'. Any kind of self-sacrifice has difficulty evolving because it is vulnerable to 'cheating'. Those who cheat reap the benefit contributed by those who sacrifice. This is a genuinely difficult obstacle and the theorists are correct to emphasize this kind of thinking. The evidence is strong, however, that programmed death *did* evolve; if our understanding of the way in which evolution works makes this seem implausible, then it is the understanding that must change, we must not discredit the evidence that is plainly before us.

In Chapter 7, I offer my own theory about how programmed death may have evolved in semelparous animals.

...and Cephelopods and Cicadas

Less well known than the Pacific salmon, but just as fascinating and compelling in its story, is the octopus. Octopuses are the geniuses of the invertebrate world. Their brains are far larger than any other invertebrate and comparable in size to some mammals'. The octopus does not have a separate head and the brain wraps like a blanket around the animal's esophagus. Much intelligence is distributed in nerves of the tentacles. Nevertheless, octopuses can learn complex tasks, they cooperate with one another, have been observed to play and even to trick one another for selfish ends.

They live a short time, a few months to a few years, depending on the species; and they die after reproducing once. The female guards and cares for her eggs, but if conditions are not right for her brood, she may eat them. If she decides the time is propitious, not only does she refrain from eating her eggs, the female stops eating altogether. Her mouth seals over. She will die within days after the eggs hatch, but her death is not induced by starvation. We know this because there are two endocrine glands called 'optic glands'* whose secretions control mating behavior, maternal care and also: death. The optic glands can be surgically removed and the octopus then lives longer. If one optic gland is removed, the female doesn't eat, but still lives an extra six weeks. That seems to be how long it takes to die of starvation. If both optic glands are removed, then the octopus does not lose its mouth and resumes eating after the eggs hatch. She then regains strength and size and can live up to 40 weeks more [17-19].

The female's behavior in consuming her own eggs is very difficult to understand from the vantage of neo-Darwinian theory. She is at the end of her life in any case and will have no legacy. Under different circumstances, the octopus can be a devoted mother. Sometimes she will carefully guard the eggs against sea predators and fungal infections; the longest observed maternal vigil was over four years [20]. Both guarding the eggs and eating them may be part of a population regulation program, octopus style. The shellfish on which the octopus depends are a finite, renewable resource and the animals may be adjusting their population size so as not to threaten the food supply for succeeding generations. If the octopus population is indeed being actively managed by the animal's behavior, it makes the evolution of a death program easier to understand. More on this theme in Chapter 6.

The cicada also has to 'worry' about population control and the danger of killing off the trees on which it depends for food, but its life cycle strategy is very different from the octopus. Larvae of the longest-lived variety of cicada live in the ground seventeen years before they come out to mate and die. Is it plausible that the larva is growing as fast as it can and that seventeen is exactly how many years it takes to make a full-grown cicada, on a best efforts basis? I think it more plausible that the purpose of the cicada's Rip van Winkle act has more to do with the trees than with the larva. Cicadas swarm in the spring and can completely denude the trees in an area. Refraining from an annual attack on the trees may be essential to the long-term viability of the cicada, but a fleecing every seventeen years is an insult that most trees can endure and survive.

The cicadas get another benefit from emerging all at once, rather than a few at a time each year. Birds feed on cicadas and will gorge themselves during cicada season. If the cicadas staggered their appearance, they could support a much larger bird population, which is not a good outcome for (collective) cicada fitness. But in a swarm, they overwhelm the birds' appetites: the birds' consumption saturates while cicadas are still plentiful. The cicadas avoid providing the birds with a steady diet and thus find safety in numbers.

All the leaf-eating and the denuding are the work of the young cicadas, not the parents. The adults are interested only in laying eggs. Once nature has invested seventeen years in creating a fertile adult cicada, you would think she would be motivated to maximize her return by keeping the cicada alive, eating, laying eggs, reproducing as many times as possible before the end of the season. But this is not the cicada's way. The male dies promptly after mating. The female dies after depositing

---

* The name of the gland comes from the fact that the gland has a nerve link to the animal's eye and lighting plays an active role in timing the gland's primary secretions, which lead to sexual maturity.

her eggs under the bark of a twig. Neither of them eats in the adult stage, but they don't starve to death. Their bodies dry up as they become inactive, suggesting that their deaths are genetically programmed.

Mayflies have independently adopted a similar strategy, though on a shorter time scale. Mayfly larvae live in the water for a full year, eating algae and diatoms, hiding from predators under rocks and sediment. Somehow, they coordinate their maturity, so that one spring day, they all emerge as adults to mate, lay eggs and die. (How do they manage to agree on the day? There is no known means of communicating or coordinating behavior [21].) Even though they are quite vulnerable to predation as adults, nature has not left their fate to depend on chance encounters. Death is part of the program and follows within hours after reproduction.

In the face of these diverse examples, the theoretical literature on semelparity must seem overly abstract and vague. All of it starts with the idea that natural law somehow imposes the choice between reproduction "now" and saving resources for reproduction later, an assumption for which there is not an iota of direct evidence. In fact, as I've tried to show in this section, there is considerable inferential evidence to the contrary. When pressed with the evidence, some neo-Darwinists will concede that there is, indeed, an appearance of programmed death, but that semelparity constitutes at most a limited exception to the rule, which has been able to evolve because these animals have exhausted all reproductive capacity and so have nothing left to lose [8]. As Medawar [22] said (in a different but related context), this argument "canters twice round the perimeter of a vicious circle".

Variations on a Semelparous Theme

I said that semelparity cannot work for birds or mammals, because they need to care for their young. Therefore they cannot afford to reproduce all in one burst, let alone to die afterward without nurturing their offspring into independence. But that does not mean that aging cannot come suddenly.

Albatrosses show us another style of sudden aging and death. They don't reproduce in a burst—quite the contrary, they stay with their mates and lay just one egg every year or two, investing heavily in each chick. Over four decades, they lose little if any of their fertility with age. Nor does their death rate rise gradually with time. But suddenly, some time after age forty, the death rate spikes. The birds die suddenly and mysteriously, usually before the age of 50 years and without any signs of aging that biologists have been able to discover [23-25]. Detecting signs of mortality acceleration in a population of albatrosses was a *tour de force*, finally achieved in 2006 [26].

In a similar vein, the arctic *guillemot* shows no signs of age for the first 35 years, then drops dead. The sea bird looks like a miniature penguin, but it lives at the wrong pole. It can fly as well as swim. Kyle Elliott studied their life cycle for his dissertation and comments, "Despite the prediction that survival should decrease at higher latitudes, many of the longest-lived warm-blooded animals live in the polar regions" [27]. This appears to be an exception to the oft-cited theoretical prediction [2, 28] that high rates of incidental mortality ought to drive evolution of shorter lifespans.

Naked mole rats (NMR) are an exotic and obscure species from the desert of East Africa which became darlings of gerontological research once it was discovered that they have extraordinarily long lifespans. Though they are no bigger than a mouse, they live ten times longer. Like albatrosses, NMRs seem to be lifelong procrastinators: they do all their aging "at the last minute". Unlike mice, they are not susceptible to cancer. Their tissues remain elastic, their arteries resilient and their muscles strong. There is no increase in mortality over the first 27 years of life [29]. They have solved the problem of skin aging by adopting the appearance of a wrinkled old troll beginning at birth. But in zoos and laboratory colonies, somewhere around age 30, they are found to die without warning, of unknown causes. NMR colonies are eusocial (only the queen reproduces), so the effect of mortality on an individual's fitness is less direct than in the case of the albatross and guillemot referenced above.

Post-Reproductive Lifespan

Menopause is Darwinian death, as fitness suddenly drops to zero. Even a few years ago, it was thought that menopause was unique to humans and perhaps a few other highly social mammals: primates, elephants and whales. Not so. Many mammals and birds outlive their reproductive organs and become Darwinian orphans. Opossums [28], parakeets [30] and quail [31] don't care for their grandchildren, but all these animals can live long enough to lose their fertility in the wild. Female sturgeons run out of eggs and consequently cease to lay them. More puzzling: the nematode *C. elegans* runs out of sperm at a time when they have unfertilized eggs left in their bodies [32]. Aside from rare males, *C. elegans* are hermaphroditic and capable of self-fertilization. Eggs are much larger cells, including nutrients to jump-start the next generation's growth, whereas sperm are tiny packets of genetic material only. Metabolically, sperm are cheap and eggs are expensive. If Mother Nature were economizing, sperm is not the place she would be tempted to skimp. This little fable suggests that perhaps natural selection has some other goals in its sights than simply maximizing reproductive potential. One hint is that *C. elegans* is exquisitely adapted for population homeostasis, with a lifespan that is highly plastic in response to environmental cues and the ability to 'hibernate' as a *dauer* during periods of drought or food scarcity. One of the biggest existential threats to the worms' viability is that a crop of re-awakening dauers may be too large for the available food supply and the worms exhaust the available food before any of them has grown to reproductive maturity. I have speculated [33] that both the limit on lifespan and the presence of post-reproductive worms in the population may be adaptations that help stabilize populations.

One of the most thorough and careful demographic surveys involved guppies on the Caribbean island of Trinidad and post-reproductive life was detected [34]. It is difficult to census these animals in their native habitat, so these studies are open to question; but conversely, it is also possible that these surveys are just the tip of an iceberg and that, as some ecologists have argued [35], post-reproductive life is very common in nature.

From the neo-Darwinian perspective, life without reproduction serves no purpose and should quickly disappear, as the body evolves to invest its resources more fruitfully. One of the original predictions of Williams [2] in proposing the pleiotropic theory of aging was that "[t]here should be little or no post reproductive period in the normal life-cycle of any species". If post-reproductive lifespan is real and general, then this undercuts the neo-Darwinian presumption every bit as much as programmed aging does.

What evolutionary purpose could be served by keeping animals around when their fertility and even their parental behaviors are ended? My hypothesis (with Charles Goodnight) is that the post-reproductive animals form a demographic buffer that helps to stabilize population levels over time [33]. In times of famines or disease, the old, infertile animals are the first to succumb and since this has no effect on the community's breeding capacity, the population is poised for a quick recovery. More about this to come in Chapter 7.

"Normal" Aging: What Determines the Lifespan?

Land mammals and birds are the animals most familiar to us and among these iteroparity is the norm. But there is a huge range of lifespans even among animals that are otherwise quite similar. Mice may live two or three years in the protected environment of captivity; their biological cousins the naked mole rats are the same size and have similar metabolisms and slower metabolic rates, yet they live 20-30 years. Bats are of comparable size with much faster metabolisms and they live 30-50 years.

Across similar species, larger animals live longer than smaller animals. They take longer to develop and mature, so perhaps the extra time reflects a higher investment in each offspring that is produced. But within a given species, the opposite is true. Thus rats don't live as long as pigs and elephants live much longer still. But Chihuahuas live a lot longer than St Bernards or Greyhounds [17]. How might this principle apply to people? The jury is still out. Some authors conclude that taller people live longer [36], while others cite data that shorter people enjoy longer life [37]. The answer remains ambiguous because it is so difficult to separate genetics from the effects of nutrition and medical care in childhood, which can lead to both greater height and longer lifespan.

In natural settings, death rates are always matched to birth rates and maturation times, so that the population can remain steady over time. In a way, this is a tautology: those animal species with low birth rates and short lifespans disappeared a long time ago, because they were not able to sustain themselves. But the opposite is also true: species that live too long and reproduce too prolifically suffer almost as swift and sure a demise, because their numbers quickly overwhelm the available food resources and famine can wipe out a species faster than its prey can grow back. (Chapter 6 contains some dramatic case histories.)

Methuselahs of the Forest

Long life requires both a low base mortality rate and also a slow rate of aging, so that mortality remains low. Most of the longest living things on earth are trees.

Trees that live hundreds of years are too common to enumerate. Even many smaller plants can live for centuries. Harsh environments seem to breed longevity, with desert, mountain and arctic climates taking top honors. In arid, rocky areas of the American Midwest, Bristlecone pines are common. Up to 4,800 annual rings have been counted in their trunk wood [38]. Giant sequoias are larger, but not older. The oldest sequoias are thought to be 'only' 3,000 years. The association with harsh environments makes a rough kind of evolutionary sense: When the odds for your offsprings' survival to maturity are low, you are motivated so much the more to cling to life. In Chapter 4, we shall see that, among animals, those that live in arctic environments have some of the longest lifespans, but also the highest proportions of death caused by senescence. Thus in harsh environments, it seems that nature has kept a firmer hand on the demographic tiller.

Aspen groves may look like forests of independent trees, but aspens propagate underground, like mushrooms and new trees grow up from roots, without seeds*. Some groves are thought to be tens of thousands of years old [39]. Nevertheless, we may not be able to point to any chunk of wood on a particular tree and demonstrate that it has been around from the beginning. Should Aspens count as ancient? On the affirmative side, the grove is a single organism that has grown without sexual recombination from a single seed. You might want to protest that this tree is like George Washington's original hatchet, of which the handle has been replaced a few times over the years and a new head has been substituted. But on a finer scale, we, too, are all like George Washington's hatchet: the cells in our bodies are recycled and replaced from one week to the next (blood, skin cells) or from one decade to the next (some nerve cells).

The Pando Grove in Utah has been called the world's oldest living thing [40]. A single Aspen plant, its shoots and roots range over about half a mile. There is one root system, linking a mass of trees estimated at 6,000 tons. The entire grove grew from a single seed about 80,000 years ago.

...and Elders of the Deep

There are no known examples of animals living thousands of years, but many with lifespans over 100.

Sturgeons have been found to live over 150 years. Females carry a finite stock of eggs and become infertile when they run out [17]. Sharks are cartilaginous fish, even more ancient than sturgeons and with a mythology all their own. In the Orient, shark fin soup is an expensive delicacy, consumed for health and longevity. In the West, shark cartilage is sold as a dietary supplement for arthritis. Is it true that sharks are free from aging? The answer is unclear. Some smaller sharks live to a venerable age. The dogfish grows to a maximum size of 15 or 20 pounds, but may live 80-100 years [41]. Aging in larger species has not been detected and it is a legitimate speculation that they continue to grow all their lives, with no biological limit and no aging.

---

* Occasionally, they spread via flowers and seeds as well. This is important for long-distance dispersal and for maintaining diversity through sex.

Galapagos tortoises can live over 150 years in the wild. One subspecies from Pinta Island is represented by a single ancient male, who was taken into captivity in 1972, in an attempt to help him breed. After 36 years in captivity, he successfully fertilized eggs of two closely-related females in 2008. Zoo-keepers of the world mourned the death of "Lonesome George" in the summer of 2012, world-weary at the tender age of 100 [42].

The Rougheye Rockfish grows in deep, cold water off the North American West coast, from San Diego up through the Aleutians, down the Asian Coast to Japan. In life at the bottom, light is absent, food and oxygen are scarce, temperatures are low. (Because of high pressure and salinity, the temperature can actually be below zero Celsius, which we normally think of as the freezing point of water.) Everything happens more slowly down there and the Rockfish life cycle unfolds at a relaxed and leisurely tactus. Lifespans have been reported over 200 years [43]. It is the arrogance and folly of human opportunism that we have been netting these elder statesmen of the deep and marketing them for food, so that they are now endangered and very slow to regrow.

Guessing the ages of marine life can be an inexact art, because annual temperature cycles are much less pronounced in the ocean, so the annual growth rings that are common in land species may be missing [43]. We don't know for sure how to tell a whale's age and it was a surprise in 2008 when a bowhead whale was captured with a 130-year-old harpoon tip lodged in its back [44]. It is likely the whale was over 200 years old.

Intuition based on our experience may suggest to us that whales and elephants (80 year lifespan) seem less impressive than tiny lichens and sea urchins with comparable life expectancies. There is a scientific basis for this intuition, both in experiment and in theory. Among animals with a given metabolic plan, larger size is associated with slower metabolism and longer lifespan. The simplest reason for this is quite heuristic—that with the same metabolic rate, producing more cells can take longer. So development and maturity happen more slowly, reproduction happens more slowly and the species needs a longer lifespan. In reality, it is more complicated than that. There are physical theories that almost work [45], indicating why metabolic rates are actually lower for the larger animals, amplifying the need for extra time. These same theories become more speculative when they suggest how lifespan should be connected to size*. Of course, the physical theory also has trouble accounting for the anomalies, like naked mole rats that live so much longer than other rodents and man, another outlier who lives far longer than comparably sized mammals. From our perspective, we should not be surprised that physical theories fail to provide a basic understanding of lifespans and aging rates. We concluded in Chapter 2 that there is no physical necessity for aging and that its explanation must be sought in biology—and perhaps not even in individual metabolisms, but in ecological relationships and population dynamics.

---

* Mathematically, there is a power law connecting the two and the standard theory gets the exponent almost right.

Animals that Don't Age at All

Other animals do not seem to age at all, even though their typical lifespans are short because of predation and other hazards.

Hydra are primitive invertebrates with radial symmetry—a mouth on a stalk, surrounded by oversized tentacles, living in ponds and streams. Under a magnifying lens, they look a bit like (but are unrelated to) tiny squids. With their tentacles, they snare "water fleas" and other tiny crustaceans, on which they feed. Hydra have been studied for four years at a time, starting with specimens of various ages collected in the wild and they do not seem to die on their own or to become more vulnerable to predators or disease with age [46].

In the human body, there are certain cells that are sloughed off and regenerated continuously; blood cells, skin and the stomach lining are examples. The hydra's whole body is like this, regenerating itself from stem cells every few days. Some cells are sloughed off and die, but other cells grow into hydra clones that bud off from the stalk-body when they are large enough to make it on their own. This is a primitive style of reproduction, without sex. The hydra can also reproduce sexually.

One recent article [47] claims that the hydra does indeed grow older and shows it by slowing its rate of cloning. The author suggests that perhaps clones inherit their parents age and so these "youngsters" do not seem to do any better than their aging parents. The hypothesis is that only sexual reproduction resets the aging clock. If this is true, then the hydra's style of aging is a throwback to "replicative senescence" in protists. There is a sense in which, every time a cell divides, the daughter cells inherit the mother's age. We'll look at telomere biology in Chapter 3.

Some clams and oysters do not seem to get any 'closer to death' as they get older. The name *quahog* may sound exotic, but the clam to which it refers is likely as not to be the one in your clam chowder. It gets larger with each year of life and annual growth rings make its age easy to determine. They have been found to live up to 400 years [48, 49], though they commonly fall prey to starfish at any age and we do not know how long they might live in a protected environment [50]. That is to say, if chowder clams age at all, their aging has yet to be measured.

Sea urchins are spiny, primitive animals that are *sessile*—rooted in the sea floor like plants. It is difficult to find very old sea urchins in nature because they are food for fish and mammals, but it is possible to collect statistics for urchin populations and ask whether the old ones have a higher statistical risk of death than the young ones. This analysis indicates that sea urchins do not weaken or lose function with age, so far as we can tell [17]. In confirmation of this idea, the oldest sea urchins have been carbon dated at over a century [51].

Tarantulas can take up to 10 years to reach maturity. The males are subject to aging but, at least in some species, females seem not to age. Some species of tarantulas have lived 20 years in captivity with no sign of senescence [17]. No less an authority than the Guiness Book lists the oldest fully documented tarantula at 49 years.

A Fountain of Youth where Only Queens can Drink

Bees have an interesting tale to tell us, because of the difference between workers and queens. Queen bees are genetically the same as worker bees. When a new hive is begun, the nurse bees will select—arbitrarily as far as we can tell—one larva to be fed on "royal jelly". The combination of nutrients in royal jelly triggers a program in the developing bee that causes her to grow not into a worker, but a queen bee instead, with overdeveloped gonads that give her a whole new shape. The queen makes one flight at the beginning of her career, during which time she might mate with a dozen different drones and store their sperm inside her for many years to come.

The fully-grown queen is too heavy to fly. She lays eggs at a prodigious rate of about 2,000 per day. (A day's worth of eggs may weigh more than the queen herself.) She is attended continually by specialized workers who feed her, remove her waste and transmit her pheromonal messages to the rest of the hive.

Worker bees have short lifespans. They live only a few weeks and die of old age; they do not just wear out from broken body parts and the rough-and-tumble worlds in which they fly. Worker bee mortality has been measured at different ages and it increases with the same Gompertz (exponential) function typical of other animals [52].

Queen bees, despite the fact that they have identical genes to the workers, show no signs of getting weaker with age. They can continue to live and lay for years. If the hive is healthy and stable, the queen may occasionally live for decades. The absolute limit on her lifetime arrives when the sperm she acquired in her maiden flight runs out. At that point, she may continue to lay eggs, but they are unfertilized and can only grow into drones. The depleted queen is assassinated by the same workers that formerly attended her. They gather about and sting her to death [53, 54].

The most natural interpretation of this saga is that rapid aging is programmed into the bees' metabolisms, but the aging program can be turned off entirely by interventions (royal jelly) early in the bee's life.

There are other examples where the same genes can lead to long or short lifespans, always dependent on ecological roles or social factors. Close cousins of the 200-year-old rockfish that live in shallower waters have never been observed to live past 13 years [55]. This raises the question why the longer lifespan was not available in the evolutionary trajectory of the 13-year variety.

Strongyloides ratti is a parasitic nematode that infects rats by burrowing through the skin [56]. While inside the rat, female worms produce clones that can either remain within the host or find their way out with the feces. Those that remain in the host are all females, while those that enter a free-living stage can be male or female. The free-living developmental path is triggered by the lower temperature outside the rat [57]. Diversity in the genome is provided by mating in the free-living stage. The *Strongyloides* life cycle and genetics have other oddities, but for our purpose the salient point is that the parasitic form and the free-living form are morphologically similar, but the free-living form ages and dies within five days, while within a host, the worm can live more than a year [58].

What do we Mean by 'Aging in Reverse'

Most striking and counter-intuitive are cases in which aging progresses in reverse. If we use the demographer's definition of aging as mortality acceleration, then growth that leads to greater strength and lower mortality fits the definition of "negative senescence". In most trees and some animals, mortality rates can decline over an extended time. Fertility also commonly increases as a plant or animal continues to grow larger. This may seem unexceptional to our intuition, because we think of it as a continuation of the growth to maturity; but it can be problematic for theories in which reproductive fitness is strictly maximized. There is a fitness bonus for early reproduction and so it is to be expected that natural selection favors a shift in reproduction to the earliest age that is physically possible.

A developing thesis in this book links aging to the need for population control in animals. Plants, as primary producers, have much less necessity for population control and this explains why we observe all the examples of extreme longevity and most examples of negative senescence in plants. Negative senescence is common in plants, rare in animals.

The oldest sequoias living today are over 3,000 years old and over 350 feet tall (about one inch per year). A giant sequoia produces about hundreds of millions of seeds over its lifetime. The oldest and largest trees are not only greatly resistant to fire, winds and erosion, they also produce the greatest quantity of seeds. So sequoias meet both criteria for negative senescence and can remain on this trajectory for many hundreds of years. Only for the very largest and oldest trees do mortality rates begin to rise.

Sequoias are unique for their size, but not their longevity. The giant Cypress in Tule, Mexico is 2,000 years old and it is quite ordinary for trees to live for centuries. There simply hasn't been enough study to know whether aging in trees is the rule or the exception. Data must be compared for large numbers of trees over long periods of time. But examples abound for the plasticity of aging in trees. In other words, when trees seem to be slowing down with age, they can be induced to fresh spurts of growth by pruning of buds. And it is well-known that branches can be cut from old fruit trees and induced to grow roots of their own. These trees seem to have an entirely new lease on life, with the vigor and lifespan of a tree grown from seed. This behavior contrasts with animals that can regenerate in the manner of plants. An arm can be amputated from a starfish and the arm will grow into an intact starfish; but in this case the regenerated starfish remembers its age. If the original starfish was old, the regenerated animal will have a short remaining lifespan. This idea of inherited age reminds us of the hydra (p 20) when it reproduces clonally and some microbes. The underlying mechanism probably has to do with telomeres, as explained in Chapter 3.

A Mathematical Proof that Aging is Inevitable

There is a long and embarrassing history in the sciences of 'proofs' that things cannot possibly be otherwise than they are. A prominent and astute theoretical biologist, William Hamilton fell into this trap in 1966.

Hamilton "proved" mathematically that reverse aging was not possible. A good scientist will make clear and testable predictions; a great scientist makes bold predictions based on close reasoning from fundamental principles. Hamilton's 'proof' was in this latter category. Right in his abstract, he claimed "that senescence is an inevitable outcome of evolution," which "cannot be avoided by any conceivable organism". Hamilton was smart and courageous enough to make bold predictions. To his further credit, he was honest and confident enough to change his perspective late in his life, after experiment had proved him wrong.

(Hamilton's career was cut short in 2000 when he died at age 63, after contracting malaria on a research trip to the Congo. Richard Dawkins, who popularized 'Hamilton's Rule' in his book on *The Selfish Gene* [59], has never reformed his thought and continues to be an articulate and influential salesman for the ideas that Hamilton abandoned in his maturity. Dawkins has become the world's best-known neo-Darwinist.)

Hamilton's "proof" was derived within the context of the prevailing theory of his day. "Genetics" was still an abstraction, because the implications of Crick's decryption of the genetic code [60] had not yet been assimilated and "epigenetics" was still decades in the future. It was conventional to assume that every gene came with a time stamp, determining at what age it was to be expressed. The origin of aging was sought in differential selection pressure on genes that are time-stamped for different ages. In retrospect, it is too easy for us to apprehend the absurdity of the assumption that the present strength and fertility of an organism might be a function solely of the genes expressed in that moment, without reference to the organism's history of growth and development. But it was within such a paradigm that Hamilton formulated his proof.

He distinguished two types of genes that might have a favorable or unfavorable impact on present fitness. With more mathematical formalism than was really required, he demonstrated the intuitively reasonable proposition that, with advancing age, there is less selection pressure for favorable mutations and less selection pressure against unfavorable mutations. This was the crux of his proof.

Williams had proposed his theory of aging in 1957 [2], based on the idea that there are genes that have benefits to fitness at one time of life, while exacting a cost in fitness at other times. The (hypothetical) existence of genes that have mutually antagonistic effects at two different times in a life cycle was accepted as plausible. If such genes exist, they would put nature in a bind, demanding a price later in life for enhanced fertility or other benefits earlier. By the time Hamilton was writing this classic paper, eight years after Williams, the existence of such 'pleiotropic' genes was no longer questioned and the authority in the 29-year-old Hamilton's reasoning was beyond challenge.

The other prevailing theory was based on accumulation of mutations that are masked from natural selection because they only act at late ages, after most individuals have reproduced and died (of non-age-related causes). Hamilton demonstrated mathematically what Medawar had proposed 15 years earlier, based on heuristic reasoning. The later that such genes are scheduled to act, the smaller is the force of selection against them.

It is interesting that Hamilton's proof was valid for either of the two prevailing theories. Therefore, the discovery of exceptions—animals and plants that defied this "proof"—should have been taken as evidence calling into question both prevailing theories. Historically, that's not what happens. Biologists realize that Hamilton must have been wrong, but they have not taken the next step, to analyze his proof and to guess which of the assumptions that went into it were mistaken.

Revisiting the Proof in Light of the Evidence

Hamilton was thinking mathematically while avoiding the elephant in the room. The particular elephant he missed was the effect of size. Species that grow throughout their lifetimes and have no fixed size commonly meet both criteria for negative senescence (rising fertility, falling mortality).

James Vaupel, director of the Max Planck Inst in Rostock, Germany, is the foremost demographer of our time. He is best known for documenting the steady rise in human lifespan in the developed world [61], which has proceeded at a remarkably even pace for over 160 years. Perhaps it was just to make a point that Vaupel worked with his student Annette Baudisch to create their own 'proof' in counterpoint to Hamilton's. In a provocative 2004 article [7], they offer a general proof that *aging is impossible*. It is ruled out by the same evolutionary theory from which Hamilton had reasoned, so that the ability to survive must always increase with age. Vaupel is not an advocate for programmed aging or group selection; however he reminds us that population biology is an experimental science, where theory is always on shaky ground.

The assumptions that go into Vaupel's proof are not only very reasonable—they closely parallel the reasoning in Hamilton's proof. In addition to genes that demand a tradeoff (the subject of Williams's pleiotropy), there are (more normally) genes that produce reinforcing effects at different stages of life—growth genes, for example. Larger size is a defense against predation. Larger size means more resources are available for reproduction. Based on the existence of such generalized growth genes, Baudisch and Vaupel constructed a proof that they must always be promoted by natural selection, leading inevitably to negative senescence.

Hamilton's proof shows that aging must always evolve. Vaupel and Baudisch's proof shows that it is impossible for aging to evolve. I suspect that this delicious irony was exactly the goal that they had set in their sights. But Vaupel is, by background and inclination, a demographer. He collects and analyzes statistics about population and mortality. He is not a theorist in the tradition of Hamilton, seeking to create grand, unifying frameworks for understanding evolution. So Vaupel is content to sow doubts amid Hamilton's assurance and leave us with the paradox. (Neither Vaupel nor Baudisch is an advocate of programmed aging.)

If we are at all theoretically inclined, we might try to examine the wreckage and ask what went wrong in both these proofs—because clearly both proofs are fallacious. There are, in nature, both creatures that grow weaker with age and creatures that grow stronger with age, examples of increasing and decreasing mortality rates over extended periods in the lifespan. Presumably these life histories were molded in a process of natural selection. A conservative solution to the paradox would be to broaden the set of genes that we assume natural selection has for raw material. The difference between Hamilton's result and Vaupel's must derive from the fact that they started with different assumptions about the universe of genes on which natural selection operates. If Hamilton assumed one kind of gene and got one result, while Vaupel assumed another (more plausible, I think) kind of gene and argued to an opposite conclusion, then it should be possible to restore to nature her freedom to ordinary aging or non-aging or reverse aging if we simply allow that both kinds of genes are available.

What both proofs have in common is the neo-Darwinian definition of fitness as measured by individual reproductive success and we will come soon enough to question this assumption. I will argue in Chapter 6 that in fact nature is not optimizing 'reproductive value'; reproductive value is only one ingredient in nature's recipe for fitness. Another assumption shared in the two proofs is a background of environmental and demographic stasis. But natural population cycles are frequently deep and violent. In fact, the risk of extinction for entire populations is the missing ingredient in the recipe for natural selection and it frequently operates in direct opposition to the traditional brand of selection, which maximizes individual reproduction. More about this in Chapter 6.

Stranger and Stranger

Blanding's turtle is a species of box turtle common in the American Midwest. At two to three pounds full-grown, it is not impressively large. It matures slowly, in decades and afterward it does not keep growing, but it does continue to increase its fertility and decrease its mortality. A population of Blanding's turtles has been under observation by the University of Michigan Biology Department for over 50 years [62]. As far as they can tell, the oldest turtles in the field are not dying any faster than the young adults and they are laying just as many eggs. So the best field evidence available is that Blanding's turtle does not age.

When lobsters molt, they shed the evidence from which we might deduce how old they are. The best indication of a lobster's age is its size and when lobsters over 40 pounds have been caught, it is presumed they are many decades in age. There is no evidence of tumors or tissue degradation in large animals and the size of their gonads suggests they grow more fertile with age. In short, lobsters are a candidate for negative senescence, though the present state of field studies leaves room for doubt [63].

So far, all examples we have seen of reverse aging fit the technical definition. In addition, there are a few truly odd cases in which all the features of maturation as well as aging seem to be reversible and the aged adults reverts to a larval stage.

In 1905, Dutch biologist Peter Stoppenbrink [64] was studying the life cycles of *planaria*, a kind of flatworm, a fraction of an inch long, common in fresh water ponds. He noted that when the animals were starved, they consumed themselves, systematically, beginning with the most expendable organs (sex), proceeding to the digestive system (not much use in a famine), then muscles. The worms got smaller and smaller, until the most precious part—the brain and nerve cells—were all that remained. Stoppenbrink reported that when he started to feed the worms again, they grew back, rapidly regenerating everything they had lost. Most striking: the re-grown worms looked and acted like young worms and had the life expectancy of a young adult. When their cohorts who had not been starved began to die of old age, the starved-and-re-grown worms were still thriving. This trick could be performed again and again. As long as Stoppenbrink kept starving and re-feeding the worms, they went on living without apparent signs of age.

Carrion beetles (*Trogoderma glabrum*) live on carcasses. Like many insects, they hatch with a maggot-like body and metamorphose by shedding outer layers into the adult form. The beetle goes through larval stages, looking like a grub, then a millipede, then a water glider before assuming adult morphology as a six-legged beetle. A pair of entomologists [65] working at the University of Wisconsin in 1972 isolated the sixth stage larvae (almost ready to become adults) in test tubes and discovered that without food they regressed to stage-five larvae. Deprived of food for many days, they would shrink and regress backward through the stages until they looked like newly-hatched maggots. If feeding was resumed, they would go forward again through the developmental stages and become adults with normal lifespans. Stranger and stranger: the scientists found they could manipulate the beetles' development with food alone, allowing them to mature up to stage six, then starve back down to stage one, over and over again. The beetles normally live only eight weeks, but with alternate feeding and starving they were kept alive more than two years, before living out normal lifespans as adults. Do the beetles ever perform this trick in the wild? Someday, some patient naturalist will watch closely enough to be able to tell us; until then, I am guessing that this capacity would not have evolved unless it had survival value in the natural world.

There is a jellyfish species that apparently does the beetle one better, giving new meaning to the concept of a 'life cycle'. Jellyfish reproduce parthenogenically, breaking off polyps that begin to grow and develop into next-generation jellyfish. Most will die after reproducing. But the *Turritopsis nutricula* has evolved a trick to cheat death: after spawning its polyps, the adult *Turritopsis* regresses and becomes again a polyp, ready to begin its life cycle anew [66, 67]. This is accomplished by turning adult (differentiated) cells back into stem cells. Normal development is a one-way street from stem cells to differentiated cells, but biochemists have recently succeeded in turning differentiated cells back into stem cells in the lab (Chapter 8). Perhaps they have something to learn from Turritopsis.

There is evidence for negative senescence in humans, but only at very late ages. Mortality rises exponentially through much of the lifetime, but at advanced age it can level off, a 'mortality plateau'. For several animals observed in captivity, mortality rates have been observed to plateau late in life [68-71]. The phenomenon is striking in worms and flies and perhaps it can be observed in humans, though this remains controversial [72]. (And ever unflappable theoretical biologists have offered a mathematical proof that mortality plateaus must occur as a necessary consequence of the inexorable mathematics of natural selection [73].) There is not a lot of demographic data available for human beings over the age of 102, but what there is suggests that they are not more likely to die than humans at age 100 or 101.

The thin statistics even suggest they may be less likely to die and if that is so then we can say that humans, too, are subject to reverse aging. The inference is complicated, however, by the effect of experimental selection. The people who live to 102 have extraordinary genetics, even more so than the people who live to 100. It may be that the reason for the observed mortality plateau is merely the effect of an age sieve that leaves standing a progressively more robust set of individuals. The only way to be sure would be to repeat the study with a cohort of genetically identical humans, controlling also for lifestyle and environment.

Survey of the Range of Aging Patterns in Nature

Baudisch and Vaupel have gone on to survey the diversity of aging patterns in nature. Baudisch has introduced a useful separation of the shape of the aging curve from the time scale. The most obvious differences in aging patterns involve time scale. An insect may age and die over a few days and a turtle over a few centuries. Baudisch's innovation [74] is to remove time scale so that the shapes of diverse aging curves can be compared, even when they unfold on very different scales. The time axis is rescaled to a standard measure, taken as the age at which 95% of all individuals have died. What remains is a survival curve that may fall slowly or precipitously or it may even have periods where it levels out. Fertility, too, can be plotted on a relative scale and its relation to mortality can be observed.

Working with other members of their lab at the Max Planck Institute in Rostock, Germany, Baudisch and Vaupel published the first fruits of their survey in 2014 and the results are summarized in 48 scaled plots. The blue line plots fertility over a lifetime: how many offspring are produced per unit time; the red line plots mortality: what is the probability per unit time of an individual dying? (There is also a shaded background which shows percentage of surviving individuals.) The graphs are all stretched out or compressed in time so that each box contains one lifetime, whether that be a day or a decade.

Both vertical and horizontal axes in these plots are on a logarithmic scale. With this representation, the shaded triangles bordered by a straight descending line (diagonally downward) correspond to constant actuarial mortality or zero aging. Curves that are convex or humped correspond to normal aging, while curves that are concave upward connote negative senescence.

The top row codifies the life plan that is most familiar to us, because it is ours. Fertility peaks in early life, then declines. For females, it declines to zero. Mortality is modest for a long while, then it climbs steeply and everyone dies. This is the story we take for granted. It is the form of aging shared by humans, guppies and certain sea birds. Note that fertility drops away while most of the population remains alive and this is true not only for modern humans but also hunter-gatherers and guppies.

The next line shows life plans that are similar, but where mortality rises more slowly, so that age of death is spread out over time. This row contains some familiar mammals like deer, lions and orcas, but it also contains water fleas and bdelloid rotifers, microscopic creatures famous (at least to biologists) for having survived hundreds of millions of years without genetic exchange.

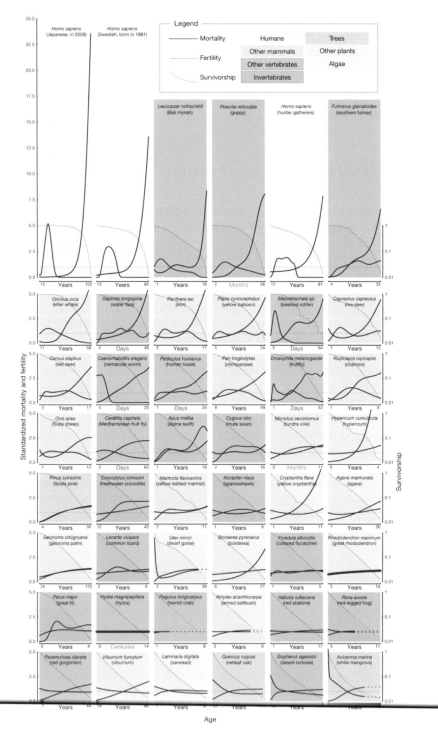

Figure copied from Jones et al., 2014, *Diversity of Aging Across the Tree of Life.*

Further down are stranger and less familiar life plans. The middle of the chart includes some life plans in which fertility and mortality both remain almost constant, corresponding to no demographic aging and no fertility curtailment. "Negligible senescence" is not an intimation of immortality; it says something about the *change* in the mortality rate and not the rate itself. Negligible senescence in natural habits is, in fact, what we would expect from Medawar's premise that senescence is invisible to natural selection, because almost no one in nature dies (or loses fertility) because of senescence. In one row of the chart, but not elsewhere, we see Medawar's prediction realized.

In the bottom rows, we see cases where fertility rises as mortality falls through most of the lifespan. According to evolutionary theory, metabolisms aren't supposed to be able to do this. The whole reason for aging is (according to theory) the necessity for compromise. Hamilton [1], following Williams, [2] accounts for aging as a sacrifice of longevity for fertility. Why are some species but not others compelled to this compromise?

Of special significance is post-reproductive lifespan. Human females go right on living after they have lost their fertility. This is supposed to be explained by the need to care for her grandchildren. But in this chart are several other species that also outlive their fertility, including elephants and ground squirrels but also worms and guppies that do not care for their young at all, let alone their grandchildren. This poses a problem for evolutionary theories of aging, because maintaining the body through an extended lifespan is always presumed to be costly in one way or another—that's why the body skimps on the job and the body is permitted to deteriorate with age. Why, then, would the body take the trouble to preserve itself for a time when it was unable to reproduce, useless to the species and invisible to evolution? Post-reproductive lifespan violates another of Williams's [2] predictions.

Another core prediction of all the theories of aging is that low background rates of mortality should be associated with long lifespans. This hypothesis has been adduced as an explanation for the fact that bats live longer than mice and it was confirmed in Austad's classic study of island opossums [28]. Indeed, this is a common prediction of all the currently accepted theories of aging. The reasoning behind it is perfectly generic: Assuming that natural selection operates to increase fitness by lengthening lifespan, the force of natural selection is high when many individuals are surviving to old age and low when background mortality prevents most individuals from attaining old age.

And yet, in this survey, there seems to be no association one way or the other between background death rate and senescence. As I write (2015) the Vaupel lab at Rostock is still engaged in collecting data for a broader survey of animals and plants, but this early sample suggests that there may be no evidence for faster senescence where background mortality is higher.

Proposed Theoretical Resolution by Baudisch and Vaupel

Baudisch and Vaupel have recognized this impending falsification of the evolutionary theory of aging for several years. In 2012, they wrote:

The classic evolutionary theories of aging provide the theoretical framework that has guided aging research for 60 years. Are the theories consistent with recent evidence?

At the heart of the theories lies the observation that the old count less than the young: Unfavorable traits are weeded out by evolution more slowly at higher ages; traits that are beneficial early in life are selected for despite late life costs; and resources are used to enhance reproduction at younger ages instead of maintaining the body at ages that do not matter much for evolution. The decline in the force of selection with age is viewed as the fundamental cause of aging. It is why, starting at reproductive maturity, senescence—increases in susceptibility to death and decreases in fertility—should be inevitable in all multicellular species capable of repeated breeding. Yet, this is not the case. Increasing, constant and decreasing mortality (and fertility) patterns (see the figure) are three generic variants that compose the rich diversity of life trajectories observed in nature. For vertebrates, reproductive trajectories are commonly hump-shaped and death rates may start rising much later than reproductive maturity. Thus, a new view on the fundamental causes of aging is needed to explain the clash of theory and data [75].

Conservatively, but anomalously, they have sought a resolution of this dilemma within the context of the popular Disposable Soma theory, which is based on resource tradeoffs. According to the Disposable Soma theory, animal metabolisms are evolved to maximize their fitness through a combination of fertility and longevity, but both fertility and longevity require food energy, so the metabolism is forced to compromise, accepting some limits on both. They propose that the wide-ranging patterns of aging (and non-aging) in nature might be explained by adaptation to different environmental threats and different kinds of metabolic constraints. "What is decisive is the 'option set' of a species, which can be summarized by the feasible combinations of survival and reproduction at all ages over the lifespan. Option sets differ widely: For some species, extra investment in repair and maintenance substantially reduces fertility; for other species there is little impact; for yet other species enhanced repair and maintenance decrease current but increase future fecundity. The details of such option sets shape age patterns of growth, fertility and mortality" [75].

At the head of this chapter, I claimed that the diversity of natural patterns of aging belies the notion that there can be anything constraining the progression of evolution toward whatever life history schedule is optimal (by nature's definition of fitness which may differ from the one assumed in classical population genetic theory). Baudisch and Vaupel have their ready answer: there is not one universal constraint, but a variety of constraints in different species, in different environments. The diversity of aging schedules is to be explained by the diversity of resource constraints, metabolic constraints, physical and environmental constraints,

The advantage of such a model is that different kinds and degrees of metabolic tradeoffs can lead to the full range of patterns of mortality observed in nature. The disadvantage is that the theory then completely loses its predictive value and says only that "anything is possible". The model takes a particular species's tradeoff profile for input and generates as output a senescence curve, such as is plotted by Jones et al. [5]. For any pattern of mortality in a particular species, some tradeoff profile can be hypothesized that will generate the right curve. The theory would be a substantive, testable hypothesis if the tradeoffs could be independently derived from fundamental considerations of biochemistry. Shanley and Kirkwood [76] attempted such a model for lactating mice in particular, constrained by availability of food energy. They emphasize the predictive successes of the model in their write-up; but in many respects, their model output is seriously at odds with reality [77] and fails spectacularly when it is extended even modestly, to encompass mice that are not lactating.

Baudisch and Vaupel go on to say that aging in nature has a richness and diversity that these simple theories do not begin to address. "theories to explain the ultimate evolutionary causes of the varieties of ageing…are in their infancy" [5].

I take this as an invitation.

Summary

"All living things are subject to gradual deterioration over a lifetime, which eventually leads to catastrophic failure".

This is the traditional belief about patterns of aging in nature which Wiesmann, Medawar, Williams and early theorists sought to explain from fundamental principles of metabolism.

But a broader survey of nature reveals a different pattern. Nature has been able to do pretty much anything she wants with the metabolism of aging and the trajectory of mortality that comes from that metabolism. Aging curves and fertility curves have all different possible shapes and the shape seems to be independent of the time scale on which aging unfolds. Plants and animals, small size and large seem to be well-mixed in the chart based on the shape of aging trajectories, with no hard-and-fast rules. Dramatically different aging styles remind us of nature's diversity. The big picture suggests that attempts to demonstrate that "aging is inevitable" are misguided.

Traditional evolutionary theory is based on the idea that aging is bad for the fitness of the individual and that natural selection should always work against aging. If most living things suffer decline with age, leading to death, this must have taken place despite natural selection. There must be some genetic constraints or physical limitations or conditions beyond control of the genome. In theory, there is a single process of optimizing reproductive potential, operant for all living creatures and the universe of aging modes can all be explained by different environmental circumstances and differences in available genes.

On its face, this seems like a dubious claim. Natural selection is capable of crafting a huge range of lifespans and rates of aging (including non-aging and negative aging). The burden of proof should be on the theories to demonstrate that a (hypothetical) mayfly that lived 1,000 years would actually have a lower reproductive output than the (common) variety that lives for a day.

Some patterns emerge from the data:

- Long lifespans are generally but not always associated with larger size. This almost certainly has a deep basis in physics [45], thus it need not command an evolutionary explanation.
- Long lifespans are usually but not always associated with long development times. This has a basis both in physics and in demography.
- Many more plants than animals exemplify negligible senescence, as well as negative senescence. This observation *does* beg an evolutionary reason.

One of the keystone predictions of all the evolutionary theories is that where the background death rate is high, the lifespan should be short. The number of exceptions to this rule ought to be raising eyebrows.

References

1. Hamilton, W.D., *The moulding of senescence by natural selection.* J. Theor. Biol., 1966. **12**(1): p. 12-45.
2. Williams, G., *Pleiotropy, natural selection and the evolution of senescence.* Evolution, 1957. **11**: p. 398-411.
3. Gavrilov, L.A. and N.S. Gavrilova, *The reliability theory of aging and longevity.* J. Theor. Biol., 2001. **213**(4): p. 527-545.
4. Orgel, L.E., *The maintenance of the accuracy of protein synthesis and its relevance to ageing.* Proc. Natl. Acad. Sci. U.S.A., 1963. **49**: p. 517-21.
5. Jones, O.R., et al., *Diversity of ageing across the tree of life.* Nature, 2014. **505**(7482): p. 169-173.
6. Administration, S.S., *Acuarial life table.* 2010: Washington, DC.
7. Vaupel, J.W., et al., *The case for negative senescence.* Theor. Popul. Biol., 2004. **65**(4): p. 339-51.
8. Kirkwood, Thomas B.L. and S. Melov, *On the programmed/non-programmed nature of ageing within the life history.* Curr. Biol., 2011. **21**(18): p. R701-R707.
9. Schneider, J.M. and Y. Lubin, *Intersexual conflict in spiders.* Oikos, 1998. **83**(3): p. 496-506.
10. Roff, D., *The Evolution of Life Histories.* 1992, New York: Chapman and Hall.
11. Kirkwood, T., *Evolution of aging.* Nature, 1977. **270**: p. 301-304.
12. Kirkwood, T.B. and D.P. Shanley, *The connections between general and reproductive senescence and the evolutionary basis of menopause.* Ann. N.Y. Acad. Sci., 2010. **1204**: p. 21-9.
13. Molisch, H., *The Longevity of Plants.* 1938, Lancaster, PA: Science Press.
14. Cockburn, A., *Living slow and dying young: senescence in marsupials, In: Marsupial biology: recent research, new perspectives*, N. Saunders and L. Hinds, Editors. 1997, University of New South Wales Press: Sydney. p. 163-171.
15. Oakwood, M., A.J. Bradley and A. Cockburn, *Semelparity in a large marsupial.* Proc. R. Soc. Lond. B. Biol. Sci., 2001. **268**(1465): p. 407-411.
16. Crespi, B.J. and R. Teo, *Comparative phylogenetic analysis of the evolution of semelparity and life history in salmonid fishes.* Evolution Int. J. Org. Evolution, 2002. **56**(5): p. 1008-20.
17. Finch, C.E., *Longevity, Senescence and the Genome.* 1990, Chicago: University of Chicago Press.

18. Wodinsky, J., *Hormonal inhibition of feeding and death in octopus: control by optic gland secretion.* Science, 1977. **198**: p. 948-95.

19. Fahy, G., *Precedents for the biological control of aging: postponement, prevention and reversal of aging processes*, In: *Approaches to the Control of Aging: Building a Pathway to Human Life Extension*, G.M. Fahy, et al., Editors. 2010, Springer: New York.

20. Robison, B., B. Seibel and J. Drazen, *Deep-sea octopus (Graneledone boreopacifica) conducts the longest-known egg-brooding period of any animal.* 2014.

21. Edmunds Jr, G.F. and C.H. Edmunds, *Predation, climate and emergence and mating of mayflies*, In: *Advances in Ephemeroptera Biology*. 1980, Springer. p. 277-285.

22. Medawar, P.B., *Uniqueness of the individual.* 1957.

23. Ricklefs, R.E., *Intrinsic aging-related mortality in birds.* J. Avian Biol., 2000. **31**(2): p. 103-111.

24. Nisbet, I.C.T., *Detecting and measuring senescence in wild birds: experience with long-lived seabirds.* Exp. Gerontol., 2001. **36**(4-6): p. 833-843.

25. Lecomte, V.J., et al., *Patterns of aging in the long-lived wandering albatross.* Proc. Natl. Acad. Sci. U.S.A., 2010. **107**(14): p. 6370-5.

26. Catry, P., et al., *Senescence effects in an extremely long-lived bird: the grey-headed albatross thalassarche chrysostoma.* Proc. Biol. Sci., 2006. **273**(1594): p. 1625-30.

27. Elliott, K., *The Arctic Phoenix.* InfoNorth, 2011. **64**(4): p. 497-500.

28. Austad, S., *Retarded senescence in an insular population of Virginia opossums.* J. Zool. London, 1993. **229**: p. 695-708.

29. Buffenstein, R., *Negligible senescence in the longest living rodent, the naked mole-rat: insights from a successfully aging species.* Journal of Comparative Physiology B, 2008. **178**(4): p. 439-445.

30. Holmes, D.J. and M.A. Ottinger, *Birds as long-lived animal models for the study of aging.* Exp. Gerontol., 2003. **38**(11-12): p. 1365-75.

31. Ottinger, M.A. and J. Balthazart, *Altered endocrine and behavioral responses with reproductive aging in the male Japanese quail.* Horm. Behav., 1986. **20**(1): p. 83-94.

32. Goranson, N., J. Ebersole and S. Brault, *Resolving an adaptive conundrum: reproduction in Caenorhabditis elegans is not sperm-limited when food is scarce.* Evol. Ecol. Res., 2005. **7**(2): p. 325-333.

33. Mitteldorf, J. and C. Goodnight, *Post-reproductive life span and demographic stability.* Oikos, 2012. **121**(9): p. 1370-1378.

34. Reznick, D., M. Bryant and D. Holmes, *The evolution of senescence and post-reproductive life span in guppies (Poecilia reticulata).* PLoS Biol., 2006. **4**(1): p. e7.

35. Cohen, A.A., *Female post-reproductive life span: a general mammalian trait.* Biol. Rev. Camb. Philos. Soc., 2004. **79**(4): p. 733-50.

36. Finch, C.E., *The Biology of Human Longevity.* 2007, Burlington, MA: Elsevier.

37. Samaras, T.T. and H. Elrick, *Height, body size and longevity.* Acta Med. Okayama, 1999. **53**(4): p. 149-69.

38. Lanner, R.M. and K.F. Connor, *Does bristlecone pine senesce?* Exp. Gerontol., 2001. **36**(4-6): p. 675-85.

39. Kemperman, J. and B. Barnes, *Clone size in American aspens.* Cana. J. Bot., 1976. **54**: p. 2603-2607.

40. Sussman, R., C. Zimmer and H.U. Obrist, *The Oldest Living Things in the World.* 2014, University of Chicago Press.

41. Saunders, M.W. and G.A. McFarlane, *Age and length at maturity of the female spiny dogfish, squalus acanthias, in the strait of Georgia, British Columbia, Canada.* Env. biol., 1993. **38**: p. 49-57.

42. Edwards, D.L., et al., *The genetic legacy of lonesome george survives: giant tortoises with Pinta Island ancestry identified in Galápagos.* Biol. Conserv., 2013. **157**: p. 225-228.

43. Cailliet, G.M., et al., *Age determination and validation studies of marine fishes: do deep-dwellers live longer?* Exp. Gerontol., 2001. **36**(4-6): p. 739-64.

44. George, J.C.B., J.R., *Two historical weapon fragments as an aid to estimating the longevity and movements of bowhead whales.* Polar Biol., 2007. **31**(6): p. 751-754.

45. West, G.B., J.H. Brown and B.J. Enquist, *A general model for the origin of allometric scaling laws in biology.* Science, 1997. **276**(5309): p. 122-126.

46. Martinez, D.E., *Mortality patterns suggest lack of senescence in hydra.* Exp. Gerontol., 1998. **33**(3): p. 217-25.

47. Estep, P.W., *Declining asexual reproduction is suggestive of senescence in hydra: comment on Martinez, D., "Mortality patterns suggest lack of senescence in hydra." Exp. Gerontol., 33, 217-25.* Exp. Gerontol., 2010. **45**(9): p. 645-6.

48. Schöne, B.R., et al., *Climate records from a bivalved methuselah.* Paleogeography, Paleoclimatology, Paleoecology, 2005. **228**: p. 130-148.

49. Abele, D., et al., *Imperceptible senescence: ageing in the ocean quahog Arctica islandica.* Free Radic. Res., 2008. **42**(5): p. 474-80.

50. Thorarindsottir, G.G., K. Gunnarsson and E. Bogason, *Mass mortality of ocean quahog, Arctica islandica, on hard substratum in Lonafjordur, north-eastern Iceland after a storm.* Biodiversity Records, 2008.

51. Ebert, T.A. and J.R. Southon, *Red sea urchins can live over 100 years: confirmation with A-bomb ^{14}C.* Fish. Bull., 2003. **101**(4): p. 915-922.

52. Remolina, S.C., et al., *Senescence in the worker honey bee apis mellifera.* J. Insect. Physiol., 2007. **53**(10): p. 1027-33.

53. Butler, C.G., *The method and importance of the recognition by a colony of honeybees (A. mellifera) of the presence of its queen.* Transactions of the Royal Entomological Society of London, 1954. **105**(2): p. 11-29.

54. Cambray, G., *To Bee or not to Bee – swarming season is here.* Science in Africa, 2006 (Oct, 2006).

55. Hicks, A.C., C. Wetzel and J. Harms, *The status of rougheye rockfish (Sebastes aleutianus) and blackspotted rockfish (S. melanostictus) as a complex along the US West Coast in 2013.* Draft dated, 2013. **6**(24): p. 2013.

56. Abadie, S.H., *The life cycle of Strongyloides ratti.* The Journal of parasitology, 1963: p. 241-248.

57. Minato, K., et al., *Effect of temperature on the development of free-living stages of Strongyloides ratti.* Parasitol. Res., 2008. **102**(2): p. 315-319.

58. Harvey, S. and M. Viney, *Sex determination in the parasitic nematode Strongyloides ratti.* Genetics, 2001. **158**(4): p. 1527-1533.

59. Dawkins, R., *The Selfish Gene.* 1976, Oxford: Oxford University Press.

60. Crick, F., et al., *General nature of the genetic code for proteins.* 1961: Macmillan Journals Limited.

61. Oeppen, J. and J.W. Vaupel, *Demography. Broken limits to life expectancy.* Science, 2002. **296**(5570): p. 1029-31.

62. Congdon, J.D., et al., *Hypotheses of aging in a long-lived vertebrate, Blanding's turtle (Emydoidea blandingii).* Exp. Gerontol., 2001. **36**(4-6): p. 813-27.

63. Klapper, W., et al., *Longevity of lobsters is linked to ubiquitous telomerase expression.* FEBS Lett., 1998. **439**(1-2): p. 143-6.

64. Stoppenbrink, P., *Der einflul herabgesetzter ern/ihrung auf den histologischen bau der siilwasser-tricladen.* Z. Wiss. Zool., 1905. **79**: p. 496-574.

65. Beck, S.D. and R.K. Bharadwaj, *Reversed development and cellular aging in an insect.* Science, 1972. **178**(66): p. 1210-1.
66. Bavestrello, G., C. Suommer and M. Sara, *Bi-directional conversion in Turritopsis nutricula.* Sci. Mar., 1992. **56**(2-3): p. 137-140.
67. Piraino, S., et al., *Reversing the life cycle: medusae transforming into polyps and cell trans differentiation in Turritopsis nutricula.* Biol. Bull., 1996. **90**: p. 302-312.
68. Barinaga, M., *Mortality: overturning received wisdom.* Science, 1992. **258**(5081): p. 398-9.
69. Brooks, A., G.J. Lithgow and T.E. Johnson, *Mortality rates in a genetically heterogeneous population of Caenorhabditis elegans.* Science, 1994. **263**(5147): p. 668-71.
70. Carey, J.R., et al., *Slowing of mortality rates at older ages in large medfly cohorts.* Science, 1992. **258**(5081): p. 457-61.
71. Vaupel, J.W., T.E. Johnson and G.J. Lithgow, *Rates of mortality in populations of Caenorhabditis elegans.* Science, 1994. **266**(5186): p. 826; author reply 828.
72. Gavrilov, L. and N. Gavrilova, *New developments in the biodemography of aging and longevity.* Gerontology, 2015. **61**(4): p. 364-371.
73. Mueller, L.D. and M.R. Rose, *Evolutionary theory predicts late-life mortality plateaus.* PNAS, 1996. **93**(26): p. 15249-15253.
74. Baudisch, A., *The pace and shape of ageing.* Methods in Ecology and Evolution, 2011. **2**(4): p. 375-382.
75. Baudisch, A. and J.W. Vaupel, *Getting to the root of aging.* Science (New York, NY), 2012. **338**(6107): p. 618.
76. Shanley, D.P. and T.B. Kirkwood, *Calorie restriction and aging: a life-history analysis.* Evolution Int. J. Org. Evolution, 2000. **54**(3): p. 740-50.
77. Mitteldorf, J., *Can experiments on caloric restriction be reconciled with the disposable soma theory for the evolution of senescence?* Evolution Int. J. Org. Evolution, 2001. **55**(9): p. 1902-5; discussion 1906.

3

Aging is not Caused by Accumulated Damage

Synopsis

The best-accepted evolutionary theories of aging are about tradeoffs and pleiotropy. But much of the gerontology community isn't buying them. Instead, there is a great deal of literature based on damage, stochastic processes and loss of order. Perhaps the best-accepted evolutionary ideas are just too strange and counter-intuitive or perhaps the analogy with physical wear and chemical degradation are just too seductive. In any case, the idea that bodies wear out in a way analogous to machines is too prevalent to be ignored and that is the reason for this chapter.

This is a thermodynamic view of aging that has been discredited since Clausius first quantified the notion of entropy [1] and Weismann published his insights into aging [2]. Physicists agree that there is no thermodynamic necessity for aging. Evolutionists agree that the cause and reason for aging must be sought in terms of natural selection. But many biologists, medical scientists and educated non-scientists have been tempted to understand aging through deceptive analogies to wear and degradation of inanimate machines.

> *Everything wears out over time. Nothing lasts forever. This is the second law of thermodynamics. The body is made of ordinary matter, so it must lose its order over time. Damage accumulates on a one-way street. Aging is inevitable.* (This is not a quote)

If stated in this way, the theory is subject to criticism and analysis and the argument falls apart. But it is seldom stated explicitly; instead, it remains in the background, an implicit influence that has misled many researchers and channeled their thought in unproductive directions. For this reason, I include this chapter which endeavors to dispel a persistent confusion.

Undeniably, many aspects of aging, e.g. oxidative damage, somatic mutations and protein cross-linkage are characterized by increased entropy in biomolecules. However, it has been a scientific consensus for more than a century that there is no physical necessity for such damage. Living systems are defined by their capacity to gather order from their environment, concentrate it and shed entropy with their waste.

Organisms in their growth phase become stronger and more robust; no physical law prohibits this progress from continuing indefinitely. Indeed, some animals and many plants are known to grow indefinitely larger and more fertile through their lives. This fact alone should silence any argument from "physical necessity".

The same conclusion is underscored by experimental findings that various insults and challenges which directly damage the body or increase the rate of wear and tear have the paradoxical effect of extending lifespan. Hyperactive mice live longer than controls [3] and worms with their antioxidant systems impaired live longer than wild type [4].

Finally, if the enormous range of natural aging rates—at least six orders of magnitude—is not sufficient reason to discredit the idea that aging is inevitable, then certainly the existence in nature of organisms that do not age at all must be a disproof [5, 6].

Fundamental understanding of aging must proceed not from physics but from an evolutionary perspective: the body is being permitted to decay, because systems of repair and regeneration that are perfectly adequate to build and rebuild a body of ever-increasing resilience are being held back, at the same time that some affirmative modes of self-destruction have been re-purposed to destroy the body [7, 8].

Introduction

It is an idea so common, so embedded in the thought process of gerontologists and medical practitioners that it is seldom questioned: Aging is a physical process of deterioration, as damage accumulates faster than it can be repaired. At least since the Renaissance, scientists and philosophers, poets, doctors and laymen have adopted this understanding of aging. It remains the basis of a great deal of medical and gerontological research today.

But despite its ubiquity and commonsense appeal, this idea was thoroughly discredited by physicists of the nineteenth century and their analysis remains cogent. Evolutionary biologists, who claim the high ground in understanding of deep causes in biology, have for the last century regarded damage as a result, not a cause of aging.

History of Thermodynamics

The idea that order spontaneously and universally dissolves to disorder is very old, but it was not until 1850 that this notion was codified quantitatively as the Second Law of Thermodynamics. Clausius [1, 9] is credited with incorporating entropy as a quantitative physical variable. He distinguished ideal 'reversible' processes from the 'irreversible' processes that take place in the real world and demonstrated that ideal processes conserve entropy, while in real systems, entropy must always increase.

The Second Law of Thermodynamics is sometimes stated thus: *In any closed physical system, the entropy will increase, until it attains its maximum value.*

The state of the system in which entropy realizes its maximum value is called 'equilibrium'.

The second law explains why a rock tumbles down a hill, turning its potential energy of gravitation into low-grade heat. Metal fatigue and oxidation are familiar examples of irreversible processes, in which entropy accumulates.

But the law applies only to closed (isolated) systems and it is possible for processes to accumulate information in one object, while entropy is dispersed elsewhere. For example: As a pool of water evaporates, the liquid can cool (lower entropy) because the gas disperses, with higher entropy that more than compensates.

Living things have taken this loophole in the Second Law and developed it as a specialty. The ongoing ability to gather free energy from the environment and concentrate it as order within, while discarding entropy as waste is a defining property of living systems. Every multicellular organism is capable of growing from seed into a fertile adult. Typically, the mortality risk of the adult is lower than the immature stage and certainly the fertility is (by definition) higher. So growth and development constitute "negative aging" in both the biological and the thermodynamic senses.

There is no theoretical reason this process could not continue indefinitely*. The organism could continue to grow larger, more fertile and more resistant to mortality of all sorts after it attained maturity and some, in fact, do just this [5, 6]. For an explanation of senescence, we should be appealing to evolutionary theory, not to thermodynamics.

Weismann's Role

If living organisms wore out like machines, there would be no need for an evolutionary account of aging. But multicellular life succeeds in the remarkable feat of constructing a complex system from fragments found in the environment, using only a genetic blueprint – only to fail at the seemingly much more modest task of maintaining the completed soma in reasonable working order. In the generation after Darwin, Weismann articulated the essential biological conundrum of aging and sought an explanation not from physics but from evolution. Weismann is credited with the first evolutionary theory of aging, but his departure from physical wear and tear was not so clean. His original theory [2] was based on a presumption that damage to the adult soma was unavoidable and that damage must accumulate over time.

Weismann backed away from this theory later in his life and wrote instead of the loss of immortality in somatic cells, as it became an unnecessary luxury. But it was not until Medawar that the essential logical flaw in Weismann's original hypothesis was articulated: "Weismann assumes that the elders of his race are worn out and decrepit—the very state of affairs whose origin he purports to be inferring—and then proceeds to argue that because these dotard animals are taking the place of the

_____

* There are, however, reasons from physical scaling that make growth beyond a certain size a competitive liability, especially for land animals that must be able to carry their own weight.

sound ones, so therefore the sound ones must by natural selection dispossess the old" [10].

Medawar realized full well that there is no thermodynamic necessity for wear and damage to accumulate. He sought not a physical explanation for aging, but an evolutionary explanation, grounded in the declining force of natural selection with age. The evolutionary community has not looked back and today there is broad agreement that aging cannot be explained as a physical necessity, but must be understood like every other biological phenomenon in terms of natural selection.

Is Somatic Repair a Difficult or Expensive Process?

Tooth wear is an example of true damage accumulation leading to senescence of the elephant. Elephants can grow six full sets of teeth in a lifetime, but if he should outlive his last set of teeth (and some have been found in nature to do so), he will become toothless and must starve to death [11]. It is a strange wear-and-tear theory that can explain how it is that the elephant's capacity for regeneration ends after its sixth set of teeth.

It has been argued (most famously by Hamilton [12]) that repair of the adult organism cannot be perfect and that errors in repair and maintenance must inevitably accumulate, leading eventually to the organism's demise. This is also a premise of the Disposable Soma theory of Kirkwood [13]. But the reasoning is logically flawed, as Vaupel [5] has demonstrated. There is nothing perfect about a freshly-minted adult and the maintenance of that adult is not a process that demands perfection. For example, when a bone is broken, it knits back together in a few weeks' time. The bone was not perfect before it was broken and it is not perfect after it heals. But mended bones are stronger than the original and will not break again in the same place. Bone repair may be said to be better than 100% efficient and clearly requires a finite amount of free energy.

The mammalian body is equipped with an impressive array of repair mechanisms, from the molecular level up to the tissue level. Proteins are recycled into constituent amino acids when they become damaged; it is only in aged animals that this process becomes inefficient [14]. DNA is constantly monitored and repaired. Under-performing mitochondria are eliminated and replaced under control of the cell nucleus [15]. And whole cells are routinely destroyed via apoptosis and replaced when they become damaged [16]. All these processes are adequate in youth to maintain the organism without loss of function and they fail progressively *as a result* of aging, causing aging damage to progress. But their efficiency in youth attests to the fact that aging is not *caused* by shoddy repair.

Loose analogies may suggest that at some point in the life of an organism, damage accumulates to the point where repair of the organism is energetically more costly than replacement through reproduction. This idea is implicit in the foundation of the Disposable Soma theory [17-19]. Our experience with man-made appliances lends credibility to the idea; but many of the reasons that a ten-year-old car can be replaced more cheaply than it can be repaired do not have analogs in the world of biology: Autos must be dismantled before they can be repaired and re-assembled afterward, while for biological organisms repair themselves from the inside out.

Auto manufacturers price the new car with a low profit margin and overcharge for replacement parts, since the customer has nowhere else to go. Auto repair is purchased at market rates for European or American labor, while cheap Asian labor and cheaper robots are used by factories in which the autos originate. Thus we should not expect our intuitions about automobiles to apply to living bodies.

The energetic cost of repairing an aging soma are substantially less than the total energetic cost of reproducing one new adult. Repairing DNA and stringing together amino acids are both processes with low intrinsic thermodynamic costs and both have been highly optimized for energy efficiency. In contrast, the cost of anabolism is quite substantial and the cost of reproduction is magnified by high mortality rates of the immature. For example, a female mouse consumes twice as much food energy while pregnant and lactating [20]. All this suggests that an enormous quantity of resource has been consumed in order to create a single mature adult and evolutionary pressure to protect and preserve that investment ought to be correspondingly high.

Almost all plants and many animals can regenerate. The process is expensive relative to repair, but cheap compared to the full cost of reproducing a new adult individual. Starfish have legendary capacity for regeneration and half a starfish can readily grow back its other half. Yet starfish age with a life expectancy of about eight years and a starfish regrown from a fragment remembers its age. Zebrafish [21] and some amphibians [22, 23] retain the ability to regenerate limbs. Porpoises and other sea mammals have the capacity to heal from severe wounds without scarring [24]. A few vertebrates and many lower animals are capable of regenerating whole body parts after dismemberment [23]. Full limb regeneration in mammals is rare and limited to the very young [25, 26].

Recent research indicates that in other mammals, the capacity to regenerate remains, but is actively suppressed by expression of certain genes and micro RNAs [27-29]. Heber-Katz [30, 31] has shown that scarless healing is latent in mice and can be switched back on by suppressing the gene *p21* or by blocking the degradation of HIF-1α [32]. *Lin28a* is a widely-conserved gene that is turned off early in mammalian development, but which can be re-activated with the result that the RNA *let7* is upregulated and regenerative ability is strongly enhanced [33].

This is clear *prima facie* evidence that the power to regenerate has been scaled back early in life by an epigenetic program. How, then, do researchers close to this field understand what they have observed in terms of the evolutionary provenance of this program and the animal's fitness? It has become conventional, almost *de rigeur*, to seek a connection to cancer. The implication, if spelled out, would be that each species is evolved for long life and maximum viability and that natural selection has balanced the expression of factors suppressing regeneration at exactly that point where the risk of cancer is exceeded by the risk of injury unhealed.

> We speculate that the total dose of *let-7* is evolutionarily determined via regulation of the expression levels of individual *let-7* members and is postnatally maintained at a level that can suppress cancer, but which also allows for adequate levels of mammalian regenerative capacity [34].

But the theory is seldom spelled out. It is noted that genes for growth are turned up in cancer cells and the converse inference—that growth genes promote cancer—is left unstated. Subjected to analysis, the idea that regeneration is suppressed in order to protect against cancer may not seem so clear or intuitive. A cancer cell has escaped control of the central metabolism and it competes with other cancer cells for rapidity of growth. It is no surprise that in the course of somatic evolution, cancer cells come to express growth hormones. But the etiology of cancer is not about growth; it is about escape from the governance of the central metabolism. It is clear that cancer leads to expression of growth factors, but it is less clear that expression of growth factors leads to cancer.

Usually the tradeoff is described only in theoretical terms, but Wu et al. [34] demonstrate the antagonistic dynamic experimentally for the case of the *Lin28/let7* system. Early in life, the onset of *Lin28* expression ties up and degrades the micro RNA *let7*, which has the result of depressing the whole body's ability to regenerate. Wu et al. report an increased risk of cancer in a mouse model that has been triply genetically modified to induce liver cancer in a high proportion of animals. Why was the enhanced cancer rate not seen without the deletion of three other genes? Why hasn't the body evolved an adaptive ability to upregulate *let7* in response to extensive tissue injury, such as a severed appendage?

The beneficial and detrimental roles of *Lin28* derive from two separate chemical actions [35]. Why are these two functions not divided between two separate enzymes, so their respective expressions might be separately optimized? Antagonistic pleiotropy only makes sense if we think there are basic physical constraints blocking evolution's path toward a solution that divides and conquers. But in fact the history of life is replete with examples in which a gene is duplicated and the two copies continue to evolve for separate, specialized purposes. Where this has not happened, we might be justified in asking, why not?

Why should antagonistic pleiotropy be so difficult to observe?

Somatic Mutations

There is an exception to the thesis that all damage is avoidable and in any case should be easily and cheaply repaired. This occurs in somatic mutations, where genetic information may be irretrievably lost. This process certainly occurs, but whether it has observable consequences for real organisms and whether it is related to the phenotype of aging is unknown. Curiously, somatic mutation is out of fashion and seldom mentioned nowadays as a primary cause of aging.*

Somatic cells are descended directly from a single gamete that contained a pristine copy of the organism's genome. When mutations inevitably occur in this lineage, they affect all descendant cells further down the line. The problem can only be resolved by a process of selection, weeding out cells with damaged genomes. It is not known whether such a mechanism exists for stem cells in modern mammals.

---

* This is mutation accumulation, but it is not the well-known "Mutation Accumulation Theory of aging". The standard theory by this name is about mutational load: mutations accumulate in the germ line over evolutionary time because the speed of natural selection is less than the rate at which new deleterious mutations occur. The Mutation Accumulation Theory should not be confused with the phenomena of somatic mutations discussed in this section.

The Hungarian-American physicist Leó Szilárd first proposed [36] that somatic mutations were the cause of aging in 1959. Szilárd had difficulty accounting for the accelerating onset of senescence and the fact that the range of lifespans around a species mean is typically narrow. Szilárd's intellectual heir was Leslie Orgel, who theorized [37] not about copying errors (mutations) but transcription errors. The attraction of the Orgel theory was that transcriptional errors could conceivably affect, among other things, the faculty of transcription itself, so that the process has the potential to be self-reinforcing. Self-reinforcing processes tend to follow an exponential progression, beginning very slowly and finishing in an avalanche. This would explain the rapid onset of aging and narrow range of lifespans that Szilárd's mutational theory failed to account for.

Orgel's theory was abandoned when experimental evidence failed to support it. Rabinovitch and Martin tested the idea in mice using a virus that is sensitive to accuracy of macromolecular synthesis and found no difference between young and old mice [38]. And direct tests of the hypothesis in cell colonies indicate that transcription errors do not increase in frequency as a lineage ages [39].

Szilárd's theory of copying errors also suffers from lack of experimental support. The theory predicts that tissues that are self-renewing on a short time scale should be a central locus of failures with age. But in humans, organs that have low rates of cell renewal (e.g., the heart and brain) are among the most vulnerable with age. Conversely, kidney epithelial cells undergo substantial mutation accumulation [40], but there is no indication that this results in increased mortality. The immune system is the only organ with a high turnover rate that is also a hot spot for aging problems, but the immune system is a special case in that B-cells *depend on* mutation in order to maintain their sensitivity to a diverse universe of antigens.

Szilárd formulated his theory at a time when stem cells were unknown and he imagined that terminally differentiated somatic cells were the reservoir for their own renewal. In fact, the mechanism of stem cells substantially mitigates the problem of somatic mutation and this may, in fact, be related to the evolutionary reason that stem cells are deployed by the body instead of simply allowing terminally differentiated cells to clone themselves [41].

Soon after the discovery of stem cells, Cairns [42] speculated that they divided with asymmetric partition, retaining the old strand of DNA in the stem cell line to minimize the accumulation of copying errors. In the intervening years, some evidence for this hypothesis has been discovered, but, curiously, it is still not known whether stem cells consistently pass a second-generation copy to each daughter cell and thus retain a "master copy" of DNA throughout the life of the soma. However, it is known that copying errors can be reduced as low as one mutated base in 10^{14} cell divisions [43] and that very large, long-lived animals with large mass and high cell count (e.g., bowhead whales) have successfully adapted to avoid greater cancer risk from somatic mutations [44, 45]. The latter observation is sometimes referred to as "Peto's Paradox" [46].

In lab worms and in fruit flies, calorie restriction extends lifespan, but has no effect on somatic mutations [47]. In an early experiment by Cal Harley [39], it was reported that genetic errors did not measurably increase in fibroblast cells cultured from fetal, young and old donors. Rodents and humans repair DNA with similar efficiency, despite the 30-fold difference in lifespans.

In theory, loss of information in DNA is a one-way street ("Muller's Ratchet" [48]) and logically it must accumulate over time. On the other hand, DNA repair mechanisms must exist with sufficient reliability to preserve the germ line over evolutionary time, a far more stringent requirement than to keep somatic mutations from causing problems during a single lifetime. There is every indication that humans and model organisms have evolved DNA repair machinery such that DNA damage is not a factor in aging, in practice. Although there remain proponents of a role for DNA damage in human aging [49], the modern view is that this is not an important cause of aging.

Mutations in the mitochondrial DNA have also been the subject of speculation as a primary origin of aging damage [50]. This is an attractive hypothesis because mitochondrial DNA must survive in a highly oxidizing environment and mitochondria reproduce at a much more rapid rate than do cells. Furthermore, it was thought possible that mitochondria reproduce in a competitive environment, so that they may be subject to selection not for efficiency of their function for their cell, but for their (selfish) rate of growth and reproduction. This combination appeared to offer the means, the motive and the opportunity to resolve the mystery of aging.

However, ingenious experiments by Hayashi [51] have indicated that mitochondrial reproduction takes place not in a competitive environment, but under tight regulation from the cell nucleus. Damaged mitochondria do not reproduce excessively (like an intracellular cancer), but are efficiently weeded out and destroyed. Somehow, the internal evolution of mitochondria is managed and directed for the benefit of the whole cell and mitochondrial selfishness is not permitted to prevail. Perhaps the most telling result is that there are no more DNA mutations in mitochondria derived from old cells compared to young cells [52].

Enthusiasm for somatic mutations as a cause of aging comes from several progeria syndromes deriving from higher copy error rates. In humans, defects in the *LMNA* gene lead to abnormalities in chromosome replication and Hutchinson-Gilford progeria [53, 54]. In mice, alteration of the DNA polymerase gamma gene affects proofreading, leading to early onset of symptoms that resemble aging [55]. But there are no known modifications of these genes or their pathways that extend lifespan; and study of these progerias has not yet translated into understanding of normal aging. Why might improperly copied genes lead to syndromes that mimic aging if old age is not caused by improperly copied genes? I suggest that an answer might be sought in the epigenetic basis for aging. Later in this book, I entertain the thesis that aging is programmed through altered epigenetics and especially the unmasking late in life of genes that are not expressed in youth. Copy errors caused by progeria mutations are more likely to occur in regulatory regions than in genes, simply because genes constitute a small fraction of all DNA. It may be that defective regulatory regions lead to the unmasking of some of these same detrimental genes.

In summary: at one time, there were sound theoretical reasons to believe that somatic mutations, including mitochondrial mutations, might make an important contribution to aging. But exploration of this hypothesis has led to evidence that the role played by somatic mutations is peripheral to aging in the genetic wild type.

Theories of Oxidative Damage

It is sixty years since Denham Harman [56] first proposed that aging is caused by progressive damage to the body's chemistry from the reactive oxygen species (ROS) that are an inescapable byproduct of respiration. The theory has inspired thousands of research projects and continues to have great currency today. The ongoing attraction of the theory is that there is broad evidence that oxidative damage to key proteins accompanies aging. Extensive experimentation has explored the use of antioxidants as an anti-aging intervention, both in the laboratory and in human epidemiology. The results of these studies have been disappointing, with the largest studies actually showing *increased* mortality for subjects ingesting antioxidants [57]. The emerging picture of the relationship between oxidation and aging is complex: peroxide is an important signal in the pathways connected to apoptosis [58, 59]. Apoptosis has two faces: it is both an essential mechanism for cleansing the body of infected, cancerous and damaged cells and also implicated in the wasting of sarcopoenia [60, 61], the loss of brain cells in Alzheimer's [62, 63] and Parkinson's diseases [64-66]. The body's important antioxidants are expressed at lower levels with age, which both accounts for the observed increase in oxidative damage [67, 68] and suggests that oxidative damage is secondary effect rather than a root cause of aging.

Theories of oxidative damage are elegant and attractive, but some of the experimental results seem almost to mock the predictions of the theory. Physical activity generates copious free radicals and yet high levels of physical activity are generally associated with longer, not shorter average lifespans. Hanson and Hakimi [3] report on a genetically modified mouse that has extra mitochondria. These mice are phenomenally active, eat much more than wild type and burn it all up, yet they live almost two years longer than wild type and remain reproductively active two years longer. Two of the body's most essential antioxidants are superoxide dismutase (SOD) and unbiquinone. Mice in which one copy of the gene for SOD has been knocked out have half as much SOD in their tissues and measurements of oxidative damage to DNA show that it is far higher than controls; yet the heterozygous *Sod2*+/– mice lived slightly longer than controls [69]. SOD knockout worms also have extended lifespan, coupled with enhanced markers of oxidative stress [70].

CLK-1 is a gene originally discovered in worms [71], inactivation of which increases lifespan by an average 40%. Double mutant worms lacking both CLK-1 and DAF-2 have lifetimes extended fivefold [72]. The homologous gene in mice is MCLK1 and its deletion also leads to enhanced lifespan [73]. There are CLK-1 homologs in yeast and flies as well and both can be manipulated to live longer when CLK-1 is suppressed [73]. The action of CLK-1 is essential for synthesis of ubiquinone and as a result, CLK-1 mutants are *less* able to quench the ROS products of mitochondrial metabolism – yet they live longer [74, 75].

Naked mole rats live eight times longer than mice of comparable size, though the latter seem to be better protected against oxidative damage [76, 77]. And lifespans of mice are generally a few years, while bats for decades, despite a higher metabolic rate and greater load of mitochondrial ROS [78].

The laboratory of Arlan Richardson at the Barshop Institute of the University of Texas reports on the results of an eight-year, systematic study of a wide variety of genes coding for antioxidant enzymes. For each target gene, they studied both knockout mice and mice with extra copies of the gene and assayed lifespans under standard conditions. The only intervention that affected lifespan was the SOD1 gene. They published their study under the provocative title, "Is the oxidative stress theory of aging dead?" [79]. Circling for the wounded beast, LaPointe and Hekimi draw a parallel conclusion from their own experiments in an article titled, "When an aging theory ages badly" [80].

It is certainly true that much of the damage we associate with senescence can be traced back to oxidative damage from ROS created as a byproduct of mitochondrial processes; but biochemical protections could be adequate to protect against these hazards with essentially perfect efficiency and the body dials down these protections with age. The mass of evidence points to the conclusion that oxidative damage is a symptom, not a cause of aging.

Pre-Senescence, Negligible Senescence, Negative Senescence and Post-Senescence

If aging were a process of stochastic damage, then that damage would be accumulating inexorably, regardless of species, of environment or time of life. The many examples of non-aging and reverse aging described in Chapter 2 attest to the fact that aging is not a physical necessity.

All multicellular life is capable of building itself up from seed. During the process of growth, aging is typically absent. In fact, if aging be defined demographically as increasing mortality rates along with decreasing fecundity, then the early period of growth is a time of negative senescence.

Summary

The idea that aging is simply physical deterioration, with no need of any other explanation has been around a long time and it continues to seduce scientists and the general public. But there is no physical necessity for aging. The Second Law of Thermodynamics says that entropy must increase in a closed system, one that does not interact with its environment. But all living things must be capable of gathering order from their environment, concentrating it and dumping entropy back out with their waste. This principle has been well-understood and accepted by evolutionary biologists for over a century.

The idea that an organism could live indefinitely without accumulating damage is not simply a theoretical possibility. Some living things manage to avoid aging entirely, while others age quite suddenly and precipitously. Some living things can regenerate body parts when injured. All living things can build themselves up from seed to form a perfect whole. This is a far more difficult feat than repair. If an animal does not repair chemical and physical damage as it occurs, this is not because it is difficult, but because the repair process has evolved to be less efficient than it could be. Indeed, there are many examples of animals that can regenerate injured body parts.

There are many manifestations of aging that look like accumulation of damage. Lipofuscin accumulates in cells; epigenetic programming becomes less specific and more random; cartilage in joints and discs in the spine wears down. There are two reasons to regard these as part of an aging program, rather than as inevitable failure of the body's best efforts to maintain itself. First, there are ways in which the body is pouring fuel on the fire. Second (from Chapter 1) when the body is stressed, it appears able to slow or to mitigate this damage. Thus we should not regard accumulated damage as an inevitable result of physics, but rather as a result of the active (mostly epigenetic) suppression of repair mechanisms.

Oxidative damage is associated with the biological processes that generate energy. Biochemists have proposed this as a promising general theory of aging. The trouble with this theory is that it does not account for the enormous differences in oxidative damage from one species to the next. Paradoxically, the chemical repair process is found to be most efficient in some animals with the shortest lifespans. It may be that oxidative damage is an important mode of aging, but why some species should allow it some of the time, while others manage to avoid it entirely, is a challenge for evolutionary biology.

References

1. Clausius, R., *On the motive power of heat and the laws which can be deduced from it for a the theory of heat.* Annalen. der. Physik. und. Chemie, 1850. **79**: p. 368-397, 500-524.
2. Weismann, A., et al., *Essays upon Heredity and Kindred Biological Problems.* 2d ed. 1891, Oxford: Clarendon Press. 2 v.
3. Hanson, R.W. and P. Hakimi, *Born to run; the story of the PEPCK-cmus mouse.* Biochimie, 2008. **90**(6): p. 838-42.
4. Ayyadevara, S., et al., *Remarkable longevity and stress resistance of nematode PI3K-null mutants.* Aging Cell, 2008. **7**(1): p. 13-22.
5. Vaupel, J.W., et al., *The case for negative senescence.* Theor. Popul. Biol., 2004. **65**(4): p. 339-51.
6. Jones, O.R., et al., *Diversity of ageing across the tree of life.* Nature, 2014. **505**(7482): p. 169-173.
7. Longo, V.D., J. Mitteldorf and V.P. Skulachev, *Programmed and altruistic ageing.* Nat. Rev. Genet., 2005. **6**(11): p. 866-72.
8. Skulachev, I.V., *Phenoptosis: programmed death of an organism.* Biochemistry (Mosc.), 1999. **64**(12): p. 1418-1426.
9. Clausius, R., *On a modified form of the second fundamental theorem in the mechanical theory of heat, In: The Mechanical Theory of Heat,* T.A. Hirst, Editor. 1867, van Voorst. p. 111-135.
10. Medawar, P.B., *An unsolved problem of biology.* 1952, London,: Published for the college by H. K. Lewis. 24 p.
11. Moss, C., *Elephant Memories: Thirteen Years in the Life of an Elephant Family.* 1988: University of Chicago Press.
12. Hamilton, W.D., *The moulding of senescence by natural selection.* J. Theor. Biol., 1966. **12**(1): p. 12-45.

13. Kirkwood, T., *Evolution of aging.* Nature, 1977. **270**: p. 301-304.

14. Knight, J.A., *The biochemistry of aging.* Adv. Clin. Chem., 2000. **35**: p. 1-62.

15. Yoneda, M., et al., *Marked replicative advantage of human mtDNA carrying a point mutation that causes the MELAS encephalomyopathy.* Proc. Natl. Acad. Sci. U.S.A., 1992. **89**(23): p. 11164-8.

16. Izyumov, D.S., et al., *"Wages of fear": transient threefold decrease in intracellular ATP level imposes apoptosis.* Biochim. Biophys. Acta, 2004. **1658**(1-2): p. 141-7.

17. Carranza, J., et al., *Disposable-soma senescence mediated by sexual selection in an ungulate.* Nature, 2004. **432**(7014): p. 215-8.

18. Shanley, D.P. and T.B. Kirkwood, *Calorie restriction and aging: a life-history analysis.* Evolution Int. J. Org. Evolution, 2000. **54**(3): p. 740-50.

19. Cichon, M. and J. Kozlowski, *Ageing and typical survivorship curves result from optimal resource allocation.* Evol. Ecol. Res., 2000. **2**(7): p. 857-870.

20. Millar, J.S., *Energy reserves in breeding small mammals*, In: *Reproductive Energetics in Mammals*, A.S.I. Loudon and P.A. Racey, Editors. 1987, Clarendon Press: Oxford, UK. p. 231-240.

21. Poss, K.D., L.G. Wilson and M.T. Keating, *Heart regeneration in zebrafish.* Science, 2002. **298**(5601): p. 2188-2190.

22. Morrison, J.I., et al., *Salamander limb regeneration involves the activation of a multipotent skeletal muscle satellite cell population.* The Journal of cell biology, 2006. **172**(3): p. 433-440.

23. Brockes, J.P. and A. Kumar, *Appendage regeneration in adult vertebrates and implications for regenerative medicine.* Science, 2005. **310**(5756): p. 1919-1923.

24. Zasloff, M., *Observations on the remarkable (and mysterious) wound-healing process of the bottlenose dolphin.* J. Invest. Dermatol., 2011.

25. Han, M., et al., *Limb regeneration in higher vertebrates: developing a roadmap.* The Anatomical Record Part B: The New Anatomist, 2005. **287B**(1): p. 14-24.

26. Yokoyama, H., *Initiation of limb regeneration: the critical steps for regenerative capacity.* Development, growth & differentiation, 2008. **50**(1): p. 13-22.

27. Bedelbaeva, K., et al., *Lack of p21 expression links cell cycle control and appendage regeneration in mice.* Proc. Natl. Acad. Sci., 2010. **107**(13): p. 5845-5850.

28. Aguirre, A., et al., *In vivo activation of a conserved microRNA program induces mammalian heart regeneration.* Cell Stem Cell, 2014. **15**(5): p. 589-604.

29. Zhang, Y., et al., *Inhibition of the prostaglandin-degrading enzyme 15-PGDH potentiates tissue regeneration.* Science, 2015. **348**(6240).

30. Heber-Katz, E., et al., *Spallanzani's mouse: a model of restoration and regeneration.* Curr. Top. Microbiol. Immunol., 2004. **280**: p. 165-89.

31. Heber-Katz, E., et al., *Conjecture: can continuous regeneration lead to immortality? Studies in the MRL mouse.* Rejuvenation Res., 2006. **9**(1): p. 3-9.

32. Zhang, Y., et al., *Drug-induced regeneration in adult mice.* Sci. Transl. Med., 2015. **7**(290): p. 290ra92-290ra92.

33. Shyh-Chang, N., et al., *Lin28 enhances tissue repair by reprogramming cellular metabolism.* Cell, 2013. **155**(4): p. 778-792.

34. Wu, L., et al., *Precise let-7 expression levels balance organ regeneration against tumor suppression.* Elife, 2015. **4**: p. e09431.

35. Huang, Y., *A mirror of two faces: Lin28 as a master regulator of both miRNA and mRNA.* Wiley Interdisciplinary Reviews: RNA, 2012. **3**(4): p. 483-494.

36. Szilard, L., *On the nature of the aging process.* Proc. Natl. Acad. Sci. U.S.A., 1959. **45**(1): p. 30-45.

37. Orgel, L.E., *The maintenance of the accuracy of protein synthesis and its relevance to ageing.* Proc. Natl. Acad. Sci. U.S.A., 1963. **49**: p. 517-21.

38. Rabinovitch, P.S. and G.M. Martin, *Encephalomyocarditis virus as a probe of errors in macromolecular synthesis in aging mice.* Mech. Ageing Dev., 1982. **20**(2): p. 155-63.

39. Harley, C.B., et al., *Protein synthetic errors do not increase during aging of cultured human fibroblasts.* Proc. Natl. Acad. Sci. U.S.A., 1980. **77**(4): p. 1885-9.

40. Martin, G.M., et al., *Somatic mutations are frequent and increase with age in human kidney epithelial cells.* Hum. Mol. Genet., 1996. **5**(2): p. 215-221.

41. Pepper, J.W., K. Sprouffske and C.C. Maley, *Animal cell differentiation patterns suppress somatic evolution.* PLoS Comput. Biol., 2007. **3**(12): p. e250.

42. Cairns, J., *Mutation selection and the natural history of cancer.* Nature, 1975. **255**(5505): p. 197-200.

43. Anderson, S.M.B.J., *The fungus Armillaria bulbosa is among the largest and oldest living organisms.* Nature, 1992. **356**: p. 428-431.

44. Caulin, A.F. and C.C. Maley, *Peto's paradox: evolution's prescription for cancer prevention.* Trends Ecol. Evol., 2011. **26**(4): p. 175-182.

45. Roche, B., et al., *Natural resistance to cancers: a Darwinian hypothesis to explain Peto's paradox.* BMC Cancer, 2012. **12**(1): p. 387.

46. Peto, R.R., et al., *Cancer and aging in mice and men.* Brit. J. Cancer, 1975. **32**(4): p. 411-426.

47. Edman, U., et al., *Life span extension by dietary restriction is not linked to protection against somatic DNA damage in Drosophila melanogaster.* Aging cell, 2009. **8**(3): p. 331-338.

48. Muller, H.J., *Artificial transmutation of the gene.* Science, 1927. **66**: p. 84-87.

49. Vijg, J., *Aging of the Genome: The Dual Role of DNA in Life and Death.* 2007: OUP Oxford.

50. De Grey, A.D., *The Mitochondrial Free Radical Theory of Aging.* 1999, Austin, TX: Springer/Landes. 212 p.

51. Hayashi, J., et al., *Nuclear but not mitochondrial genome involvement in human age-related mitochondrial dysfunction. Functional integrity of mitochondrial DNA from aged subjects.* J. Biol. Chem., 1994. **269**(9): p. 6878-83.

52. Hashizume, O., et al., *Epigenetic regulation of the nuclear-coded GCAT and SHMT2 genes confers human age-associated mitochondrial respiration defects.* Sci. Rep., 2015. **5**.

53. Prokof'eva, V., et al., *Cellular DNA repair, proliferative activity and biochemical characteristics in the human premature aging syndrome (progeria).* Tsitologiia, 1982. **24**(5): p. 592-603.

54. Prokocimer, M., R. Barkan and Y. Gruenbaum, *Hutchinson–gilford progeria syndrome through the lens of transcription.* Aging Cell, 2013. **12**(4): p. 533-543.

55. Bailey, L.J., et al., *Mice expressing an error-prone DNA polymerase in mitochondria display elevated replication pausing and chromosomal breakage at fragile sites of mitochondrial DNA.* Nucleic Acids Res., 2009: p. gkp091.

56. Harman, D., *Aging: a theory based on free radical and radiation chemistry.* J. Gerontol., 1956. **11**(3): p. 298-300.

57. Virtamo, J., et al., *Incidence of cancer and mortality following alpha-tocopherol and beta-carotene supplementation: a postintervention follow-up.* JAMA, 2003. **290**(4): p. 476-85.

58. Skulachev, V.P., *Programmed death phenomena: from organelle to organism.* Ann. N.Y. Acad. Sci., 2002. **959**: p. 214-37.

59. Skulachev, V.P. and V.D. Longo, *Aging as a mitochondria-mediated atavistic program: can aging be switched off?* Ann. N.Y. Acad. Sci., 2005. **1057**: p. 145-64.

60. Marzetti, E. and C. Leeuwenburgh, *Skeletal muscle apoptosis, sarcopenia and frailty at old age.* Exp. Gerontol., 2006. **41**(12): p. 1234-8.

61. Pistilli, E.E., J.R. Jackson and S.E. Alway, *Death receptor-associated pro-apoptotic signaling in aged skeletal muscle.* Apoptosis, 2006. **11**(12): p. 2115-26.

62. Su, J.H., et al., *Immunohistochemical evidence for apoptosis in Alzheimer's disease.* Neuroreport, 1994. **5**(18): p. 2529-33.

63. Vina, J., et al., *Mitochondrial oxidant signalling in Alzheimer's disease.* J. Alzheimers Dis., 2007. **11**(2): p. 175-81.

64. Mochizuki, H., et al., *Histochemical detection of apoptosis in Parkinson's disease.* J. Neurol. Sci., 1996. **137**(2): p. 120-3.

65. Lev, N., E. Melamed and D. Offen, *Apoptosis and Parkinson's disease.* Prog. Neuropsychopharmacol. Biol. Psychiatry, 2003. **27**(2): p. 245-50.

66. Chinta, S.J., et al., *Environmental stress, ageing and glial cell senescence: a novel mechanistic link to Parkinson's disease?* J. Intern. Med., 2013. **273**(5): p. 429-436.

67. Linnane, A.W., et al., *Human aging and global function of coenzyme Q10.* Ann. N.Y. Acad. Sci., 2002. **959**: p. 396-411; discussion 463-5.

68. Tatone, C., et al., *Age-dependent changes in the expression of superoxide dismutases and catalase are associated with ultrastructural modifications in human granulosa cells.* Mol. Hum. Reprod., 2006. **12**(11): p. 655-60.

69. Van Remmen, H., et al., *Life-long reduction in MnSOD activity results in increased DNA damage and higher incidence of cancer but does not accelerate aging.* Physiol. Genomics, 2003. **16**: p. 29-37.

70. Van Raamsdonk, J.M. and S. Hekimi, *Deletion of the mitochondrial superoxide dismutase sod-2 extends life span in Caenorhabditis elegans.* PLoS Genet., 2009. **5**(2): p. e1000361.

71. Johnson, T.E., P.M. Tedesco and G.J. Lithgow, *Comparing mutants, selective breeding, and transgenics in the dissection of aging processes of Caenorhabditis elegans.* Genetica, 1993. **91**(1-3): p. 65-77.

72. Lakowski, B. and S. Hekimi, *Determination of life span in Caenorhabditis elegans by four clock genes.* Science, 1996. **272**(5264): p. 1010-1013.

73. Liu, X., et al., *Evolutionary conservation of the clk-1-dependent mechanism of longevity: loss of mclk1 increases cellular fitness and life span in mice.* Genes Dev., 2005. **19**(20): p. 2424-34.

74. Aguilaniu, H., J. Durieux and A. Dillin, *Metabolism, ubiquinone synthesis and longevity.* Genes. Dev., 2005. **19**(20): p. 2399-2406.

75. Lapointe, J. and S. Hekimi, *Early mitochondrial dysfunction in long-lived Mclk1+/– mice.* J. Biol. Chem., 2008. **283**(38): p. 26217-27.

76. Andziak, B., T.P. O'Connor and R. Buffenstein, *Antioxidants do not explain the disparate longevity between mice and the longest-living rodent, the naked mole-rat.* Mech. Ageing Dev., 2005. **126**(11): p. 1206-12.

77. Andziak, B., et al., *High oxidative damage levels in the longest-living rodent, the naked mole-rat.* Aging Cell, 2006. **5**(6): p. 463-71.

78. Finch, C.E., *Longevity, Senescence and the Genome.* 1990, Chicago: University of Chicago Press.

79. Perez, V.I., et al., *Is the oxidative stress theory of aging dead?* Biochim. Biophys. Acta, 2009. **1790**(10): p. 1005-14.

80. Lapointe, J. and S. Hekimi, *When a theory of aging ages badly.* Cell. Mol. Life Sci., 2009. **67**(1): p. 1-8.

4

Three Prevailing Theories and their Failings

Do We Really Need Three Theories?

There are three standard theories of aging, and most scientists in the field see no inherent conflict among them. The three together have survived so many empirical contradictions largely because weaknesses of each are reported as if they were strengths of the others. All three describe aging as an accident or side-effect of evolution, and they all start with the idea that natural selection does not care as much what happens to an individual once its genes have been passed to the next generation. Aging could then be simply a matter of non-evolution—genetic drift—or it could be that there is a kind of devil's bargain, where the individual gains some positive fitness attribute early in life in exchange for the seeds of failure later on. There are logical and experimental problems with each of the three.

First is Mutation Accumulation (MA). Most people who hear the name for the first time assume that it is a wear-and-tear theory, concerned with somatic mutations during a lifetime. But in fact, the MA theory is about genetic load. Very few animals get old in the wild, so aging is (almost) invisible to evolution. Even without aging, most animals will be killed by a predator or die of disease or starvation before reaching old age. Mutations that happen to cause problems at late ages creep into the genome because there is no selection against them. A strong argument against this is that there are genes with large effect on aging that have been around for a long time and are closely related from one species to the next. This is the signature of evolution at work, not a recent, chance set of mutations that would be different for each species, if MA were the correct paradigm. Even more fundamentally, the premise that few animals die of old age in nature has been falsified by many field studies.

The second theory is called Antagonistic Pleiotropy (AP). It says that aging is caused by genes that enhance fertility early in life, but that cause problems later in life. The best evidence against it is that when fruit flies are bred for longevity, their fertility goes up. Hence whatever genes are causing aging, they cannot be enhancing fertility. More generally, a great deal of evidence has been collected that supports the idea that there are indeed pleiotropic genes controlling lifespan. What is missing is evidence that these tradeoffs are unavoidable and that there is no available path to longevity that does not involve curtailing fertility or some essential aspect of early viability. In fact, there are many examples of genes in wild-type animals that cut life short with no known pleiotropic benefit. This suggests that pleiotropy is not the root cause of aging and that the observed pleiotropic genes might command an alternative explanation.

The third theory goes by the name Disposable Soma (DS), but it is really about the body's energy budget. The theory says that there is not enough food energy to do everything the body needs to do—to forage and to compete for mates and to run a metabolism and to reproduce and also to repair the cells that get damaged. The damage is not repaired perfectly because there is not enough energy, and there is not enough energy because of this grand compromise. The best evidence against this theory is that animals that eat less actually live longer. If aging is caused by a shortage of food energy, you would have to expect that the body would age more slowly when there is more food energy available, but exactly the opposite is true.

The DS theory is often classed as a special case of Antagonistic Pleiotropy. Both AP and DS theories are based on enforced tradeoffs that limit the organism's ability to optimize different aspects of its fitness simultaneously. The difference is that in classical AP, the tradeoff is genetic, enforced over evolutionary time, while in DS, the tradeoff is metabolic and is enforced during an individual's lifetime.

Medawar and Mutation Accumulation

The earliest evolutionary explanation for aging was in a 19th century classic by August Weismann [1]. Around the turn of the century, Weismann disavowed his own theory of aging and for fifty years thereafter there was a theoretical vacuum in the field. To be sure, there was a vague discomfort with the disparity between Darwin's struggle for existence and the ubiquity of aging, but no one stepped forward to fill the void. During this era, though, the theoretical foundation for population genetics as a quantitative science was being laid by Lotka, Wright, Haldane, Dobzhansky and most prominently, R.A. Fisher. With the clear predictive power of the New Synthesis, aging appeared as an obvious and stark anomaly.

Peter Medawar was born in Brazil of a Lebanese mother and British father, raised poor, 6-foot-5, and came to Britain to attend Oxford. He was never awarded a PhD during his lifetime and legend has it that it was because he declined to pay the £25 diploma fee. At age 36, in 1951, Medawar had just accepted a promotion to faculty at University College, London and had already discovered how to make one animal tolerate a skin graft from another, work that laid the foundation for grafting human organs in coming decades and earned him the 1960 Nobel Prize. Medawar offered an Inaugural Lecture at his new academic home, proposing a solution to what he called *An Unsolved Problem of Biology* [2].

Medawar's monograph, based on the lecture, is ripe with a deep understanding of demography, of human gerontology, of simple exponential mathematics and the characteristic wit and colorful language for which he was known. His chief innovation was to realize that "the force of natural selection declines with increasing age". He invokes a time before aging when animals died randomly of hazards in the wild. After maturation, their rate of mortality was constant, by Medawar's assumption. The same percentage of them would die each day (or each year). If half of all rabbits die in the first year, then only ¼ are left after two years, ⅛ after three years and so on, until the number remaining in the eighth year is less than 1%. If an individual's fitness is measured by the number of offspring it leaves behind, its fitness depends twice as much on what happens in the first year than in the second, because half the animals never make it to the second year.

In Darwin's conception, random mutations are constantly arising, and natural selection is continually weeding out the bad ones and promoting the good ones. In any given population, at any given time, there is a certain number of mutations spread through the population that are detrimental but not lethal and have arisen too recently to have been eliminated. This is a well-studied phenomenon classically called "mutational load" or "genetic load" [3, 4]. By Medawar's reasoning, the genetic load of mutations acting late in life is expected to be far higher than the load of mutations acting early in life. Thus all systems may be expected to fail progressively with age, because there has been little natural selection to keep the body healthy at such ages. At an age where no individuals survive in nature, there is no selective benefit for continued life and we should not be surprised if the system fails catastrophically.

This formulation in terms of genetic load was implicit in Medawar's monograph, but not stated in this way until an article by Edney and Gill [5] several years later.

Critiquing Medawar from a Modern Vantage

Reading stories about Medawar and reading from his extensive contributions to popular science, it is impossible not to have affection for this man and to hold him in high regard. And his theory of aging does him proud. Based on the understanding of science that he inherited, Medawar's insights were the logical next step. But we have learned a great deal since 1951, learned about aging, genetics and ecology—the latter science barely recognized in Medawar's time. The main thing that Medawar could not have known is that many animals survive in the wild long enough to die of old age, so that senescence takes a substantial bite out of fitness. This pulls the floor out from under his argument.

Medawar's model is framed in a stable environmental background. He assumes that the background mortality rate is static in time, so that the same proportion of the population succumbs with each passing year. He could hardly have done otherwise, since population dynamics as a science was completely undeveloped in his day. The quantitative science of evolution had made headway during the first half of the century by making several simplifying assumptions, and one of them was to think about one individual at a time, with the environment held constant. Nevertheless, if we were to presume to update Medawar's thought experiment about a world before senescence, we might note that predominant sources of mortality in the wild are very sensitive to population density. Thus the background death rate would not likely be constant (without consequence) but varying cyclically or even chaotically with population fluctuations. I believe this is a central insight that profoundly changes evolutionary dynamics and opens the study of evolution to a range of phenomena that have been observed but never explained. It is the basis of the Demographic Theory, which I will develop in detail in Chapter 7.

Medawar leaves out an important, if technical, perspective that strengthens his argument. Fertility early in life contributes more to individual fitness than equivalent fitness at a later age, and not simply because some will die before they reach the later age. It is because of the potential for your children to have children, accelerating the penetration of your genes into the population. The best-accepted theoretical measure of fitness, promoted but not invented by Fisher, is the Malthusian parameter r. It is a kind of weighted average of fertility over a lifetime, with early fertility counting for more than later fertility in a self-referential computation. Taking this effect into account doubles the force of Medawar's claim that "the force of natural selection declines with increasing age".

Medawar's argument is framed in terms of an assumption that particular genes control fitness at particular times of life. Writing just before Watson and Crick's discovery of the way in which DNA carries genetic information, he made a reasonable assumption about genes and time. Today, we know that the lion's share of the genome is devoted to binding sites, promoters and repressors, which collectively determine when and where each gene is expressed. The word "epigenetics" had been introduced by Waddington [6], but only as a theoretical construct; nothing was known about the timing or regulation of gene expression when Medawar offered his Inaugural Lecture, let alone the specifics of histones, methylation and acetylation in promoter regions that are now understood to be the mechanistic basis of epigenetics.

If Medawar had been able to pursue his theory in light of present knowledge of epigenetics, he might have concluded that epigenetic regulation would tend to randomize at late ages, there being no selection pressure to assure that epigenetic factors remain properly tuned. Indeed, we do see some tendency to stochastic dysregulation of epigenetics at late ages in humans (the best-studied species) [7]. But what Medawar would never have anticipated is that there are also regular epigenetic changes in the body over time that seem not to be in the body's best interest [8]. Antioxidants and protective chemistry are dialed down late in life and destructive inflammation is dialed up epigenetically.

Mutation Accumulation—Three Dealbreakers

It detracts nothing from Medawar's achievement that he did not anticipate future discoveries, but it reflects badly on those of us who have clung to the Mutation Accumulation theory after experimental findings have made it untenable. There are three such findings, both dating from the 1980s and 1990s. First, the fitness cost of senescence in the wild is too high for senescence to survive in a "selection shadow". Second, the genetic basis of aging is ancient and well-ordered, not recent and random as we would expect from a theory of mutational load. Third, there is a measure of population diversity for a particular measure called the *additive genetic variance* which, in Fisher's theory, measures the effect that selection has had in shaping that trait; it has been found that the additive genetic variance for mortality late in life is not only very low, but decreases with age. This is the signature of a trait that has been shaped by natural selection and it is inconsistent with the hypothesis of random mutations.

High Cost of Senescence in the Wild

All the theories of aging are premised on the assumption that nature has permitted aging to evolve because it does not cost very much, in the sense that its effect on fitness is small. But for the Mutation Accumulation theory in particular, this assumption is its very core. When the theory was being developed, it was assumed that animals in the wild seldom die of old age because disease or starvation or a predator or an accident gets to them first. This makes aging so much easier to understand, and since Medawar's book [2] it was thought, based on a general view of the way the biosphere works, that it must be so: few animals in nature die of old age.

But since about 1990, the relevant field studies have been done, charting the demographics of animals in the wild. The question has been asked: what percentage of animals die because of aging? The numbers are surprisingly high.

It is important to pose the question in this way, rather than simply to ask how many animals 'die of old age'. That answer has to be very low. Even for humans, protected by civilization, this is true. Old people die of cancer or heart disease or diabetes at much higher rates than young people, though they are not literally dying of old age. Old people die of infections like influenza, though young people seldom do. Pneumonia, the 'old man's friend,' is rarely a mortal risk for people under 70.

Death from aging of animals in the wild is like this, but because the environment is more hazardous, it tends to happen at an earlier age. There are no hospitals or antibiotics, predators are ever-present, and what is more, there is often tight competition for food. When animals suffer age-related deaths in the wild, it is usually not because they lose all their faculties and keel over dead; rather they are just beginning to lose their competitive edge and they can no longer feed themselves. Or they may lose just enough of their speed that they become vulnerable to predators that cannot catch their younger, faster relatives. This, too, must be counted as a fitness cost of aging, as proposed quite early by Williams [9].

By this definition, aging has been found responsible for a substantial proportion of all the animal deaths in nature. Promislow first made this finding when collecting and reviewing studies of natural mammal populations [10]. Ricklefs cited Promislow and collected further examples and added studies of birds [11]. No one had thought before to ask the question whether aging was a factor in these animals' deaths, but collectively the data had a story to tell. If, as expected, there were few animals in nature attaining to old age, then skulls and skeletons of young animals would predominate in these collections; at older ages, there would be fewer and fewer of them left alive. But, in fact, what Ricklefs found was, in one species after another, it was the older animals that predominated. There were actually more old animals than young adults represented in this diverse collection of remains. From curves of death count versus age, it is an easy matter (in principle) to compute a logarithmic derivative and impute a rate of increase in mortality. This in turn implies an answer to the question, what is the toll of aging on the population? In the data of Ricklefs, there was not a single species for which aging was negligible. Only in rabbits and squirrels did aging account for less than 10% of deaths. For larger animals, the numbers ranged widely from 20% through an astounding 80%. In sables, African buffalo, and alpine sheep, more than 70% of the animals were living long enough for aging to be a decisive factor in their deaths. For most species, the number was in the range 20-60%.

In the chart below, I have computed the percentage of deaths attributable to aging for each species, based on the data and methodology of Ricklefs [11]. The chart does not appear in this form in his publication. The first four data columns represent parameters fitted to a Weibull curve, for which Ricklefs claims the best overall fit. In the last column, I have computed P_s, the percentage of deaths that would not have occurred but for senescence, based on integration of the Weibull curve, according to the formulas

$$l_x = e^{-\{m_0 x + [\alpha/(\beta+1)]x^{\beta+1}\}}$$

$$P_s = \int_{x=0}^{\infty} ax^{\beta} l_x dx,$$

also provided by Ricklefs.

		Mo	α	ω	β	Ps
Rhesus monkey	Macaca mulatta	0.087	1.21E-05	0.059	3.00	17.41%
Chimpanzee	Pan troglodytes	0.055	4.22E-06	0.045	2.99	23.01%
Lion	Panthera leo	0.032	2.52E-04	0.126	3.00	42.30%
Sable	Martes zibellina	0.28	5.42E-04	0.153	3.01	11.91%
Fur seal	Callorhinus ursinus	0.051	8.60E-05	0.096	2.99	51.55%
Ringed seal	Phoca hispida	0.063	1.07E-05	0.057	3.00	26.26%
African elephant	Loxodonta africana	0.04	1.70E-06	0.036	3.00	26.09%
Zebra	Equus burchelli	0.057	7.72E-05	0.094	3.00	47.08%
Hippo	Hippopotamus amphibius	0.03	5.30E-06	0.048	3.00	46.04%
Elk	Cervus elaphus	0.05	1.60E-04	0.112	2.99	57.16%
Caribou	Rangifer tarandus	0.076	2.00E-03	0.212	3.01	63.69%
African buffalo	Syncerus caffer	0.026	8.50E-05	0.096	3.00	71.01%
Alpine sheep	Ovis dalli	0.049	8.35E-04	0.17	3.00	69.48%
Chamois (alpine antelope)	Rupicapra rupicapra	0.219	1.98E-03	0.211	3.00	28.36%
African deer	Kobus kob thomasi	0.206	3.40E-03	0.242	3.01	35.20%
African topi	Damaliscus korrigum	0.175	1.00E-02	0.32	3.04	50.58%
Squirrel	Tamiasciurus hudsonicus	0.437	2.05E-03	0.21	3.00	9.48%
Rabbit	Sylvilagus floridanus	1.225	1.32E-01	0.60	2.99	9.66%
Swan	Cygnus columbianus	0.036	3.89E-05	0.079	3.00	56.52%
Gull	Larus canus	0.098	2.99E-05	0.074	3.00	20.53%
Sparrow hawk	Accipiter nisus	0.201	1.84E-03	0.207	3.00	30.63%
Little penguin	Eudyptula minor	0.195	3.13E-04	0.133	3.00	17.57%
Puffin	Puffinus tenuirostris	0.08	1.12E-04	0.103	3.00	38.43%
Pied flycatcher	Ficedula hypoleuca	0.748	3.35E-03	0.241	3.00	3.49%
Great tit	Parus major	0.756	3.43E-03	0.242	3.00	3.43%

The implied impact on fitness is huge. If fitness is measured by r, then, a proportion of senescent deaths does not translate directly into a fixed reduction in fitness, but a range of values can be computed using some reasonable curves for survival and fertility. 20 to 60% senescent deaths corresponds to a bite out of fitness that is about 12 to 45%.

What is the Impact of Aging on Fitness?

We have said that in field studies, the percentage of deaths attributable to senescence is typically in the range 20-30%. How does that translate into an impact on fitness? This is an interesting question and it has an interesting non-answer.

The measure of fitness that classically has the best theoretical support is the "Malthusian parameter," denoted r. r is an exponential rate of increase and it is computed with the same mathematics as return on investment is computed in finance. It is a time-weighted sum over the offspring that an individual produces, but the time weighting is according to r itself. Hence r can only be computed implicitly, as solution to the Euler-Lotka equation,

$$1 = \int_0^\infty e^{-ra} \ell(a)b(a)da$$

in which the integral is over all ages, $\ell(a)$ is the proportion surviving to a given age and $b(a)$ is fertility at that age. r is computed implicitly as the value that leads to an integral equal to unity.

r is a rate of population growth, hence it is zero on average in a stable ecosystem over an extended period of time.

We wish to ask what percentage change in r is produced if life is cut short when (for example) 20% of a cohort remains alive. But if r is zero to begin with, then any change in r amounts to an infinite percentage change in fitness.

So we may try to reframe the question to admit a meaningful answer. Without the time-weighting, what is the change in the number offspring produced (R_o) if the lifespan is cut off while 25% remain alive? The answer depends on details of other assumptions implicit in the calculation. For example, should we use a mortality curve that is flat, corresponding to no aging? Or steeply rising, corresponding to a Gompertz curve?

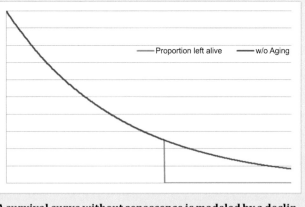

Proportion left alive — w/o Aging

A survival curve without senescence is modeled by a declining exponential. To add 25% senescent deaths in a way that has minimal impact on r, cut off the survival curve on the right at the point when 25% remain alive.

Is the decline in fertility with age to be treated as a given, in which case the impact of early deaths on reproductive fitness may be small or even zero? Or is fertility senescence part of the metabolic decline that we are trying to explain, so its impact should be added to whatever we compute to be the net fitness impact of 25% senescent deaths?

Further, we may attempt to modify the calculation of R_o in the direction of r by weighting early fertility more heavily than later fertility. We might take the original r or the final r (after the curve is modified for senescence) to determine an exponential weighting curve for weighting fertility.

I have performed a range of calculations with these different assumptions and I find no case in which the impact on fitness is negligible. The range of 12% to 45% that I claim above comes from the most conservative assumptions, using the lifespan cutoff model pictured in the figure and a weighting factor that counts early fertility more heavily than late fertility.

Evolutionary biologists are accustomed to studying cases in which natural selection has found some clever ways to add a fraction of 1% to the reproductive output of one species or another. By comparison, the potential reward for solving the aging problem is enormous. If 80% of sable deaths are attributed to old age, that means that only 20% are dying of external causes. A hypothetical sable that did not age would live five times as long, leaving five times as many offspring, and would be overwhelmingly favored by natural selection, based on classical reasoning.

Ricklefs was able to find these answers by scouring the biology journals for old data, collected with other purposes in mind. A few years later, a young Canadian researcher named Russell Bonduriansky thought to ask the same question more systematically and intensively for a single species. For his thesis project at the University of Toronto, he set out to study a species of antler flies that was copiously available in the parks of Ontario [12]. The fact that the flies lived less than two weeks made the project manageable, but their tiny size posed a challenge for marking and tracking individual flies. Nevertheless, Bonduriansky was able to follow 600 flies through their lifespan, keeping their identities straight all the while and recording how long each one lived. Conclusion: he estimated the fitness cost of old age for these tiny, short-lived flies at about 20%. For such a fragile and ephemeral species, this was a complete surprise and the result made headlines for the young researcher in *Nature*.

In later reviews, Promislow emphasized the radical implications for evolutionary theory of these and other studies, documenting the high cost of aging in the wild [13, 14]. This fact alone falsifies the MA theory and it places tight constraints on the two remaining theories as well.

The Persistence of Aging Genes

The details that separate closely-related species from one another are encoded in genes of recent origin. But there are also genes for core biochemical functions of the cell that are common to all eukaryotic life, and these have persisted for hundreds of millions of years [15]. These include genes for the basic chemistry of life, for copying and transcribing DNA, for burning sugar, and for regulating pH and salinity. These systems are part of the core metabolism necessary for the maintenance of life.

How long a gene has been around and how widely it is copied through the biosphere are closely-related markers of a gene's functional importance. Thus it was a substantial surprise and a blow to evolutionary theory when the discovery came to light in the 1990s of a common genetic basis for aging across widely-separated taxa [16, 17]. Some genes related to aging are just as old and just as widely distributed as the ancient, essential genes that are at the heart of cell metabolism. Every gene that has been preserved and transmitted over hundreds of millions of years performs some function of central importance. The fact that genes for aging are comparably old and comparably related across the biosphere is an indication that natural selection has regarded aging as an essential life function. Nature has guarded the mechanism of death just as faithfully as she has preserved the chemical basis of life. Keeping death under genetic control has been treated as an essential priority, as judged by the tenacity and fidelity with which aging genes have been preserved over the æons.

CLK-1 was described in the last chapter, a gene with homologs in yeast, worms, flies and mice, whose deletion extends lifespan in all these lab models. The best-known case of lifespan genes that have been conserved is the gene family that responds to insulin and IGF-1. IGF-1 stands for "insulin-like growth factor". Insulin is one of the body's central signaling hormones, with many related functions. (Insulin is produced in the pancreas and a shortage of insulin is diagnosed as Type I diabetes. Weakness in the body's response to insulin produces the symptoms of Type II diabetes.)

The most familiar role of insulin is to regulate sugar in the bloodstream. Digestion of our food produces sugar that is pumped into the blood for the body's fuel. If we are eating a lot and not very active, then an insulin signal will tell the body to stop generating sugar and to store the fuel as fat. IGF-1 is a similar hormone that circulates in the bloodstream and controls growth and body-building. Both insulin and IGF-1 have long-term as well as short-term effects. One of the long-term effects is to modulate the rate of aging. Insulin and IGF-1 are part of the machinery that tells the body to age more slowly when there is a fuel deficit (lots of exercise; little food intake). Evidence for this mechanism is widespread over several species that have been studied- hence this was the first candidate for a conserved gene that controls aging [18].

In *C. elegans*, the sole receptor for insulin/IGF-1 is the gene *daf2*. The *daf2* gene is necessary for development and worms without it die in the embryonic stage, but worms with impaired *daf2* have extended lifespans. Some worms with modified *daf2* have other markers of starvation—for example, their metabolisms slow, they stop reproducing temporarily, and they go into a kind of hibernation. But other *daf2* mutants live longer without these side-effects [17]. Fruit flies may not conform to our idea of a higher life form, but compared to roundworms, they are vastly larger and more complex; of course, the evolutionary relationship between worms and flies is not at all close. So how surprising was it to discover that flies had genetic mechanisms that closely paralleled the worms' insulin/IGF-1 signaling pathways and that the flies' lifespans can be extended by genetic manipulation of these same genes [19]?

(Yeast cells are far more primitive than either worms or flies. Though they have a response to calorie restriction that has been studied extensively, the response is not mediated by insulin/IGF-1 [20, 21].)

The biology of mammals is more complex. Mammals also rely on signaling from insulin and IGF-1, but the story of lifespan seems to be less straightforward. Mice that have been put on restricted diets in the lab live longer and blood tests show that, like worms and flies, they produce less IGF-1.

This family of closely-related genes that regulate aging in animals whose last common ancestor is half a billion years old indicates that there is something very basic about aging. Of course, the metabolisms of yeast, mice, worms, and flies are very different and the physiology of aging is very different. The fact that the same genes can affect lifespan in these widely-separated species tells us that aging is controlled from the top down. It is not a simple matter of accumulated damage at a low level, spread out over many systems; more accurately, it may be manifested as an accumulation of damage to many systems, but this damage is permitted to happen at a rate that is under central control. The insulin/IGF-1 genes that regulate aging must sit atop a cascade of chemical signals that control the rate at which damage is permitted to accumulate at the lowest levels [18, 21].

What is more, the close relationship among genes that regulate aging in such different organisms is an indication that natural selection has treated aging as an adaptation. Natural selection evidently regards aging regulators as sufficiently important that she keeps their form and function, even as everything around them is evolving and deeply transforming in many other ways.

In addition to insulin/IGF-1, there are other aging mechanisms and other genes that have been conserved from very primitive life forms through mammals. In Chapter 5, we will describe the two mechanisms for aging that exist in protists: telomeres and apoptosis. It has been known for a long time that humans retain these genetic pathways and have adapted these mechanisms. But only in the last few years has it been clear that both these mechanisms contribute in important ways to human aging.

Additive Genetic Variance

Fisher's fundamental law of selection says that when natural selection for a quantitative trait is strong, the average value of the trait changes faster. That much should be obvious. A less obvious part of the same law says that the rate of change is also proportional to the variance in that trait itself. This is because selection can only work to the extent that there are phenotypic differences from which to select. For example, if everyone were the same height, it wouldn't matter whether there was a selective advantage to being taller or shorter. Only when individuals have a range of different heights can natural selection operate to select an optimal height.

Over time, these two factors—variance and strength of selection—become locked in a reciprocal relationship. If selection for a certain trait is strong, then it will eliminate all but the "best" version of that trait, so that the population variance for that trait becomes quite narrow. Conversely, if different phenotypes are all roughly equivalent in the eyes of natural selection, then random variation will spread the population out among those possibilities and the variance will be broad.

It follows that you can study the variance of a trait within a natural population to determine how strongly natural selection has been operating on that trait. For example, if you find different rabbits in Georgia that are black, white, or brown, then you conclude that all of these forms must be about equally fit, so selection has not differentiated among them. But if you find that all the rabbits in Alaska are white, you may suspect that in Alaska there is a selective advantage to being white.

This suggests an experiment that could determine whether aging is an adaptation under strong selection or an artifact, accident, or "spandrel" in the colorful metaphor of Gould and Lewontin [22]. If natural selection for the death rate from aging is strong, then the variance in the death rate should be very low. If natural selection has been operating to assure death by a certain age, then the variance in death rate should get lower and lower as the age (and the death rate) gets higher and higher. And indeed, variance of the mortality rate becomes lower and lower with increasing age, as impending death becomes a certainty.

This is a commonplace observation, for which no experiment should be necessary. It is obvious that there is much more variance in the death rate for young (but mature) animals than there is later on, when imminent death is a certainty. A middle-aged animal has many possible fates; an aged animal but one. The middle-aged individual may die sooner or later, but the animal near the end of its natural lifespan will almost certainly die quickly. This is a strong indication about the variance in the death rate and the way it changes with age. One may object that it is not an absolute proof, because the variance in death rate comprises two pieces: part is due to environmental factors and part to genetics. It is only the genetic part that has been shaped by natural selection and that is the subject of Fisher's theorem. But these two variances add together and both are positive numbers, so there is no way that a large variance in mortality at late ages could be masked. Thus this simple observation—that death at advanced ages is statistically quite certain—this one observation can be interpreted using Fisher's theorem to tell us that aging is no accident and no side-effect, but a direct result of the action of natural selection.

To turn this idea into a scientific measurement is trickier than it may seem. Separating genetics from environment from chance requires a special experimental design and a very large initial population, so that by the time most of them have died, there are still enough left to determine a statistical trend. The formal experiment was properly conducted by a team of four scientists at the University of Minnesota in 1996 [23, 24], using tens of thousands of flies to measure and compare death rates. They devised an experimental design that statistically separated heredity from environment as a cause of death. To accomplish this, they worked with 256 separate clonal populations, each cloned from a single example of a wild-type fly. Thus they formalized the criteria for Fisher's theorem to apply and closed the chain of logic. Their result was the same as our informal observation: low variance for the death rate at late ages. At least for fruit flies, natural selection has affirmatively chosen programmed death at a well-defined age.

This is a shocking blow to the standard theories that grow from Medawar's big idea. All the standard theories are based on the idea that natural selection gets weaker with age and is so weak at advanced ages that selection simply does not care and lets the individuals die. In this case, we would have expected a large variance—a signature of the hypothesis that it does not matter to selection. The Minnesota finding was exactly the opposite of what was expected. The observation of low additive genetic invariance is deal-breaker for the Mutation Accumulation theory, which relies absolutely on the assumption that selection pressure weakens with advancing age.

The Minnesota Four: Why did the Experiment Have to be so Complicated?

Fisher's theorem concerns the genetic variation for a single trait in a natural, evolving population. For example, suppose the trait we were interested in was weight. We might capture a thousand flies from a natural population and weigh them. Suppose we find that the average weight was 1 mg. The variance has to do with how much a typical fly's weight departs from that average, on either the high or the low side. It measure the breadth or spread of the flies' weights around their average weight.

The Minnesota team faced the task of measuring the genetic variance for the death rate. The dilemma was that no single fly has a 'death rate', because each fly dies only once. They could record the age of each fly when it died, but that would not be the same thing. The timing of death is influenced by both heredity and environment. How could they separate out the hereditary component?

Their solution was to use intensive inbreeding, combined with early genetic engineering. (The experiment was done in 1995, when genetic engineering was quite young.) They began with a natural population with full natural variability and an inbred population of lab flies that had very little variability. They combined these to produce 100 clonal populations in 100 jars. Each jar contained about 360 flies that were genetically identical within each jar, but together the 100 jars spanned the full range of variability found in nature. Thus the 256 different, genetically homogeneous populations were created by classical methods of inbreeding, without need for biochemical genetic intervention.

Even though the flies in each jar were genetically identical, they did not all die at the same time. For each jar, enough flies died each day to establish a daily death rate and the scientists tracked the way that rate changed over time for each jar.

By comparing the way the death rates varied from one jar to another, the team was able to establish the natural genetic variance in death rate. Then by tracking that variance over time, they were able to chart the way the variance in death rate depends on age. It was all quite subtle and complex. The idea of "genetic variance in death rate" does not sound so complicated, but measuring it in practice required a good deal of ingenuity and a labor-intensive experiment.

Williams and Antagonistic Pleiotropy

In Medawar's monograph, he refers briefly to the possibility that the weakness of natural selection at late ages might not be enough to explain aging, that it might need a little help. The Mutation Accumulation theory argues that there is no selection *against* aging, but Medawar anticipated that there might actually be selection *in favor* of aging, if a cost later in life might be plausibly linked to a benefit early in life. This is the idea of a *tradeoff*, which is a staple in evolutionary theories of aging. For example, sex hormones lead to higher fertility, but the same hormones are steroids that might damage the body over time. In Medawar's words, "a heightened juvenile rate of reproduction, achieved perhaps at the expense of recurrent stress that leads later to deterioration" [2, p 20].

In 1957, George Williams [9] took this detail from Medawar's paper and ran with it. He intuited what we have described above—that even though few animals in nature actually keel over and die of old age, nevertheless early stages of senescence take a substantial toll in the wild.

The name of the theory was introduced by Michael Rose, an experimental geneticist at Irvine who actually did most to disprove Williams's theory, though he would never admit it. 'Pleiotropy' describes the situation where a single gene has two or more actions in an organism. There is a special word for this because, within the neo-Darwinian framework, it is a case requiring special treatment. Classical population genetics analyzes the effect of fitness from each gene and multiple, separate effects must be treated as an exception. However, in the real world, geneticists find pleiotropy wherever they look. Pleiotropy, indeed, seems to be the rule and it is tightly targeted genes that are the exception. (There is no word for 'one gene—one effect', but the situation is unusual enough that there should be.)

"Antagonistic pleiotropy" means that one gene carries both a benefit and a cost. Williams's insight was that if there were such genes, where the benefit comes early in life and the cost comes late, then this would handily explain aging. This idea forms the basis of the theory that has become the most popular and best-accepted theory of aging over fully half a century.

There was no understanding of how genes regulate developmental timing in 1957. (Even today, there is only sparse and rudimentary understanding of this issue.) So Williams thought abstractly in terms of genes whose action is focused on one segment of an organism's lifetime and genes that act at multiple times, perhaps in independent ways. It did not seem a shortfall of the theory that examples of such genes or of the ways in which they work were lacking. Rather, it was understood that selection would be maximizing individual fitness at every opportunity. According to well-established theory, all opportunities to maximize reproduction should be vigorously exploited in nature. It seemed natural enough that some of these would come at a cost. It was Williams's insight to realize that if the cost came late in life while the benefit accrued early, then the benefit would win out over the cost most of the time. This seemed a concise and appealing explanation for where aging comes from that fit handily into the conceptual framework of neo-Darwinism, which was Williams's own native element.

As a good scientist, Williams listed predictions of his theory—experimental tests that might be done. He was courageous enough to bet his theory on these predictions. Curiously, he did not predict explicitly that many genes would be identified which have the requisite property (conferring benefit early in life; exacting a cost later on). There was no such thing as DNA sequencing in 1957 and the prospect of cataloging genes must have seemed remote. It was natural enough in that era to think of genes as traits and Williams listed some mutant traits of laboratory-bred fruit flies that were known even then to lengthen lifespan. Why were these traits unknown in nature, though they were so easily found in the lab? There could be only one answer (within the neo-Darwinian framework) and that is that the wild-type trait carried some yet-undiscovered benefit.

He stated quite directly that the primary motive for his theory—and also the best arguments for its acceptance—were based on theory, rather than actual identification of pleiotropic genes. "[T]here seems to be little necessity for documenting the existence of the necessary genes. Pleiotropy in some form is universally recognized and no one has ever suggested that all the effects of a gene need be equally beneficial or harmful or that they must all be manifest at the same time."

Looking back at Williams's seminal paper from a distance of 50 years, I find it strange that he did not seek to ground the theory more in experiment. Why did he feel it unimportant to identify actual genes that were good candidates for pleiotropy, genes that had both a demonstrable benefit in youth and also had a clear association with some change that we commonly identify as aging? One hint concerning Williams's thinking is this: "Senescence should always be a generalized deterioration and never due largely to changes in a single system." Williams expected that the number of pleiotropic genes must be very large, since natural selection would seize every available opportunity to accelerate reproduction and there must be a large number of such opportunities, accompanied by a broad variety of late-life costs. He explicitly rejected Medawar's hypothesis, that just a few mechanisms would be discovered that underlay all the various phenomena we identify as aging. "Any such small number of primary physiological factors is a logical impossibility if the assumptions made in the present study are valid." So Williams did not propose to look for identifiable aging genes because he expected that they would be extraordinarily hard to spot, each one by itself having only an insignificant effect.

If he had written the paper a few decades later, Williams might have cited testosterone in human males as an example of a pleiotropic adaptation. Testosterone makes men stronger and sexually more aggressive. It also increases risk of prostate cancer and infectious diseases later in life. Testosterone is a steroid hormone, which means (among other things) that it dials down the body's immune response. As we age, the human immune system fails progressively, which makes us susceptible to diseases from pneumonia to cancer. So later in life, men do better with less testosterone; though early in life, testosterone plausibly leads to higher fecundity.

Through this and other means, castration substantially increases male life expectancy [25]. In Williams's theory, this is a measure of the pleiotropic sacrifice that is made in order to keep men fertile. It is a known fact that men with their gonads intact are more successful at passing their genes to the next generation than men who have been castrated.

Many examples of pleiotropy around lifespan can be found, but it does not seem to be an inevitable precondition that natural selection has been forced to work with. In other words, pleiotropy exists, but it does not have the significance that theory ascribes to it. There is evidence that aging is chosen not despite its fatal consequences for the individual, but because of them, and that pleiotropy is constructed for the purpose of helping overcome individual selection in order to keep aging in place. I mean to suggest that long-term natural selection wants to keep lifespan on a short leash and has used pleiotropy to prevail over short-term selection.

Testosterone may suppress the immune system, but it does so in the here and now. It does not work over time to produce permanent damage to the immune system. The decline of the immune system is due largely to gradual involution (shrinking) of the thymus gland [26], where the white blood cells are trained to recognized 'self' from 'other'. In fact, the immune system in young men is most effective at just the time in life when testosterone (and its concomitant sexual behaviors) are raging. And while it is true that high testosterone levels contribute to the progression of prostate cancer once the disease has initiated, testosterone can hardly be the root cause of prostate cancer, since cancer rates are minuscule just at the time in life when testosterone levels are highest. It was once thought that the deep cause of cancer was mutations in early life and that pre-cancerous cells gestate over a period of decades, which is why cancer appears so much more often in old age. But a more modern perspective is that mutations turn dividing cells into potential cancers all the time, while the immune system recognizes such cells and efficiently does away with them. The prime reason that cancer appears so much more often in old age is that the immune system is so much less capable of recognizing and eliminating the mutants in older people. Remember mice! Their cells grow no faster than ours do, but their cancers have no trouble progressing from the early stages to full-blown metastatic disease in a matter of months.

More deeply, neither Williams nor Medawar had available our modern perspective on gene regulation: that expression of genes is controlled by signaling networks of exquisite complexity; that the time and place of gene expression is adapted under the control of natural selection, just as the forms of the genes themselves are selected. Both imagined false constraints on evolution—ways in which evolution was stuck with fundamentally limited genetic machinery. Medawar imagined that each gene came with a time stamp that determined when in life it would be turned on. (Those genes that had late time stamps were defectively evolved because so many animals died before those genes could turn on and subject themselves to selection.) Williams imagined that genes were either always on or always off. (Thus, a gene that offered benefits early in life could not be turned off if it caused harm to its bearer late in life.)

Medawar and Williams were forced to speculate in the absence of our modern knowledge of genetics. Medawar was just before and Williams just after Watson, Crick and Franklin. We cannot fault them for failing to imagine the universe of promotional factors and regulatory networks, embedded so deeply in the chemistry of metabolism [27]. Unavailable to them was the knowledge that some of the genes for aging are actually turned on only late in life, so that their only effect is destructive [28]. We should lose no respect for the incisiveness of their thought, but we do need to re-evaluate the viability of their theories in light of all we know today.

Confirmation Bias

It has become commonplace for experimental geneticists to report instances of tradeoffs in the language of antagonistic pleiotropy, as if they corroborated the theory. It is incontestable that tradeoffs exist. But the theory says more than that tradeoffs exist—the theory proposes that there are no evolutionary pathways that escape the tradeoffs, and further, that these tradeoffs are the cause of the symptoms we observe as aging. There is a great deal of evidence for the existence of tradeoffs. There is little evidence for a connection between tradeoffs and the phenotypes of aging, and no evidence that the tradeoffs are unavoidable.

A confirmation bias is apparent in reportage of genetic tradeoffs. Positive findings are announced with fanfare in high-profile media, but when it seems that natural selection has shunned an opportunity to maximize individual fitness, the result is never reported as evidence against the theory, but rather as a puzzle to be resolved. When a wild-type gene is discovered that seems to offer no benefit in exchange for reduced lifespan, authors express confidence that the benefit exists, though it has yet to be discovered. Three examples:

- Working with *C. elegans* in 1988, Tom Johnson reported the first instance of a single gene that significantly extended the worm's lifespan when disabled, an aging gene which he dubbed AGE-1. He reported [29] the result together with the explanation that worms missing both copies of the AGE-1 gene laid only one fourth as many eggs over a lifetime. Johnson's discovery is still described in this way today. But a few years later, he discovered a second gene, FER-15, that had inadvertently been lost along with AGE-1. Worms with the FER-15 mutation had impaired fertility, but no extended lifespan. Worms with the AGE-1 mutation had extended lifespans with unimpaired fertility [30]. (Homozygous (-/-) AGE-1 double mutants develop slowly and have lifespans extended tenfold compared to wild type [31].)

- In 1984, Michael Rose reported first results from his long-term experiments breeding *Drosophila* for longevity. As he had anticipated, the flies with longer lifespans laid fewer eggs when young. He wrote, "The scientific significance of these conclusions is that senescence in this population of *Drosophila melanogaster* appears to be due to antagonistic pleiotropy, such that genes which postpone senescence appear to depress early fitness components. Put another way, these results corroborate the hypothesis of a cost to reproduction (Williams 1957, 1966), since prolonged life seems to require reduced early reproductive output." [32]. When continued breeding produced flies that had longer lifespans without depressed fertility, he invoked a theoretical explanation that did not imply conflict with the theory [33].

- Many studies have sought an association between female fertility and longevity in human populations. Theories of aging based on metabolic tradeoffs predict a negative correlation, while historic surveys have usually found a slight positive correlation (reviewed by [34, 35], with more recent findings by [36, 37]) But when Tom Kirkwood purported to have discovered a population and a statistical test that confirmed the predicted negative correlation, the result was headlined in Nature [38]. Kirkwood's positive result continues to be cited more frequently than the negative results, despite questions raised about the methodology [39-41] (details below, p 87).

Predictions of Antagonistic Pleiotropy

When George Williams suggested in 1957 that aging was a side-effect of fertility genes, it was a brilliant but abstract hypothesis, ahead of its time experimentally. The theory came from pure thought, but Williams made specific predictions from his theory. Of course, some of those "predictions" were actually gross observations about the phenomenology of aging, things that had been known to be true for a long time. For example, he "predicted" that animals that take longer to develop and mature should have longer lifespans. (This is true in general, but there are exceptions: remember the locust that spends 17 years maturing underground before living out its adult life in a few weeks.)

Williams also stuck his neck out to make some real predictions, some of which could not be tested for decades afterward:

1. Aging should be universal in higher organisms, absent in one-celled creatures and cloners.
2. Low adult accidental death rates should be associated with long lifespans.
3. Animals in which adults increase in fecundity should age more slowly.
4. Where there are sex differences in death rates, higher mortality in one sex should be associated with shorter lifespan.
5. When an animal's systems fail with age, everything should fail at once; no single gene or even a single system should be able to prolong lifespan.
6. After reproduction ends, there is no evolutionary pressure to keep an animal alive and so we expect that animals in nature should die promptly after they are no longer fertile.
7. The first signs of aging should appear at the time of sexual maturity.
8. In lab experiments, artificial selection for increased longevity should result in decreased vigor and curtailed fertility in youth.

And how have these predictions been borne out over the years? By and large, they have been an embarrassment, creating opportunities for industrious theorists to extend or modify the original theory time and time again. The first seven are summarized in the box on the following page; the eighth is the subject of the most direct experimental tests for the theory of Antagonistic Pleiotropy and the subject of the remainder of this section.

Seven Predictions of George Williams (1957) and how they Fared

1. Aging should be universal in higher organisms, absent in one-celled creatures and cloners.

   ✗ We know from Chapter 2 that there are some animals and many plants that do not age. Williams probably thought it was a safe bet, based on what was known in 1957, that single-celled organisms do not age. But we learned in Chapter 3 that there are two modes of aging in single-celled organisms that cannot be explained by Pleiotropy theory. Even bacteria have found a way to incorporate aging into their life cycle (also Chapter 3). None of this can be explained by Williams's theory or by the other standard and accepted theories of aging. Are we to think that aging in microorganisms evolved on a completely different basis and for a different reason than aging in multi-celled life?

2. Low adult accidental death rates should be associated with long lifespans.

? There have been some experiments that confirm this expectation and others that confound it. When opossums were transported to an island where there were no predators, they evolved longer lifespans [42]. But in Trinidad river pools where guppies are preyed upon by bigger fish, the animals actually evolve longer lifespans than nearby pools where there are no predators [43].

3. Animals in which adults increase in fecundity should age more slowly.

✓ This prediction has been borne out. But unanticipated by Williams, some animals continue to grow more fertile over their whole lives and they 'age in reverse', in the sense that their mortality rate declines from one year to the next.

4. Sex differences: higher mortality in one sex should be associated with shorter lifespan.

? This prediction has yet to be tested systematically.

5. When an animal's systems fail with age, everything should fail at once; no single gene or even a single system should be able to prolong lifespan.

✗ One of the great surprises in the field of aging genetics has been how easy it is to find single genes that can be modified to extend lifespan. Williams conceived of pleiotropy as thousands of tiny bargains in which the integrity of one bodily system after another was traded away for a little increment in fertility. Contrary to the expectations of Williams and everyone else, aging seems to be controlled in the main by a handful of genes with large effect.

6. After reproduction ends, there is no evolutionary pressure to keep an animal alive and so we expect that animals in nature should die promptly after they are no longer fetile.

✗ We are all aware of the counterexample of menopause in human females. Anthropologists like to explain this in terms of older women's devotion to the upbringing of their grandchildren. But surprise! Life after the end of reproduction turns out to be ubiquitous in the biosphere—in animals like worms and even yeast cells that do not care a whit about their grandchildren. Whales, otters, opossums, elephants, guppies, quail, parakeets, and mice have all been reported to live on after they lose their fertility [44].

7. The first signs of aging appear at the time of sexual maturity.

? It is rare for animals to show signs of aging before sexual maturity, but many begin to age only well after they have begun to reproduce.

8. See below Section (Williams's Prediction #8).

Williams's Prediction #8

8. In lab experiments, artificial selection for increased longevity should result in decreased vigor and curtailed fertility in youth.

There have been two lines of direct experimental tests for pleiotropy. Fruit flies have been the experimental animal of choice for both. First, breeding experiments have been done to see if fertility and longevity are related. The expectation was that when flies are bred for longevity, they would lose fertility in the process. Second, natural variation was used as a probe. Do the individual flies that live longest tend to lay more eggs or fewer?

Looking for Pleiotropy in Laboratory Breeding Experiments

In the first category, the marathon experiment has been carried out by Michael Rose's lab at the University of California, Irvine [32]. In the 1970s, Rose was a star student of a great British theorist of mathematical evolution, Brian Charlesworth. Rose, too, is a mathematical theorist at heart; but he also realized that what the field needed was an experimental basis for the heady science. So he set about in 1981 to create just the experiment described by Williams that would validate the central premise of the theory of pleiotropy.

As a young professor in Halifax, BC (and later Irvine, CA), Rose began breeding fruit flies for longevity. His method involved no genetic engineering but a straightforward application of the way that plants and domestic animals have been bred for hundreds of years. Beginning with a genetically diverse population, he maintained his flies in jars until 90% of them had died, then collected eggs from the remaining flies. The next generation of flies would live a little longer and he repeated the same procedure with them, as longevity progressed with each generation.

This simple experiment required no knowledge of the detailed genetics of aging. In order for the experiment to work, all that is required is that there must be some genes that affect lifespan and there must be some variation among the flies in the distribution of these genes. Internally, what must be happening is that various genes for longevity become more and more concentrated in each successive generation.

When Rose began his experiment, each generation of flies lived for four weeks. But the lifespan continued to advance, doubling to eight weeks by the time he collected his papers in a volume about *Methuselah Flies* [45] in 2004. As I write in 2015, his experiment continues, but with flies that live more than twelve weeks.

The fact that it was possible to breed very long-lived flies is perhaps a surprising result. There were certainly no flies that lived anywhere close to twelve weeks in the population that Rose began with in 1981. We imagine that what is happening is that many kinds of longevity genes were spread through the population, so that some flies had longevity gene A and some had longevity gene Z, but none had a full complement of all the longevity genes. Breeding is a (slow and laborious) way to combine these genes and gather them together in a single individual. It is this process that led to longer-lived flies than any in the initial population.

The big question in Rose's experiment—the subject of his work and the reason that he embarked on the experiment: can he detect pleiotropy? Rose fully expected that over the years, as his inbred flies lived longer and longer, they would grow less and less able to reproduce. He even imagined that ultimately, the limit on the experiment would be reached when he was able to breed flies that had super-long lifespans, but that laid no eggs at all from which he could breed a next generation.

Two years into the experiment, there was a dip in fertility and Rose rushed to publish a paper in which he announced that the signature of pleiotropy had been detected. But soon the results began to turn around. After two more years, the result was undeniable: the long-lived flies were laying more eggs than the control flies (that continued to live for only four weeks). The theory of antagonistic pleiotropy says that the genes for longevity were the same genes that depressed fertility—that is why natural selection over the æons had failed to do the job that Rose's lab had done in a few years. But the experimental result seemed paradoxical: these same genes that increased longevity were also enhancing fertility. How could that be? Where was the pleiotropy? Or, more to the point, why was it that natural evolution had failed to find these same super-fly combinations that Rose was able to breed artificially in such a comparatively short time?

Rose the theorist stepped forward with proposed answers to these questions. But he has not faced to this day the fact that the central prediction of George Williams has failed spectacularly, or to hold the theory accountable for its failure. The explanation that Rose poses for this result is that while he was breeding for longevity, he was also, incidentally and unintentionally, breeding for fertility as well. There may have been many infertile flies in that last remaining 10% of each generation. But these flies did not contribute eggs to the next generation; it was only the flies that were both fertile and long-lived that were selected by his procedure.

This is an unsatisfying answer, however, because it does not address the question how there can be such flies, that are both more fertile and longer-lived, or why it is that nature's own evolutionary process has not identified them. It does not address the fact that not only do Rose's superflies lay more eggs in old age; they are more fertile in their youth than the flies in the control bottles that live only four weeks. In the lab, the "fitness" of the flies was increased in just a few years far beyond what nature had been able to achieve in many millions of years. This suggests that nature was not really trying to increase the lifetime reproductive output of the flies—that our standard definition of "fitness" is missing something.

Perhaps this genotypic plasticity of aging is less surprising when we remember Kenyon's one-line proof that aging is programmed [personal communication, 2002]: The range of time scales for senescence across the biosphere extends from hours to thousands of years. No physical process of deterioration could act with such a variable rate, spanning six orders of magnitude; therefore the rate of aging must result from a biological program under evolutionary control.

Looking for Pleiotropy Using Variation in Wild Populations

In the second category, there have been many scientists who look for a relationship between fertility and longevity in animal populations. Instead of taking many generations to breed animals for large differences in longevity, they examine the natural variation within populations. Some animals live longer than others; some animals are more fertile than others. The Pleiotropy theory predicts that these two traits should be inversely related. The animals that live longer should tend to leave fewer offspring and the animals that leave the most offspring should tend to have shorter lifespans. When statistics are compared, this effect would appear as a negative correlation between lifespan and fertility.

The best design was by the same four scientists at the University of Minnesota mentioned above and the work was performed in the context of their study of the genetic variance of aging. Their experiment, described above, had 100 bottles of fruit flies, where the flies within each bottle were all genetically identical to each other. They tracked both fertility and death rates day by day, so the results were complicated. Their main finding was that there was more positive than negative correlation between longevity and fertility—the opposite of the theoretical prediction.

Here is a little irony of the field that you are now in a position to appreciate. You know that there are two 'standard' theories for the evolutionary origin of aging: Mutation Accumulation and Antagonistic Pleiotropy. The Minnesota Four tested both of these when they studied the variation among their 100 jars of fruit flies. One paper focused on genetic diversity, to test the Mutation Accumulation theory. It was written up with Daniel Promislow as the first author [23] and he concluded that the results were inconsistent with Mutation Accumulation, so this should be interpreted as a suggestion that Antagonistic Pleiotropy was probably the right theory. The second paper focused on correlations between fertility and longevity, to test for Antagonistic Pleiotropy. It was written up with Marc Tatar as the first author [24] and he concluded that the results were inconsistent with pleiotropy, so Mutation Accumulation was probably the right theory.

The Minnesota Four working with flies was the only group to take the time and expense to create hundreds of clones for each of the different genetic varieties they studied. But dozens of other experimenters have done the easier thing and studied existing genetic variation in natural populations where each individual is unique. The only drawback of this approach is that it does not separate the random environmental effects affecting each individual from the genetic effects unique to it; so all correlations would tend to be diluted. Still, we might expect that a correlation so strong that it is responsible for all of aging should easily be detected. But overall, there is no pattern. Some of these studies claim to see a positive correlation, some a negative correlation, and some see no correlation at all [46 p 204].

Pleiotropy Exists, but is not the Cause of Aging

Overall, theorists who summarize the data always tend to take a forgiving view and report that Pleiotropy theory has been partially confirmed and we do not yet understand the exceptions. I disagree. I think that if Antagonistic Pleiotropy were really the deep cause of aging in the biosphere, then these correlations would be the very source of aging. The correlations would have to be very large and very consistent. They would jump from the page in any experimental report. The fact that results are so inconsistent and often go in the wrong direction tells us that pleiotropy is real and it sometimes has an effect, but it cannot be the deep cause of aging. An honest report would be that pleiotropy sometimes modifies the rate of aging.

Allocating the Energy Budget to Maximize Fitness: The Disposable Soma Theory

The Disposable Soma theory posits that the energy cost of maintaining the body has to compete with other energy demands in the body. If this were true, then supplying the body with more food energy would cause it to live longer, when in fact experiments in Caloric Restriction dramatically demonstrate the opposite. DS theory also predicts that males should live longer than females (because they invest less energy in reproduction) and that females that do not reproduce should live longer than females that do reproduce. Demography of humans and animals fails to confirm these predictions. Why are there so many smart scientists who still believe in the Disposable Soma?

Caloric Restriction in the Context of the Disposable Soma Theory

The DS theory says that the root cause of aging is that an animal always lives in a tight energy economy. There is never enough food energy to do a perfect job of keeping the body in repair because the need to reproduce is competing for that same food energy. In the abstract, this thesis sounds more than reasonable. It is sensible and logically compelling. But in the context of the Caloric Restriction effect, it would seem to be ruled out. On its face, the DS theory is wildly out of line with the fact that animals have shorter lifespans the more they eat. Common sense tells us that if there is a compromise among competing demands on the body's energy, then an increased energy supply overall should lead to each of those allotments receiving more energy. So if energy is used for reproduction, for metabolism, and for repair, then more total energy should mean more energy for each of these uses. More food means more energy means more lifespan.

Tom Kirkwood proposed the DS theory as a young man in 1977 [47], at a time when he was not yet aware of the CR effect. Over the ensuing decades, Caloric Restriction came to be regarded as the most reliable and consistent way to extend animal lifespans. Kirkwood did not retreat from his theory, but in 1999, together with his student Daryl Shanley, he published a computational model [48], that attempts to reconcile DS theory with the CR phenomenon for the case of lactating female mice. The gist of the model is that in the CR state, females do not reproduce and do not lactate. But if they are fed just enough to support a pregnancy, then the energy they spend on reproduction is actually more than the food energy increment that restored their fertility. Shanley and Kirkwood demonstrate that in this limited range when fertility depends on food intake, the net effect of food intake is a drain on energy.

In the Kirkwood/Shanley model, when the mouse has access to increased energy, she is programmed to put *all* of that energy increase into reproduction and then to dip into the allocation for repair, to steal even more energy and devote that to reproduction, too. Reproduction is linked to an on/off switch. When there is insufficient food energy for reproduction, then all available energy goes into repair; as soon as reproduction becomes possible, then the allocation for repair and maintenance is raided, so that lifespan is most curtailed when energy for repair is most abundant. Conversely, just when the total energy supply is lowest, the body shunts all available energy into repair and that turns out to be much more energy than was possible when food energy was plentiful.

This thesis was published prominently and is cited uncritically even today, because it is the only way to "save" the Disposable Soma theory. But there are many things wrong with the idea. First, the model was worked out in quantitative detail for lactating female mice, because they use an enormous amount of energy in nourishing their young. In Kirkwood's theory, the energy from all that milk becomes available for keeping the body in good repair if reproduction is turned off. But the numbers do not work for most other animals—including male mice. Male mice devote much less energy to reproduction than female mice and their fertility suffers only marginally when they are put on caloric restriction; yet on caloric restriction, they live as long as females. Where are these male mice getting the energy dividend to allocate to repair? Even for female mice, Kirkwood's numbers only work out if they are reproducing and lactating, but the CR experiments are always done with mice that are caged separately, so they do not get a chance to mate or reproduce. Kirkwood's theory compares mice that eat more and reproduce to mice that eat less and do not reproduce. But experiments in caloric restriction are always done comparing mice that do not reproduce with other mice that do not reproduce. Only the quantity of food is different. So according to Kirkwood's DS theory, the animals that are fed more should be expected to live much longer—opposite to what is observed.

There is another essential problem with the Kirkwood model: If we accept the idea of the on/off switch, then the longest lifespans should be for animals that are fed *almost* enough to support reproduction. We should expect lifespan to *decrease* gradually as food is restricted, until a point is reached where the decision is made to shut down reproduction; then there should be a sharp increase in lifespan. If food is restricted further, then the decrease in lifespan ought to resume its downward trend. But the fact is that lifespan increases smoothly over a wide range of calorie restriction: the less the animal is fed, the longer it lives (see graph p 1). In mild caloric restriction, the mouse is still reproducing and yet it manages to live longer. In the most extreme caloric restriction, food intake is far below the threshold for reproduction. On the lean side of that threshold, calories can be restricted more and more and still the animal lives longer and longer, even as fertility holds steady at zero (so there is no reservoir of reproductive energy to be raided for repair).

This is a straightforward case where our common sense agrees with the rigorous scientific analysis. Life extension from CR is the best-studied and most robust experimental manipulation of aging and the results are utterly incompatible with Kirkwood's Disposable Soma theory.

Details on Reproduction and Lifespan

Theory says that there should be a powerful inverse relationship between reproduction and lifespan. Both the DS and AP theories make this prediction, though their reasons are subtly different. Both are based on compromises involving longevity and fertility. In the AP theory, fecundity (potential reproduction*) is controlled by genes that have a pleiotropic effect on aging and natural selection has created genomes that promote fecundity at the expense of longevity. In the DS theory, fertility (actual reproduction) requires energy (calories) that is subtracted from the energy available

---

* Demographers refer to the capacity to reproduce as fecundity and the rate at which women actually reproduce as fertility. Biologists frequently use the opposite convention, saying that fertility is the capacity and fecundity is the realization. Here I use the demographers' convention.

for repair and maintenance of the soma. Hence the DS theory implies a cost of reproduction, both in humans and animals, males and females. The DS theory but not the AP theory predicts that an individual's life should be curtailed by the process of producing offspring; the more offspring, the shorter the life expectancy.

Caleb Finch summarizes the evidence for a cost of reproduction in his encyclopedic *Longevity, Senescence and the Genome* [49] thus: There is a great deal of evidence that animals die *in the act* of reproducing (as many women used to die in childbirth, right through the 19th century). But there is no evidence that those who survive have foreshortened lifespans. Finch interprets this to mean that reproduction entails an immediate mortality risk that bears no relationship to aging. The most comprehensive recent study on the subject looked at zoo animals, living in a protected environment and with well-documented ages and fertilities. Ricklefs et al. [50] looked at 18 species of mammals and 12 birds and found marginal evidence for a positive relationship between parity and lifespan (i.e., the opposite sign to the correlation predicted by DS theory).

Reproduction and Lifespan—What about People?

Complementing animal studies are historic and actuarial studies of humans. The disadvantage of working with humans is that controlled experiments are excluded. Compensating for this is the fact that there are copious hospital records on the health of huge numbers of humans and the power of statistical methodology can extract from these evidence about correlation and possibly, causation. Epidemiologists routinely extract public health implications from such data; theories of evolution may similarly be tested. There are also historical studies, based on databases of births and deaths over the centuries.

In humans, it is frequently claimed that eunuchs live about 10% longer, based on folk evidence and stories handed down from the royal courts of old [51], though this has been disputed [25]. In the twentieth century, there is only one study [52], based on institutionalized men from the American age of eugenics, when the mentally retarded and others with birth defects were commonly neutered, for the good of the gene pool. The study found that men in institutions who were castrated died at older ages compared to similar men who were not. The difference was primarily in middle-aged deaths from infectious disease; a large proportion of the institutionalized men died in this way and those who had been castrated escaped that fate. There was no evidence that rates of cancer or heart disease—the primary diseases of old age—were lowered by castration.

There is no evidence that women who have hysterectomies live longer than women who do not. And fertility in women is mostly found to be positively correlated with longevity. Women who have children live *longer*, especially if they give birth later in life [53, 54]. (Studies are confounded by the effect of wealth, which is associated with both longer lifespan and lower fertility in modern times [37].) Multiple studies of historic databases have looked for correlations between women's parity and longevity, going back more than a century to the well-known statistician Karl Pearson [55]. They have found either a positive association or none.

In a large-scale contemporary study of Norwegians, Grundy and Kravdal [37] found a positive correlation between fertility and longevity. Perls [53] found a strong positive relationship with late childbearing in a study of Boston centenarians. Korpelainen [56] examined historic data from rural Finns and European aristocrats in the eighteenth and nineteenth centuries. She found positive correlations between number of offspring and lifespan in both men and women, with the (expected) negative effect only for a small sample of women over 80. Lycett [57] studied a North German historical population in the same time frame and found, again, a "reverse cost" of reproduction, particularly strong among the lower socioeconomic classes. LeBourg [58] and also Muller [54] studied French Canadian populations in this same time frame and found no evidence for a cost of reproduction (these studies and other demographic data are reviewed by LeBourg [34].) McArdle et al. [36] studied an Amish population from the eighteenth through the twentieth centuries and found a positive relationship between fertility and longevity. After removing the inverse correlation associated with long-term demographic trends, a positive correlation for men remained and the correlation for women was insignificant.

The one large-scale human study which claims to discern a negative correlation was conducted by Kirkwood himself, together with the demographer J.G. Westendorp [38]. Kirkwood's study was published prominently in *Nature*, and because it produced the theoretically expected result, more scientists continue to cite its positive results than all the other negative studies combined. The abstract at the head of the article is the only part that most scientists take time to read and the abstract emphasizes the negative relationship between fertility and longevity, but the data in the article are sliced and diced in many ways and there is only one tranche that supports this conclusion, using an obscure and inappropriate statistical test. I personally re-analyzed the data from this study and found that when the common and appropriate statistical test is used, it supports the opposite inference: that bearing children is positively associated with a woman's longevity [41], consistent with every other modern study. Specifically: instead of a standard linear regression model, Westendorp and Kirkwood chose a Poisson regression to correlate a woman's age at death with her parity. This model is only valid if the number of children per mother is Poisson distributed. In fact, the number of children in their database is far from being Poisson distributed and this leads to extreme distortion in the model's sensitivity. "This makes the result overly sensitive to a handful of women with 15 children or more who lived before 1700. When these five women are removed from a database of more than 2,900, the Poisson regression no longer shows a significant result. Bilinear regression relating lifespan to fertility and date of birth results in a small positive coefficient for fertility, in agreement with the main trend of results" reported in the past and since [41].

There is intriguing evidence in animals that the sexual organs actually extend lifespan. Unfertilized eggs have an evolutionary interest that is not identical to the mother in which they live and perhaps they try to influence their mother's metabolism in a direction that will give opportunity for an evolutionary legacy of their own. When ovaries from a young mouse are transplanted into an older female, the lifespan of the older mouse is extended [59-61].

In experiments from Kenyon's UCSF lab, two effects on a worm's longevity were segregated: the effect of sex organs and the effect of its storehouse of eggs. The worms' eggs or ovaries were separately destroyed by laser micro-surgery, so that worms could be compared with ovaries, eggs, both, or neither. Kenyon concluded that the presence of the eggs *shortens* lifespan, while the gonads tend to *lengthen* lifespan. This is the opposite of what I might have thought, based on the argument above about the separate life interest of the eggs. Both effects are quite substantial, but they cancel each other out, so that in previous experiments that had removed the eggs with the gonads, no effect on lifespan was seen [62].

The separation between eggs and ovaries has not been done in mice, but it was performed in fruit flies by Linda Partridge's lab at University College of London. Her team found a different result for flies: no life extension was observed after the flies were modified genetically so as to have ovaries but no eggs [63].

For the purpose of this chapter, the take-home message from the Kenyon and Partridge experiments is that, while we find a relationship between reproduction and lifespan, the mechanism of action is through signaling, rather than physiology. Partridge emphasized this in her report: "Traditional explanations of this 'cost of reproduction' suggest that tradeoffs between reproduction and longevity should be obligate [but] it is possible to uncouple the two traits... Our results contrast with the widely held view that it is downstream reproductive processes such as the production and/or laying of eggs that are costly to females [63]." Fertility entails no *necessary* sacrifice, as is required by the pleiotropic theories. Rather, the gonads emit hormonal signals to which the body responds in many ways, one of which is to dial up the rate of aging.

These results confirm the existence of pleiotropy, but not in a consistent way, and not connected deeply to the symptoms of aging. We shall see this pattern again and again: pleiotropy is real, but it is not an explanation for the general phenomenon of aging. It is not an unavoidable cost of fertility, not an imposed limitation, but rather a choice that natural selection has made. I'll speculate on the reason for that choice in Chapter 7. Pleiotropy is actually an evolutionary strategy for maintaining senescence in defiance of short-term, individual selection.

The Most Eclectic Version of Pleiotropy is the Most Plausible

Might there be other scarce resources than energy that have forced evolution to forge compromises? Kirkwood proposed the theory in terms of caloric energy and continues to describe it in this way. Other prominent gerontologists have adopted the spirit of Kirkwood's theory, however, applying it to generalized scarce resources, without specifying what the limiting resource might be. The general concept that the body must make compromises seems appealing; the specifics of why that might be and how it might work remain elusive.

Austad has been the foremost advocate of a variant DS theory in which the compromise between fertility and longevity is compelled by another (unspecified) scarce resource, not food energy [64]. The theory in this form escapes the Caloric Restriction evidence that is so telling against the classical DS theory. The variant DS theory remains vulnerable to the body of data cited above on fertility and longevity. Until a scarce resource is specified, the variant form of the DS theory remains a tantalizing speculation, but it is impossible to adduce evidence either in support or against it.

Common sense tells us that it is more difficult to optimize two variables simultaneously, and that increase of one quite generally results in constraints that limit the other. But common sense may be misleading us here, as there are copious examples of adaptations that increase fitness now and also increase fitness later. For example, transgenic mice with the PEPCK-C gene are found to be hyperactive, with super-endurance and also greater longevity than wild type. Females have almost twice the active reproductive period, compared to wild type [65]. Reznick found that guppies evolved in a high-predation environment evolved, as expected, faster maturity and higher fertility; unexpectedly, they also lived longer. Where is the tradeoff? Why did the guppies in the low-predation environment not evolve these traits that give every indication of offering a free lunch [43, 66]? Daphnia have also been observed to evolve faster maturity and higher fertility in response to predation, paying no apparent cost for the substantial boost in their fitness (as fitness is classically measured) [67, 68]. Examples like these are not rare [69] and they cast a shadow over *all* theories of aging that depend on a presumption of inescapable tradeoffs.

The existence of super-fit fleas and guppies seems puzzling. Why did they fail to take over the populations in low-predation environments? Reports from Reznick's experiments include a hint of an answer. He reports that he twice introduced super-guppies into the low-predation environments just a few hundred meters away and each time their numbers swelled, leading to the outbreak of a "yet unidentified infection" of a kind unknown in all his previous work [66]. This suggests that the guppies' fertility and longevity were tempered by natural selection to avoid crowding—a hypothesis that is anathema to the orthodox neo-Darwinian paradigm.

Other Tradeoff Theories—Variations on a Theme

Within the neo-Darwinian framework, only individual fitness is recognized and since aging *per se* reduces individual fitness, theorists have invoked constraints, operating outside evolution, that tie aging to other, pro-fitness traits. These constraints are always postulated to exist without direct evidence, and indeed direct evidence for constraints is very difficult to garner. (It is possible, however, to adduce evidence against a given constraint by citing instances in which the constraint is breached. Within the present neo-Darwinian culture, this is often taken as though it were evidence in favor of a different constraint.) Another necessary assumption, never justified, is that "the game is worth the candle" in the sense that whatever sacrifice the metabolism makes in exchange for aging is offering a greater benefit than the fitness cost of aging. In the early days of the tradeoff theories, 1957-1991, it was generally assumed that the cost of aging was small and that even a modest benefit could offset the lost fitness from aging. But, as we discussed above (p 70ff), the fitness lost to senescence is generally substantial (20-30% deaths attributable to senescence) and in some cases can be much higher. Thus there is another quantitative burden of proof that these theories have never been asked to satisfy, because they were the only game in town, consistent with neo-Darwinian population genetics.

There are two primary tradeoff theories described in this chapter. Classical AP is based on tradeoffs at the genetic level, operating in evolutionary time. DS theory is based on tradeoffs at the metabolic level, operating within a single lifetime. In additional to these, there are several minor tradeoff theories and variants, championed by one or another theorist.

Blagosklonny [70, 71] has argued for a kind of epigenetic inertia. "Aging and growth may be linked in such a way that growth produces aging." Even though growth comes to an end early in life, the proteins that promoted growth hang around and continue to pose a danger throughout life. The body just does not seem to be able to shut them down. Blagosklonny takes TOR as the canonical example. TOR (target of rapamycin) is a gene that is important for growth, but blocking the gene's action (with rapamycin, for example) is observed to slow aging [72-74] "[L]ife-promoting TOR signaling seems also to contain seeds of death. Aging and its manifestations such as age-related diseases appear with excessive growth-promoting signaling, when actual growth is no longer possible. Aging is not programmed, of course, but is an aimless continuation of the same process that drives developmental growth."

"Of course" lifespan cannot be programmed, as a matter of theory, hence there must be some glitch in the developmental program that keeps TOR turned on long after it has lost its usefulness.

Walker [75] makes a similar case and is more explicit both about the term "developmental inertia" and about the fact that such theories can only work if the selection against aging in nature is negligible, because in nature, "aging rarely occurs, if ever."

> Aging is the result of a design flaw in the developmental program that allows uncoordinated expression of genes, causing developmental inertia at a time when stability, not change, is essential for biological immortality.
>
> …
>
> Ultimately, continuation of part of the developmental program that forces persistent change undercuts the body's ability to sustain the optimal function needed to maintain health and vitality. Indeed, it is the continued transformation of our bodies, which was beneficial during development, that becomes detrimental after young adulthood. The reason for this dichotomy is two-fold. First, after completing the transformation from fertilized egg to young adult, there is nothing of the boy left to change. The body is complete in its mature form. Second, because the developmental program is finished, gene-directed instructions for further change are not available, such that any further change is nonprogrammed.
>
> …
>
> Because physical maturation occurs after reproductive capability is reached, there is no evolutionary mechanism to stop expression of the genes causing developmental inertia...the failure to stop developmental inertia upon completion of the developmental program is irrelevant to all other [non-human] species in which aging rarely occurs, if ever.

Long before there was understanding of epigenetics, G.P. Bidder [76] proposed that aging is triggered by the cessation of growth. "[S]enescence is the result of the specific action of the regulator after growth has stopped." Of the nature of the "regulator" or the reason it has not evolved to shut off, Bidder is silent. Brown [77] cites Bidder with approval. Brown's own theory invokes sexual selection on mate choice that favors individuals who conserve resources for the next generation. The hypothesis is intriguing, but crucial details are left nebulous. "Predation, competition among individuals of a species and other conditions, drive the individual to select for altruistic traits in their mates because such traits favor the fitness of their mutual descendants. The flexibility of the processes of Mate-Selection that derives from the effects of diploidy enables and drives the selection of altruistic traits while exacting little cost to the fitness of the selecting individual."

Holliday [78] takes a position akin to Austad, that unnamed "metabolic resources" are diverted from repair and maintenance to reproduction in a way that makes gradual aging not just expected but inevitable. He accepts Hamilton's [79] proof at face value and invokes explicitly the requirement that the fitness cost of aging be small: "On the basis of very simple and reasonable assumptions, it can be shown that the ability of complex organisms to survive indefinitely would necessarily decrease fitness." (It is interesting to note that Holliday is well-informed enough, even in 1995, to make an exceptions for "simple animals...that reproduce vegetatively.")

Atul Gawande is not an evolutionary biologist, but an MD, researcher and popular author. Even more than most other authors, he tends to focus narrowly on humans, and he seems unaware of the evidence confirming the high fitness cost of aging in the wild. "[F]or most of our hundred-thousand-year existence—all but the past couple of hundred years—the average lifespan of human beings has been thirty years or less...So when we study aging what we are trying to understand is not so much a natural process as an unnatural one [80]." Like many scientists with a broad knowledge of the physiological results of aging, but without a background either in physics or in evolution, Gawande is inclined to see aging in terms of accumulated damage and does not find it curious that such damage is *actively permitted* to accrue. In the same article, Gawande cites approvingly the Reliability Theory of Aging, as articulated by Leonid Gavrilov and Natalia Gavrilova [81].

The Gavrilovs describe aging from an engineering perspective, rather than an evolutionary perspective. The theory for which they are best known is a quantitative realization of Williams's [9] hypothesis that many systems of the body ought to fail simultaneously at the end of a lifespan. "Senescence should always be a generalized deterioration and never due largely to changes in a single system." Based on general principles of engineering and optimization, and the assumption that evolution has "designed" the body to last as long as possible subject to (unspecified) constraints and tradeoffs, they deduce that if any one system were so durable that it never wore out in a lifetime, then (unnamed) resources could profitably be diverted away from that system and invested more profitably in making the weakest link more durable. With mathematical modeling, they are able to show quite generally that if the number of independent systems is large, then the survival curve deduced from the Reliability Theory has a Gompertz [82] shape, qualitatively similar to many observed for iteroparous animals in the wild.

Among the problems with this approach to aging, we might list the following:

- Living beings differ from machines in that they have an inherent capacity for repair and regeneration. The Gavrilovs' theory does not address the primary mystery, as articulated by Williams [9]: "It is indeed remarkable that after a seemingly miraculous feat of morphogenesis a complex metazoan should be unable to perform the much simpler task of merely maintaining what is already formed."
- In common with other theories, the Reliability Theory assumes tradeoffs without specifying their nature or source, let alone attempting a quantitative accounting to demonstrate that natural selection has indeed obtained maximum fitness values by her choices.
- The sudden onset and rapid progression of senescence predicted by the theory is but one of many patterns of mortality observed in nature [49, 83], not necessarily typical. The discovery of single genes that have major effects on lifespan falsifies Williams's original prediction that aging must be essentially multi-factorial and suggests a different reason why many systems fail at once, to wit, that the failure of all these systems is coordinated in time by a single signal.

I have always found it curious that Leonard Hayflick has so firmly denied the possibility of programmed aging. Hayflick is not only a very independent scientific mind, but he also was the discoverer of cellular senescence (Chapter 5), which is arguably the clearest example of programmed aging in nature. Hayflick [84] is appropriately modest and tentative about his own theory of aging, but he repeats the discredited assumption that "Wild animals, because they rarely live long enough, do not experience aging." On this basis, he handily dismisses the need for an evolutionary account of aging.

Nick Lane has written perceptively and with a wide biological perception about many aspects of the history, and especially the origin, of life, yet he falls prey to the same fallacy about thermodynamics that fools so many biologists. "Certainly, the intractable laws of physics forbid eternal youth as firmly as perpetual motion [85]." Lane is well-informed on the topic of aging and notes, "It is a curious thing that mutations in all the life-extending genes, called *gerontogenes*, act to prolong rather than shorten lifespan. The default position [wild-type] is always shorter lifespan." He cites the specific example of a SNP mutation in human mitochondrial DNA that doubles the probability for a 100-year lifespan and greatly reduces the incidence of all diseases of old age [86, 87]. Yet Lane resists the implication that aging might be programmed, on the theoretical ground that it would be too easy for "cheating" to evolve. If gerontogenes did not have a net benefit in individual fitness, then they would long ago have been selected out of existence. Lane does not mention that pleiotropic costs have been identified for only a minority of gerontogenes [46, 88, 89].

Summary

Biology was the domain for observers of nature right through the nineteenth century and Darwin's theory of evolution was descriptive, not quantitative. Twentieth-century scientists formalized Darwin's theory with variables and equations. Ronald A. Fisher was primarily responsible for creating the scheme that we know today. He made the simplest possible assumptions: that genes were spread randomly through a population and evolved on their own, linkage playing an insignificant role. The 'fitness of a gene' was defined as its effect on the reproductive output of its bearer, averaged over all the gene combinations and all the micro-niche environments of a mating deme.

This paradigm, called "population genetics" or "neo-Darwinism," took root and became the standard mode of evolutionary theory in the twentieth century. Neo-Darwinism brought the evolutionary conundrum of aging into sharp focus: clearly by Fisher's definition, aging is a drag on fitness. How could it have evolved?

The breakthrough in answering this question came in 1951, when a renowned British biologist named Peter Medawar came up with the hypothesis: even without aging, mortality rates in nature will be high, so many animals won't make it to old age. Thus the force of natural selection is lower for the old than for the young.

From this idea grew all the theories of aging that have currency today:

- Mutation Accumulation: Perhaps the force of selection is so weak at late ages that random mutations are permitted to collect faster than natural selection can eliminate them.
- Antagonistic Pleiotropy: Perhaps there are genes that have benefits early in life (e.g., enhanced fertility) but that exact a cost later on. These genes would find their way into the genome because the benefit matters more to natural selection than the cost.
- Disposable Soma: Animals need to budget their food energy, balancing various uses like metabolism and reproduction against the cost of repairing damaged tissue and maintaining DNA. Because of the compromise, the repair and maintenance functions will never be performed perfectly, so damage is allowed to accumulate with age.

Many biologists today believe in a loose combination of these theories, invoking mutations as well as various tradeoffs to explain different aspects of aging. (Pleiotropy is an example of a genetic tradeoff and Disposable Soma is an example of a metabolic tradeoff.) Other tradeoffs have been proposed and often assumed to result from some underlying physical constraint. But the root cause of the constraint is never specified and indeed, is impossible to confirm in any practical experiment.

Concerning the "declining force of natural selection," however, a direct test of Medawar's main assumption is quite feasible and has been explored extensively since 1991. Surprisingly, surveys of animals in the wild have found that the force of natural selection is actually quite persistent and that many animals in nature do die of old age. But recognition of this fact and of its subversive effect on all the theories of old age has been slow to diffuse into the theoretical community.

References

1. Weismann, A., et al., *Essays upon Heredity and Kindred Biological Problems*. 2d ed. 1891, Oxford: Clarendon Press. 2 v.
2. Medawar, P.B., *An unsolved problem of biology*. 1952, London: Published for the college by H. K. Lewis. 24 p.
3. Muller, H.J., *Our load of mutations*. Am. J. Hum. Genet., 1950. **2**(2): p. 111.
4. Crow, J.F., *Some possibilities for measuring selection intensities in man*. Hum. Biol., 1958: p. 1-13.
5. Edney, E.B. and R.W. Gill, *Evolution of senescence and specific longevity*. Nature, 1968. **220**(5164): p. 281-2.
6. Waddington, C.H., *Canalization of development and the inheritance of acquired characters*. Nature, 1942. **150**(3811): p. 563-565.
7. Sedivy, J.M., G. Banumathy and P.D. Adams, *Aging by epigenetics—a consequence of chromatin damage?* Exp. Cell Res., 2008. **314**(9): p. 1909-1917.
8. Munoz-Najar, U. and J.M. Sedivy, *Epigenetic control of aging*. Antioxid. Redox Signal., 2011. **14**(2): p. 241-59.
9. Williams, G., *Pleiotropy, natural selection and the evolution of senescence*. Evolution, 1957. **11**: p. 398-411.
10. Promislow, D.E., *Senescence in natural populations of mammals: a comparative study*. Evolution, 1991. **45**(8): p. 1869-1887.
11. Ricklefs, R., *Evolutionary theories of aging: confirmation of a fundamental prediction, with implications for the genetic basis and evolution of life span*. Am. Nat., 1998. **152**: p. 24-44.
12. Bonduriansky, R. and C.E. Brassil, *Senescence: rapid and costly ageing in wild male flies*. Nature, 2002. **420**(6914): p. 377.
13. Bronikowski, A.M. and D.E. Promislow, *Testing evolutionary theories of aging in wild populations*. Trends Ecol. Evol., 2005. **20**(6): p. 271-3.
14. Moorad, J.A. and D.E.L. Promislow, *Evolution: aging up a tree?* Current biology: CB, 2010. **20**(9): p. R406-R408.
15. Wright, B.E., *Stress-directed adaptive mutations and evolution*. Mol. Microbiol., 2004. **52**(3): p. 643-650.
16. Curran, S.P. and G. Ruvkun, *Life span regulation by evolutionarily conserved genes essential for viability*. PLoS Genet., 2007. **3**(4): p. e56.
17. Kenyon, C., *A conserved regulatory system for aging*. Cell, 2001. **105**(2): p. 165-8.
18. Guarente, L. and C. Kenyon, *Genetic pathways that regulate ageing in model organisms*. Nature, 2000. **408**(6809): p. 255-62.
19. Tatar, M., et al., *A mutant Drosophila insulin receptor homolog that extends life span and impairs neuroendocrine function*. Science, 2001. **292**(5514): p. 107-110.
20. Longo, V. and P. Fabrizio, *Visions & reflections: regulation of longevity and stress resistance: a molecular strategy conserved from yeast to humans?* Cellular and Molecular Life Sciences CMLS, 2002. **59**(6): p. 903-908.
21. Fontana, L., L. Partridge and V.D. Longo, *Extending healthy life span—from yeast to humans*. Science, 2010. **328**(5976): p. 321-326.
22. Gould, S.J. and R.C. Lewontin, *The spandrels of San Marco and the Panglossian paradigm: a critique of the adaptationist programme*. Proc. R. Soc. Lond. B. Biol. Sci., 1979. **205**(1161): p. 581-98.
23. Promislow, D.E., et al., *Age-specific patterns of genetic variance in Drosophila melanogaster. I. Mortality*. Genetics, 1996. **143**(2): p. 839-48.

24. Tatar, M., et al., *Age-specific patterns of genetic variance in Drosophila melanogaster. II. Fecundity and its genetic covariance with age-specific mortality.* Genetics, 1996. **143**(2): p. 849-58.

25. Wilson, J.D. and C. Roehrborn, *Long-term consequences of castration in men: lessons from the Skoptzy and the eunuchs of the Chinese and Ottoman courts.* J. Clin. Endocrinol. Metab., 1999. **84**(12): p. 4324-4331.

26. Aspinall, R. and D. Andrew, *Thymic involution in aging.* J. Clin. Immunol., 2000. **20**(4): p. 250-6.

27. Davidson, E. and M. Levin, *Gene regulatory networks.* Proc. Natl. Acad. Sci. U.S.A., 2005. **102**(14): p. 4935-4935.

28. Adler, A.S., et al., *Motif module map reveals enforcement of aging by continual NF-kappaB activity.* Genes Dev., 2007. **21**(24): p. 3244-57.

29. Friedman, D.B. and T.E. Johnson, *A mutation in the age-1 gene in Caenorhabditis elegans lengthens life and reduces hermaphrodite fertility.* Genetics, 1988. **118**(1): p. 75-86.

30. Johnson, T.E., P.M. Tedesco and G.J. Lithgow, *Comparing mutants, selective breeding, and transgenics in the dissection of aging processes of Caenorhabditis elegans.* Genetica, 1993. **91**(1-3): p. 65-77.

31. Ayyadevara, S., et al., *Remarkable longevity and stress resistance of nematode PI3K-null mutants.* Aging Cell, 2008. **7**(1): p. 13-22.

32. Rose, M., *Laboratory evolution of postponed senescence in Drosophila melanogaster.* Evolution, 1984. **38**(5): p. 1004-1010.

33. Leroi, A., A.K. Chippindale and M.R. Rose, *Long-term evolution of a genetic life-history tradeoff in Drosophila: the role of genotype-by-environment interaction.* Evolution, 1994. **48**: p. 1244-1257.

34. Le Bourg, E., *A mini-review of the evolutionary theories of aging. Is it the time to accept them?* Dem. Res., 2001. **4**: p. 1-28.

35. Gavrilova, N.S. and L.A. Gavrilov, *Human longevity and reproduction: an evolutionary perspective, In: Grandmotherhood*, E. Voland, A. Chasiotis, and W. Schiefenhövel, Editors. 2005, Rutgers University Press: New Brunswick, NJ. p. 59-80.

36. McArdle, P.F., et al., *Does having children extend life span? A genealogical study of parity and longevity in the Amish.* J. Gerontol. A Biol. Sci. Med. Sci., 2006. **61**(2): p. 190-5.

37. Grundy, E. and O. Kravdal, *Reproductive history and mortality in late middle age among Norwegian men and women.* Am. J. Epidemiol., 2008. **167**(3): p. 271-9.

38. Westendorp, R.G. and T.B. Kirkwood, *Human longevity at the cost of reproductive success.* Nature, 1998. **396**(6713): p. 743-6.

39. Gavrilov, L.A. and N.S. Gavrilova, *Evolutionary theories of aging and longevity.* Scientific World Journal, 2002. **2**: p. 339-56.

40. Gavrilova, N.S., et al., *Does exceptional human longevity come with a high cost of infertility? Testing the evolutionary theories of aging.* Ann. N.Y. Acad. Sci., 2004. **1019**: p. 513-7.

41. Mitteldorf, J., *Female fertility and longevity.* Age (Dordr), 2010: p. 79-84.

42. Austad, S., *Retarded senescence in an insular population of Virginia opossums.* J. Zool. London, 1993. **229**: p. 695-708.

43. Reznick, D.N., et al., *Effect of extrinsic mortality on the evolution of senescence in guppies.* Nature, 2004. **431**(7012): p. 1095-9.

44. Holmes, D.J. and M.A. Ottinger, *Birds as long-lived animal models for the study of aging.* Exp. Gerontol., 2003. **38**(11-12): p. 1365-75.

45. Rose, M.R., H.B. Passananti and M. Matos, *Methuselah Flies: A Case Study in the Evolution of aging.* 2004: World Scientific.
46. Stearns, S.C., *The Evolution of Life Histories.* 1992, Oxford; New York: Oxford University Press. xii, 249 p.
47. Kirkwood, T., *Evolution of aging.* Nature, 1977. **270**: p. 301-304.
48. Shanley, D.P. and T.B. Kirkwood, *Calorie restriction and aging: a life-history analysis.* Evolution Int. J. Org. Evolution, 2000. **54**(3): p. 740-50.
49. Finch, C.E., *Longevity, Senescence and the Genome.* 1990, Chicago: University of Chicago Press.
50. Ricklefs, R.E. and C.D. Cadena, *Life span is unrelated to investment in reproduction in populations of mammals and birds in captivity.* Ecol. Lett., 2007. **10**(10): p. 867-72.
51. Wilson, J.D. and C. Roehrborn, *Long-term consequences of castration in men: lessons from the Skoptzy and the eunuchs of the Chinese and Ottoman courts.* J. Clin. Endocrinol. Metab., 2000. (84): p. 4324-31.
52. Hamilton, J.B. and G.E. Mestler, *Mortality and survival: comparison of eunuchs with intact men and women in a mentally retarded population.* J. Gerontol., 1969. **24**(4): p. 395-411.
53. Perls, T.T., L. Alpert and R.C. Fretts, *Middle-aged mothers live longer.* Nature, 1997. **389**(6647): p. 133.
54. Muller, H.G., et al., *Fertility and life span: late children enhance female longevity.* J. Gerontol. A Biol. Sci. Med. Sci., 2002. **57**(5): p. B202-6.
55. Beeton, M., G.U. Yule and K. Pearson, *On the correlation between duration of life and the number of offspring.* Proc. Royal Soc. B, 1900. **65**: p. 290-305.
56. Korpelainen, H., *Fitness, reproduction and longevity among European aristocratic and rural Finnish families in the 1700s and 1800s.* Proc. Biol. Sci., 2000. **267**(1454): p. 1765-70.
57. Lycett, J.E., R.I. Dunbar and E. Voland, *Longevity and the costs of reproduction in a historical human population.* Proc. Biol. Sci., 2000. **267**(1438): p. 31-5.
58. Le Bourg, E., et al., *Reproductive life of French-Canadians in the 17-18th centuries: a search for a tradeoff between early fecundity and longevity.* Exp. Gerontol., 1993. **28**(3): p. 217-32.
59. Cargill, S.L., et al., *Age of ovary determines remaining life expectancy in old ovariectomized mice.* Aging Cell, 2003. **2**(3): p. 185-90.
60. Mason, J.B., et al., *Transplantation of young ovaries to old mice increased life span in transplant recipients.* The Journals of Gerontology Series A: Biological Sciences and Medical Sciences, 2009. **64A**(12): p. 1207-1211.
61. Mason, J.B., et al., *Transplantation of young ovaries restored cardioprotective influence in postreproductive-aged mice.* Aging Cell, 2011. **10**(3): p. 448-456.
62. Arantes-Oliveira, N., et al., *Regulation of life span by germ-line stem cells in Caenorhabditis elegans.* Science, 2002. **295**(5554): p. 502-5.
63. Barnes, A.I., et al., *No extension of life span by ablation of germ line in Drosophila.* Proceedings of the Royal Society B: Biological Sciences, 2006. **273**(1589): p. 939-947.
64. Austad, S., *Why We Age.* 1999, New York: Wiley.
65. Hanson, R.W. and P. Hakimi, *Born to run; the story of the PEPCK-cmus mouse.* Biochimie, 2008. **90**(6): p. 838-42.
66. Bryant, M.J. and D. Reznick, *Comparative studies of senescence in natural populations of guppies.* Am. Nat., 2004. **163**(1): p. 55-68.
67. Walsh, M.R., D. Whittington and M.J. Walsh, *Does variation in the intensity and duration of predation drive evolutionary changes in senescence?* J. Anim. Ecol., 2014. **83**(6): p. 1279-1288.

68. Walsh, M.R. and D.M. Post, *Interpopulation variation in a fish predator drives evolutionary divergence in prey in lakes.* Proceedings of the Royal Society B: Biological Sciences, 2011. **278**(1718): p. 2628-2637.

69. Reznick, D., L. Nunney and A. Tessier, *Big houses, big cars, superfleas and the costs of reproduction.* Trends in Ecology and Evolution, 2000. **15**(10): p. 421-425.

70. Blagosklonny, M.V. and M.N. Hall, *Growth and aging: a common molecular mechanism.* Aging (Albany NY), 2009. **1**(4): p. 357-62.

71. Blagosklonny, M.V., *Aging and immortality: quasi-programmed senescence and its pharmacologic inhibition.* Cell Cycle, 2006. **5**(18): p. 2087-2102.

72. Kaeberlein, M., et al., *Regulation of yeast replicative life span by TOR and Sch9 in response to nutrients.* Science, 2005. **310**(5751): p. 1193-1196.

73. Vellai, T., et al., *Influence of TOR kinase on life span in C. elegans.* Nature, 2003. **426**(6967): p. 620.

74. Wilkinson, J.E., et al., *Rapamycin slows aging in mice.* Aging Cell, 2012: p. no-no.

75. Walker, R., *Why We Age: Insight into the Cause of Growing Old.* 2013: Dove Medical Press. 121.

76. Bidder, G.P., *Senescence.* Br. Med. J., 1932. **2**(3742): p. 583-585.

77. Brown, K. *Mate-Selection, Scale and Aging* 2014 11 May, 2014 [cited 2015 16 April 2015]; Available from: https://sites.google.com/site/limitsofgrowththeoryofaging/.

78. Holliday, R., *Understanding Ageing.* Vol. 30. 1995: Cambridge University Press.

79. Hamilton, W.D., *The moulding of senescence by natural selection.* J. Theor. Biol., 1966. **12**(1): p. 12-45.

80. Gawande, A. and K. Rockwood, *The way we age now.* The New Yorker, 2007. **30**(2007): p. 50-59.

81. Gavrilov, L.A. and N.S. Gavrilova, *The reliability theory of aging and longevity.* J. Theor. Biol., 2001. **213**(4): p. 527-545.

82. Gompertz, B., *On the nature of the function expressive of the law of human mortality, and on a new mode of determining the value of life contingencies.* Philosophical transactions of the Royal Society of London, **1825**: p. 513-583.

83. Jones, O.R., et al., *Diversity of ageing across the tree of life.* Nature, 2014. **505**(7482): p. 169-173.

84. Hayflick, L. and R.N. Butler, *How and Why We Age.* 1996, Ballantine Books.

85. Lane, N., *Life ascending: the ten great inventions of evolution.* 2010: Profile Books.

86. GONG, J.-S., et al., *Mitochondrial genotype frequent in centenarians predisposes resistance to adult-onset diseases.* J. Clin. Biochem. Nutr., 1998. **24**(2): p. 105-111.

87. Alexe, G., et al., *Enrichment of longevity phenotype in mtDNA haplogroups D4b2b, D4a, and D5 in the Japanese population.* Hum. Genet., 2007. **121**(3-4): p. 347-356.

88. Kenyon, C., *The plasticity of aging: insights from long-lived mutants.* Cell, 2005. **120**(4): p. 449-60.

89. Arantes-Oliveira, N., J.R. Berman and C. Kenyon, *Healthy animals with extreme longevity.* Science, 2003. **302**(5645): p. 611.

5
CHAPTER

Aging is Very Old

Synopsis

According to neo-Darwinian evolutionary theory, one-celled organisms cannot age. None of the standard theories describing how aging can evolve apply to yeast cells or *Paramecia*. Apparently, these microbes haven't read the theory books. Programmed death seems to be as old as the cell nucleus, that is, about two billion years.

Paramecia age via cellular senescence, which is telomere attrition. In paramecia and other ciliates, sex and reproduction are separate, unrelated functions. Reproduction occurs via mitosis and each cell division erodes the telomere. Sex is via conjugation, in which two paramecia cells exchange genetic material. Only during conjugation is the enzyme telomerase expressed, restoring full telomere length. What is the purpose of withholding telomerase? This is an unanswered question in the literature. I suggest that telomerase is withheld in order to enforce the imperative to share genes, helping to avoid the dangers of genetically homogeneous, clonal populations. Computer simulation supports the hypothesis that telomerase sequestration can evolve on this basis.

In some birds and mammals, including humans, cellular senescence contributes to organismal senescence and mortality acceleration with age. Telomere elongation in humans, as in paramecia, is associated with sex, meiosis and the creation of a new individual. This picture suggests a conserved function of cellular senescence, from ciliates to mammals.

The second ancient mechanism of programmed death is *apoptosis*. In response to an internal or external signal, a cell may shut down and begin digesting itself, chopping up its proteins, degrading its DNA. The cell membrane bubbles outward and contents of the cell are released in bite-size packets (*blebs*) that can be engulfed and digested by other cells. This is the oldest form of suicide and it has been known since the 19th century that diseased cells in our bodies undergo apoptosis. If the cell is infected, this protects us from spread of the infection and if the cell is cancerous, then apoptosis protects us from tumors.

But with age, apoptosis begins to kill healthy cells. In aging humans, apoptosis seems to be partially responsible for the muscle loss (sarcopoenia) and cognitive loss (dementia) to which we are prone. Connections exist between apoptosis and atherosclerosis, as well as female menopause.

Apoptosis has an ancient origin. In yeast colonies that are starved for nutrition, 95% of the cells will sacrifice themselves to create food for the other 5%. Apoptosis has been observed in marine algae as well.

Only in the 21st century has it been discovered, first, that microbes are subject to aging and programmed death, and second, that the two modes of programmed death in microbes are implicated in the aging of higher organisms, including humans. Evolutionary theorists have been caught off guard by both these phenomena and the field is ripe for re-evaluation.

Aging in Microbes—it Only *Looks Like* Aging in Higher Organisms

The chemical machinery for respiration in mammals—the *Krebs Cycle*—is substantially identical to the system that does the same job in protists and it is even controlled by genes that are closely related. But this is an illusion, a product of convergent evolution. There is no evolutionary relationship between respiration in protists and respiration in humans. The two functions evolved separately, at different times and for entirely different purposes.

Do you believe it?

Of course not! The idea is absurd on its face. The close chemical and genetic relationship across species is conclusive evidence that multicelled life forms inherited the Krebs Cycle intact from our single-celled forebears.

But biologists are prone to say something almost as preposterous about aging. I have spoken to prominent researchers who dismiss the idea of a genetic program for aging. When I ask, 'What about microbes?' they admit an exception. They say that aging in microbes may be a genetic program, evolved via group selection; this is possible because microbe colonies tend to be close genetic relatives, descended from a small number of founders. But, they claim, group selection in multicelled organisms is not a significant force, so aging in multicelled organisms has nothing to do with aging in microbes and it evolved for a different reason entirely.

It is not only the same function but the same mechanisms and some of the same genes that regulate aging in mammals and in microbes.

Many Modes for Senescence in Microbes

It is a safe bet that microbes have even more different ways to die of old age than all the modes of aging we observe in macroscopic organisms. Only a bit of the territory has been explored. Many microorganisms do not suffer aging—most bacteria do not age, but amazingly some do! Aging in amoebas is not observed. But yeast cells age in two different ways and *Paramecium* is the species in which replicative senescence was discovered. *Tokophrya* is a single-celled, sessile ciliate that ages in both the mode of *Paramecium* and also of yeast [1].

What can aging mean for a cell that reproduces by simple division? The very concept is suspect, because aging normally begins after the onset of reproduction, but if reproduction is a simple cell division, then there is no one left to suffer aging. Nature has found two ways to get around this and introduce aging into single-celled organisms.

The simplest is asymmetric cell division. When some microbe cells divide, one part is larger than the other. There is a clear "mother" and "daughter" cell. Budding yeast reproduces in this way and the main way in which yeast cells age is that the mother slows and then stops producing daughters after a time. Some bacteria are rod-shaped and there is a tiny asymmetry between the end of the rod where a split last occurred and the outer end, which was also an end in the previous generation. This tiny asymmetry is enough to allow aging to get a toehold: The half of the half of the half of the cell that includes the old, old, old end gradually becomes weak and eventually fails to reproduce.

The second innovation that allows aging even when the two daughter cells are identical is sex. *Protists* are eukaryotes, typically 10^5 times larger and more complex than bacteria, with cell nuclei and other organelles. Gene exchange in bacteria occurs in an un-regulated way via passing of DNA loops, called *plasmids.* But in protists, sex is in the form of conjugation, a function that demolishes the identities of two older individuals and creates from them two new individuals.

Age in protists is reckoned from the last conjugation event. Senescence accrues in a clonal lineage and age is reset when genes are exchanged to form new identities. Ciliates can reproduce several hundred times via mitosis, but all the offspring eventually become tired and stop reproducing unless they have sex. Conjugation resets the aging clock.

In addition to gradual aging, protists are also subject to a form of programmed cell death or apoptosis. In multicellular life, apoptosis subjugates the welfare of the cell to the organism. This is well understood and anticipated by classical evolutionary theory, based on individual selection. But apoptosis also occurs in yeast cells and colonies of algae. Because they are not part of a single individual, this poses a challenge for classical neo-Darwinism. Yeast cells sacrificing themselves for the benefit of a colony, while somatic cells eliminate themselves for the benefit of the individual and the common germ line. The logic and the mechanisms are closely analogous for the two cases, but orthodox evolutionary theory treats them very differently. Classically, the reproducing unit defines an individual and there can be no cooperation on wider scales (except as motivated by shared genetics). The discovery of "altruistic suicide" in yeast cells was dismissed with incredulity for a decade before the evidence was permitted into print [2].

Apoptosis has been studied since the nineteenth century and replicative senescence since the mid-twentieth century, but it is only recently that these mechanisms have been elucidated on a biochemical level and both are hot topics of current research.

Part I: Telomeres and Replicative Senescence

How Replicative Senescence was Discovered

As a microbiology grad student in the early 1950s, Leonard Hayflick learned about the longest-running experiment in biological history. Alexis Carrel had kept a cell culture alive, growing and replicating for 34 years, from 1912 to 1946. This proved that cells themselves were immortal and that aging must take place at a higher level within the organism as a whole.

Carrel was a French doctor who pioneered organ transplant operations. He moved from Paris to Chicago, where he was recruited by the Rockefeller Institute and in 1912 won the Nobel Prize for figuring out how to join blood vessels so that they would grow together and feed the transplanted organ. On a return visit to Paris, Carrel gave a presentation about his new interest: growing animal cells—including human cells—*in vitro*, outside the body, in lab conditions. He was crowing to his compatriots about the superior facilities and research environment in America. The Europeans were incensed and challenged him to demonstrate his heretical ideas.

Carrel took the dare and upon his return, set about demonstrating rigorously that cell cultures could be grown in a test tube. He sent an assistant to learn the technology for keeping them alive and started his own culture with embryonic cells from a chick heart. The experiment proved successful and he wrote about it for two years, adding to his fame and influence. Carrel, as it turned out, was articulate and well-endowed with charisma; this combined with his scientific success turned him into a celebrity and an unchallengeable authority.

Carrel passed his chick cell culture off to a colleague, Arthur Ebeling, who maintained the experiment for thirty more years. Though he had let the experiment out of his personal control, Carrel remained interested in the results and soon became an advocate for the view that individual cells could divide and grow indefinitely. Over the decades, it became a piece of the scientific canon: animals may get old, but the cells of which they are made have the capacity to grow and divide indefinitely.

Scientific canons are difficult to oppose. Others researchers were growing cell lines in the 1940s and 1950s and saw different results. They published their findings, but always attributed the death of their cell lines to special conditions and did not challenge the orthodoxy. A theory (a myth, actually) grew up that kept scientists from having to confront the contradiction: that something in the chemistry of the culture became poisoned with age and this would prevent the culture from continuing to grow, even though the cells themselves were immortal.

...And so we return to Hayflick. Just a few years out of grad school, he was recruited to head the cell culture laboratory at University of Pennsylvania's Wistar Laboratory. He designed an experiment to compare cancer cells to normal cells and he didn't think to question the scientific results he had inherited: cell lines could be grown *in vitro* without limit [3].

But he soon encountered difficulty with his cell lines. The normal cells (but not the cancer cells) would slow down and die after a year or so, corresponding to 40 cycles of growth and division. At first, he assumed that his lab technique was to blame. But after a few years of refined experiments, he was convinced that cell aging was not an artifact. At this point, he switched gears in his research. Putting cancer aside, he asked the basic question, how could he demonstrate cellular aging unambiguously?

His idea was to grow old cells and young cells in the same culture. If Carrel's claim was correct, then the poison from the old cells ought to kill both. But if the problem was endemic in the cells, the young cells might continue to grow, even as the old ones died.

But how could he tell the two cell lines apart? This was 1959, before modern techniques of biochemistry or DNA sequencing. Hayflick solved the problem with cells derived from men and women. Even though the biochemical details could not be discriminated, the difference between a full-size X and a stubby Y chromosome could be easily discerned under a microscope. Hayflick grew cells from a man's skin until they got old and their reproduction slowed. He added fresh skin cells from a young woman.

In a short time, there were only female cells in the culture, continuing to grow and to replicate. The result was clear: The 'poison' theory was dead. Somehow the cells knew how many times they had divided and slowed down with age. Once this dam had broken, it was not long before the result was replicated by multiple labs. A scientific doctrine established for decades fell quickly. Hayflick repeated his experiment using cells aged *in vivo*; he began his colony with skin cells drawn from older humans and younger humans. Cells from the older people had a shorter life time in the laboratory before they showed signs of aging. This confirmed that the phenomenon he had discovered was not some laboratory oddity: within the body, cells are aging measurably. This re-opened the possibility that the aging of an animal has its roots in processes at the level of the cell.

How Did this Happen?

For anyone seeking scientific truth from the scientific establishment, this is a cautionary tale about charisma and the power of group-think. The need for replication as an essential step in the scientific process had been honored, yet so powerful was the scientific consensus, that contradictions in the new results were explained away, side stepping the need to challenge an established dogma. Scientists are human.

Still the question remains: how could Carrel and Ebeling—good and careful scientists, both—have obtained the results that they did over such a long period of time? Hayflick was polite enough to suggest in his original paper that Ebeling's medium had inadvertently become contaminated. The nutrients that were added daily to the cell culture were derived from fertilized eggs. If occasionally the nutrient broth was not properly sterilized before being mixed into the cell culture, that would provide a fresh supply of embryonic cells that could explain the apparent longevity of the cell culture.

We will never know for certain, since "the ultimate effects of the ageing process have made it impossible for Carrel to respond in his own defense [4]." But there is a relevant anecdote from a contemporary scientist who visited Carrel's labs in 1930. Ralph Buschsbaum claimed a lab technician told him that periodically the cell line would be discovered dead, and the technicians, thinking that they had made some mistake, added fresh cultures to cover their derrières [5].

Telomeres

Once it had been established that aging takes place at the cellular level, the question was ripe: What is the mechanism? How do cells keep count of how many times they have replicated, and what process resets the counter? New biochemical techniques, including DNA analysis, would be required before the question could be answered.

In the mid-1970s, another young postdoctoral researcher, Elizabeth Blackburn of Yale (now at UC San Francisco) found direct and compelling answers to both these questions. She was working not with human or animal cells, but with single-celled *Paramecia*, a protist. Blackburn discovered that the replicase enzyme crawling along the chromosome has trouble at the end of the line. It runs out of room and cannot properly copy the last few hundred base units. The result is that every time a chromosome is copied, it becomes a bit shorter.

The chromosome must have some compensatory mechanism to assure that chromosomes do not lose information in the long run. The solution, also discovered by Blackburn, has two parts. First, there is a buffer of DNA that carries no meaningful information at the end of every chromosome. This is called a *telomere* and it is just a repeated pattern of bases—TTAGGG*, repeated in thousands of inline copies. In a functioning chromosome, the telomere tail automatically folds over on itself to give the DNA a neat termination that renders it chemically inactive, so that the double helix will not come unwound. These days, Blackburn likes to introduce her public lectures with slides showing the aglet at the end of a shoelace, preventing the lace from raveling.

The telomere protects the information-carrying part of the DNA and provides a disposable region that need not be transcribed, and contains no biochemical information. Telomeres also affect gene expression near the chromosome end [6, 7]. The telomere is typically tens of thousands of bases long and continues to function as an endcap even if a few hundred or a few thousand bases are lost in multiple generations of copying. (The chromosome in its entirety is far longer, with tens of millions of base pairs.)

The second part of the solution: how are telomeres restored? Having a buffer of meaningless DNA is a temporary expedient, but sooner or later the buffer must be rebuilt. This, too, was anticipated and solved by Blackburn in her early work on the biochemistry of the telomere. There is an enzyme which she named, logically

---

* TTAGGG is the repeated sequence in the telomeres of humans and other vertebrates. In the protists that Blackburn studied, the mechanism was the same, but the sequence is not: It's TTGGGG. There are about twenty known variant sequences, in different board families of life forms.

enough, *telomerase*, the principal* function of which is to add copies of TTAGGG to the end of a chromosome. Normally, DNA is copied to 'messenger RNA' as the chromosome sends messages out to its protein factories (called ribosomes), giving instructions for what proteins to make and how to make them. This order of nature was immortalized by Francis Crick, who named it the *central dogma of molecular biology.* But like other dogmas, it eventually encountered exceptions and was forced to be less dogmatic. Rarely, RNA is transcribed 'backwards' into DNA. The AIDS virus is an example: it is made of RNA, but it is translated with *reverse transcriptase* inside human blood cells and becomes part of the DNA.

Telomerase uses this same trick: it contains a short piece (the six bases) of RNA as part of its molecule and uses this RNA template over and over to extend the DNA tail. Telomerase is the answer to the question, how is it that the telomere grows back the length that it loses in cell replications?

If the telomere were to shrink to zero, the chromosome would start to lose real (coding) information with each additional replication. But it never gets that far. The cell detects when its telomeres are starting to get short, because chromosome end caps are misformed. When there are still thousands of bases left in the telomere, the cell already senses that it has a short telomere and it goes into a senescent mode. At first, metabolism is slowed and as the telomere shortens further, the cell becomes inactive and ceases to divide. It may begin to spew poisons that damage younger cells around it. It may commit suicide via *apoptosis*, a process described below; but in any case, it has ceased to have an active biological function and one way or another it will die.

Why Do Cells Ration Telomerase?

Telomere attrition is an ancient problem and telomerase is a well-developed solution. Every eukaryotic cell is capable of making the enzyme telomerase, but across the biosphere, some species express telomerase freely, while others keep it locked up, available only in conjugation or embryonic development.

In humans, dogs and horses (but not mice, pigs or cows) stem cells replicate without telomerase and eventually become senescent, to the detriment of the whole animal. Senescent stem cells fail to renew the body's tissues as needed and they also secrete cytokine signals that accelerate inflammaging. This is programmed death in its second-most-ancient form (after apoptosis).

Sex and Reproduction

In most higher organisms, sex and reproduction are tightly integrated, but the two functions, replication and gene sharing, had separate origins and remain distinct in most single-cell organisms.

---

* Probably not the only function of telomerase. Recent research has uncovered hints that telomerase can act as a kind of growth hormone and that telomerase can improve healing and extend lifespan even in situations where there is no use for longer telomeres. See p 118.

Almost all living things share their genes. Bacteria promiscuously trade short DNA rings called plasmids and genes pass freely across species lines. Protists share genes via conjugation, described below. The vast majority of multi-celled eukaryotes are capable of a reproductive mode with sex, even though they may also be capable of cloning or selfing. There is a handful of organisms for which no gene-sharing mechanism has yet been observed, including amoebas and most famously, the bdelloid rotifers, millimeter-scale tubular animals that live typically in ponds.

The sharing of genes has never been explained within the framework of classical neo-Darwinian theory. Benefits of gene sharing accrue to the community in the long run, while the costs are to the individual in the short run; since classical theory always adjudicates such conflicts in favor of the individual and the short run, there can be no integral account of the evolution of sex. Hence, it has become conventional to assume sexual reproduction as a given when performing population genetic calculations and to set aside the origin of sex as an unsolved problem. Sex is treated as though it were a unique and mysterious anomaly within the classical framework of population genetics [8].

Gene-sharing makes evolution proceed more efficiently because so many more gene combinations can be tried out at once. Without sex, evolution works "too efficiently" to eliminate genes that may be out of favor only temporarily. Spreading genes around helps to maintain population diversity, hedging against the danger that one genome might evolve to fixation in advance of an environmental change that would have promoted the value of some discarded genotypes. It is a powerful and robust long-term strategy to keep those variant strategies idling in the background, ready to spread rapidly through the genome when they are needed. There is a credible hypothesis that sex promotes other forms of cooperation [9].

The Imperative to Share Genes

The difference between evolution in a sexual population and an asexual population is like the difference between multitasking and working on one project at a time. Without sex, each innovation—each mutation—must arise in sequence and they accumulate one-by-one. If two innovations arise simultaneously in different individuals, there is no escape from the eventuality that one of them will be lost. But with sex, innovations can appear in different individuals, perhaps providing some intermediate benefit. Eventually, the descendants with these separate innovations may mate and the innovations are combined in a single individual [10].

Conversely, a detrimental mutation may become fixed in a clonal population, either by genetic drift or because it has hitchhiked along with a beneficial genetic variant. Once the information is lost to the population, it is lost for good. Additional information loss can only make the problem worse. Since beneficial mutations are far less common than detrimental mutations, Muller [11] theorized that the genome of a clonal population was bound to degrade in the long run, as good genes are lost to accident, one by one. This phenomenon has become known as Muller's Ratchet. Muller suggest that the purpose and evolutionary significance of sex is that it protects a population from this process. Muller's hypothesis has become an accepted part of the canon on evolution of sex, despite the fact that it is teleological and lacks a mechanistic basis [12].

Over the long haul, sex makes evolution far more efficient. In the process, sex also softens individual competition. Every individual in a community of cloners is in a winner-take-all competition, because eventually, its lineage must either die out (overwhelmingly probable) or evolve to dominate the entire population—there can be no middle ground. In a sexual community, however, some of each individual's genes will probably survive into the future and others will certainly die out and this is true for every individual.

Sex increases the individual's investment in the deme (gene-sharing community) [9]. In a sexual population, every individual has thrown in her lot with the clan. Instead of competing relentlessly in a winner-take-all tournament, the competition is spread out. The advantage is that many different combinations of genes are tried out. Some are bound to work much better than others. The disadvantage is that even the most successful gene combination is destined to be broken apart in the very next generation and only very gradually will the especially-favorable gene combinations come to be established as the new norm.

As we know from experience, sometimes there may be 'better and worse', but sometimes it is just 'two different styles'. A strategy that works better in one situation works less well in another situation. The fact that a sexual population is more diverse than a clonal population means that the clonal population can be more refined, more specialized, better competitors in a particular niche. But if anything changes, the specialized population is more vulnerable to calamity. A diverse population has a better chance of surviving and is more resistant to extinction. This, again, is a group-level advantage of sex. Undoubtedly, it has a lot to do with why sex evolved and why sex is ubiquitous in plants and animals.

Sex and No Sex are two separate evolutionary games, with separate sets of rules. The No Sex game is hard-edged competition, winner-take-all. In the Sex game, almost everyone goes home with a prize, though some prizes are bigger than others. There is much more experimentation in the Sex game than with No Sex, so there's much more innovation in the long run. Evolution with Sex can go places that No Sex may never find. There's no question, the Sex game is a better game, a more interesting game. There's good reason for throwing in your individual lot with the Sex community.

But at any given moment, an individual who is a strong competitor can gain advantage by playing the No Sex game of all-or-nothing. If one individual only is playing the hard-edged No Sex game while everyone else is playing softball, the individual without sex is very likely to wipe out the competition in the short run—then stagnate in the long run.

The game of Sex is a superior game, but only if everyone plays by the rules. Where the Sex Game is played, it is vulnerable to invasion by No Sex. The Sex game needs to protect itself from invasion by the No Sex game or Sex will die out, experimentation will languish and exploration of new niches will slow to a crawl. How can a sexual species protect itself from that mutant individual who abjures sex and challenges the community, all-or-nothing? A billion years before Augustine and Gandhi engaged in lifelong struggles with the temptation of sex, Evolution struggled with the opposite temptation—the temptation to forgo sex.

How did Sex learn to protect itself against No Sex? This has been a central question in the history of evolutionary science and there have been many answers, many ways that sexual communities are protected against the rogue mutant that refuses to share its genes. It is likely that *replicative senescence* evolved as an early answer to the question of how to enforce the imperative, *Thou shalt share thy genes!* In the genome, telomerase was cordoned off and held in reserve. Only by participating in conjugation could *Paramecia* get access to (their own) telomerase and without telomerase, the *Paramecium* lineage would slowly peter out [13].

The Problem of Males

In the world of larger animals and plants that is most familiar to us, sex and reproduction are inextricably linked. The mechanisms are so intertwined that, through habit of observation, it is difficult for us to conceive of one without the other. Eggs that are unfertilized do not even begin to implant or to develop. The need for two sexes is built right into the biochemistry, so that reproduction does not begin until there has been a meiotic event. This is evolution's way of laying down the law: if you want to reproduce, you will have to share your genes. It is heavy-handed, but necessarily so for the evolutionary program. If asexuals were permitted to compete openly with sexuals, the asexuals would wipe out the competition in short order—but then evolution would be far less robust and productive for a long time to come.

Even if we grant to evolution the necessity of sex, it is still not clear why there are two separate sexes. Why aren't we all hermaphrodites, carrying both male and female sex organs? The evolutionary advantage compared to the present state of affairs would be a full factor of two in fitness (as fitness is defined in neo-Darwinism). And the advantage would be available both for the population and for the individual.

Hermaphrodites are still compelled to share genes when they reproduce. Some hermaphrodites can fertilize themselves and then the genes within an individual's own pairs of chromosomes are shuffled. The result is an offspring that is not a clone of the parent, but neither does it benefit from the range of diversity and novelty available if genes were shared between two hermaphrodites. (Self-fertilization is called *autogamy* or sometimes *selfing*.)

Earthworms are hermaphrodites and their separate male and female organs are situated so as to make selfing mechanically impossible. Land snails, slugs and some sea mollusks are hermaphrodites. Most flowers are hermaphroditic, so that there is the possibility that pollen from a flower can fertilize its own pistil. But there are mechanical and biochemical barriers that discourage this, insuring that most of the time, most flowers do cross-pollinate.

Hermaphroditism is clearly viable and it carries an enormous fitness advantage (by neo-Darwinian accounting). Why are so few higher animals hermaphroditic? Why does evolution put up with males when they are such a drag on the all-important rate of reproduction?

Neo-Darwinian theory offers no answer to this question. Any conceivable resolution to the cost of males involves powerful group selection [14]. In fact, the cost of males is 50% of fitness and we have seen in the last chapter that the cost of aging is typically 12%-45%. So a group selective explanation for aging need not be more extreme than the explanations for evolution of sex that are already considered plausible.

I believe that dioecious sex (separation of the sexes) is common in higher animals because it provides a firewall against reversion to selfing. (Compared to sexual exchange between different individuals, selfing provides a much weaker mechanism for creating novelty and maintaining diversity). The same computational model described below (for withholding of telomerase) can be minimally modified and re-interpreted to demonstrate an advantage for separation of the sexes.

The advantage of separate sexes appears only in the long-term operation of natural selection. It is too easy for a mutation to arise that allows hermaphrodites to revert to self-fertilization or even clonal reproduction. An atavistic mutant that escaped from sex could reproduce rapidly and efficiently via parthenogenesis and would come to dominate its population in short-order. The long-term disadvantage would show up too late. Natural selection has separated the sexes as a gambit, a ploy sacrificing short-term fitness for a long-term goal. Separating the sexes means that no one individual has the biological tools to reproduce independently. This makes it much more difficult for a mutant to arise that reverts to selfing.

Hermaphroditism is the exception (among animals) because it is just too dangerous to put male and female sex organs in the same animal. This is a teleological explanation—it explains why, but not how the sexes came to be separated. But no matter what explanation we adopt for the separation of the sexes, we are stuck with the paradox that it has been costly by neo-Darwinian accounting, far more costly than aging.

In a forthcoming paper, excerpted in the box below, I make the argument quantitatively and show that separate sexes can be an ESS (an evolutionarily stable strategy, that is to say, not vulnerable to invasion by hermaphrodites or cloners). A necessary condition for this to be true is that overall population density be limited and sufficient reproductive capacity be available to sustain population at that limit, after accounting for the factor of two lost to separation of the sexes [13]. When overall population is at carrying capacity, there is, in a sense "no place to go" for any excess reproductive capacity. Thus the factor of two available to hermaphrodites offers little advantage to the community. However, by standard neo-Darwinian reckoning, the increase in individual reproductive output offers a huge within-group advantage that ought to enable any invading hermaphrodite to eliminate the competition and fix its descendants through the group in short order. Thus the model demonstrates an essential error in neo-Darwinian accounting for fitness and proper treatment of this dynamic opens the door to understanding aging, as well as many other communal adaptations.

Darwin proclaimed that nature is a struggle for survival and reproduction, but it was neo-Darwinists of the 20th century who narrowed the terms of the competition and defined 'fitness' as fecundity—a race to produce the most offspring in the least time. In defiance of neo-Darwinian theory, all the animals that we know that exist in two separate sexes are only half as 'fit' (by neo-Darwinian measure) as they could be if they multitasked as hermaphrodites. Surely this is a clue that the neo-Darwinian definition of 'fitness' is missing something. Whether or not my model is accepted as correct, the fact that so many animal species bear the "cost of males" has a message we must heed: *Selective success in evolution's competition is not dependent on maximizing reproductive output.* This is a simple and straightforward inference, but the message for classical evolutionary theory is profound.

Returning to the Topic of Replicative Senescence in Protists

The point of this exegesis has been that sex and reproduction are tied tightly together in higher organisms in order to enforce the imperative to share genes. But in the *Paramecium*, sex (conjugation) and reproduction (mitosis) are entirely separate and distinct functions. How, then, does nature enforce the imperative for protists?

In *Paramecia*, replicative senescence is the answer to this question. By rationing telomerase, evolution has placed a firewall in the path of any selfish individual that refuses to share its genes via conjugation. An errant cell that forgoes sex may make hay for a few hundred generations, but its lineage will be a dead end.

The capacity to make telomerase has to be there in the cell. In the long run, there is no life without it. But cells keep telomerase under epigenetic lock and key. In the course of ordinary metabolism, while the cell is respiring and consuming and growing, there is no telomerase. When the cell splits, reproducing two daughter cells with shorter telomeres, there is no telomerase. Only when the cell conjugates, does telomerase appear.

Two cells sidle up to one another and dissolve the cell walls between them. This creates a double cell with two cell nuclei. Then the nuclei merge into a double nucleus, with two copies of every chromosome. Within the double nucleus, corresponding chromosomes find each other and some genes cross over, so that the chromosomes that emerge contain thorough mixtures of the genes from the two parents. When the chromosome pairs separate once more, the individual identities of the two parents have been thoroughly scrambled*. Two nuclei separate once more and then the cells separate as well. The two daughter cells that emerge from the process each contain equal genetic material from the original two parent cells.

In higher organisms that are familiar to us, sex scrambles the genes from two parents to create a new offspring. But in conjugation of *Paramecia*, there are no offspring separate from the parents. The two parents themselves actually fuse and scramble their own identities to create two new individuals. Two cells come together

---

* This is a precursor to the process of meiosis in higher life forms. Multicelled animals and plants have two copies of every chromosome, one from each parent. Protists have only one copy. When two protists undergo conjugation, they are creating a jumbo nucleus with two copies of each chromosome. The crossover mechanism is a close analog to the corresponding process in meiosis and the separation of pairs of chromosomes in conjugation foreshadows the separation of chromosome pairs in meiosis.

to conjugate and two cells emerge from conjugation, but the cells that emerge cannot be identified individually with the original cells. You and I have both become 'half me and half you'.

In animals and plants, sex and reproduction have been tied tightly together so that organisms cannot revert to reproduction on their own (that is, they cannot easily mutate into a clonally-reproducing variant). In *Paramecia*, the imperative to share genes is enforced by the telomere mechanism: Natural selection has arranged that the enzyme they need to keep their telomeres from shrinking is only available during the act of exchanging genes.

Selection pressure in favor of epigenetic sequestration of telomerase is a tertiary benefit, while the cost of sequestration is a primary benefit to individual fitness. In other words, the individual's reproductive capacity is limited by replicative senescence, so its fitness takes a direct hit. But the benefit of replicative senescence is only that it prevents a potential loss of the propensity to conjugate with other cells and even loss of conjugation would have a secondary cost, as it contributes in the long run to less diversity, less evolvability. Evolvability is the rate of change of fitness and not fitness itself [15]. Despite the very direct, near-term cost and indirect, long-term benefit, it can be demonstrated that sequestration of telomerase is an ESS, with caveats as above, including a fixed carrying capacity for total population.

A Computational Model for Evolution of Telomerase Rationing in Ciliates

Why is telomerase withheld during mitosis? The effect on individual fitness is purely negative. Withholding telomerase introduces the possibility that some progeny undergo cellular senescence and fail to reproduce. There are no published suggestions of an evolutionary purpose for cellular senescence in ciliates and it is clear that none of the standard evolutionary theories of aging are germane.

Hypothesizing that cellular senescence in ciliates has an adaptive function, I have identified only one candidate for a benefit. The withholding of telomerase motivates the individual cell to share genes and helps to ensure that conjugation occurs. Conjugation is energetically costly for the individual and what is worse, it breaks up successful gene combinations that might otherwise go on to dominate the community a few generations hence. Cellular senescence acts as a firewall against individual selection that would otherwise tend to discourage conjugation. My conjecture is that cellular senescence is an adaptation to enforce the imperative to share genes.

As stated, this hypothesis is a teleological explanation and begs for a quantitative mechanistic model before it can be taken seriously. This is especially true since the cost of senescence is direct and immediate for the individual, while the benefit of senescence accrues indirectly, slowly to the community and not the individual. The benefit is not secondary, but tertiary. Primary fitness is measured by robustness and average rate of reproduction. Secondary is the enhancement of progressive evolution that is facilitated by gene-sharing. The tertiary benefit is to keep the rate of gene-sharing high and prevent evolutionary reversion, propelled by individual selection. It is only on this tertiary level that cellular senescence has positive value. How can such a remote and indirect benefit compete with a primary cost that is direct and immediate?

Model Description

The model is realized in cellular automata on a 2D grid. Food is introduced into each grid-cell in each time step and diffuses into neighboring grid-cells with a diffusion constant that is a parameter of the model. Each grid-cell may support an indeterminate number of individuals (or none). The model is initialized with one individual per grid-cell and as evolution progresses, the individuals become more efficient and population increases.

Individuals are capable of four behaviors: they may eat, die, reproduce via mitosis and conjugate with another individual in the same grid-cell.

Individuals have three genes:

- **Reproduction-threshold:** How much energy must the individual accumulate before reproducing? This is the primary fitness of the individual. Lower values correspond to greater fitness.

- **Propensity-for-conjugation:** In each time step, every pair of individuals within a cell has a probability of conjugating that is computed as the product of the corresponding genes of the two participants.

- **Senescing:** (a boolean variable, true/false) This is the gene for aging. Those individuals with the allele = 1 produce daughter cells in each replication with telomeres that are 1 unit shorter than the parent. Those individuals with allele = 0 do not lose telomere length when they replicate, thus they are never subject to senescence.

Individuals have two properties that characterize their state:

- **Energy** is accumulated by eating food and lost to metabolism and to the energetic cost of conjugation. When energy reaches the reproduction-threshold, mitosis takes place.

- **Telomere length.** Senescing individuals lose one unit of telomere with each replication; non-senescing individuals never lose telomere length.

All individuals emerge from conjugation with a full-length telomere and this length is another parameter of the model.

In each time step,

- There is a constant probability of death from **random mortality**.
- Food **energy** consumed is a constant proportion of the available food concentration in the grid-cell.
- A constant amount of **energy** is deducted for metabolism as a "cost of living".
- **Mitosis** occurs if **energy** exceeds the (gene for) **reproduction-threshold**.
- For each pair in a given grid-cell, there is a probability of conjugation. The two individuals emerge from each conjugation have, respectively, higher and lower fitness than the average of the fitness genes of the two original individuals.

The most important parameters of the model are:

- **mortality** probability per time step
- **split constant**, fitness gained or lost in conjugation
- **energy cost** of conjugation

Results

Beginning with equal numbers of senescing and non-senescing individuals randomly distributed, the senescing and non-senescing varieties first tend to self-organize into patches. In patches dominated by non-senescing individuals, the gene for propensity to conjugation evolves lower and lower, because there is an energetic cost of conjugation, which is an individual disadvantage.

This creates an early advantage and the non-senescing patches tend to grow, encroaching on the territory of the senescing individuals. But on a longer time scale, the patches of non-senescing individuals are not increasing in fitness as fast. The fitness of the senescing population eventually overtakes them.

If the grid is sufficiently large, the long-term advantage always wins out in some region and from there, the senescing variety expands to take over the grid. The larger the presumed fitness boost from conjugation, the smaller the grid size necessary to see the senescing variety prevail [13].

Micronucleus and Macronucleus

It is not essential to our story, but it is an interesting diversion that some protist cells (but not higher life forms) actually have two cell nuclei. There is a micronucleus that contains the archival copy of all the chromosomes; and then there is the macronucleus that contains many working copies. In the course of the cell's metabolism, it is the macronucleus that directs all the cell's activities. The original copies of the genes are preserved in the micronucleus, which is only active during reproduction and conjugation. Genes in the micronucleus are organized strictly onto chromosomes. Genes in the macronucleus are cut apart for easy access. The number of copies of each gene is proportional to the amount of activity that gene needs to contribute to the cell's metabolism.

After reproduction, the micronucleus fortifies the macronucleus with new gene copies.

After conjugation, the two macronuclei are destroyed and digested! This is so new instructions can be read from the new library of genetic material. New macronuclei are created separately in each daughter cell, with faithful copies of that daughter's genes.

The process of disassembling the macronucleus foreshadows apoptosis (programmed cell death, see below). Much of the chemical machinery is common between apoptosis and this stage of conjugation, especially enzymes that dissolve the nuclear membrane, cut up the DNA and recycle it.

Why do Adult Humans Sequester Telomerase?

In humans, it is roughly true that the replicative lifetime of our cells was already determined in early stages of the embryo. Telomeres are about 20 kilobases in length shortly after fertilization when telomerase activity spikes, declining to 10 kb at birth because of the rapid pace of cell replication in utero. Childhood and growth consume another 5 kb pairs and the adult's remaining 5 kb must last a lifetime.

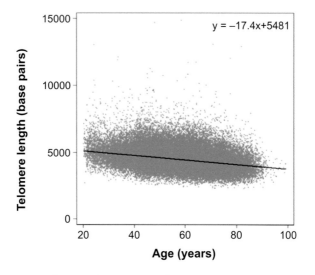

Figure from Rode, 2015, supplementary materials [16].

As soon as the story of telomerase was fleshed out and the Hayflick limit explained, the question was posed, why is telomerase rationed? In 1990, a young Carol Greider, fresh from the work that was to win her and her thesis advisor a belated Nobel prize [17], was the first to float the idea that the reason that man and most other mammals have evolved with short telomeres is to help protect against cancer. Independently in 1991, a senior geneticist with more established credibility, Ruth Sager proposed the same hypothesis [18] with more detail, citing circumstantial evidence. Their hypothesis was that the individual (and her stem cells) are provided before birth with long enough telomeres to last a lifetime. By limiting telomere length, the organism is protecting against cancer later on. Uncontrolled cell proliferation of cancer would be checked when a malignant cell line ran out of telomere and became senescent. This evolutionary hypothesis gained credibility when it was discovered a few years afterward that approximately 80 to 90% of human cancers have mutated so as to express telomerase freely. Today, the hypothesis is well-established and invoked without citation in many papers on telomere biology. Campisi writes, correctly, "The senescence response is widely recognized as a potent tumor suppressive mechanism [19]." Widely recognized, to be sure, but perhaps not accurately perceived. In fact, there is clear evidence and logic to the contrary.

In 2003, technology became available for the first time to do a retrospective study correlating human telomere length with mortality. Cawthon [20] used twenty-year-old blood samples preserved by a local Utah hospital to measure telomere lengths for 143 subjects, all about 60 years old at the time the blood was drawn and he looked for correlations with morbidity and mortality over the ensuing 20 years. The result was a striking relationship, easily significant in his small sample: Short telomeres predict higher morbidity and mortality; longer telomeres (at the same age) predict longer life expectancy. This posed (or should have posed) a serious crisis of credibility for the cancer protection theory of telomerase rationing. The theory had been based on the premise that rationing telomerase was cost-free to the individual, because his telomere length was sufficient to avoid any effect of cell senescence on whole-organism senescence. The hypothesis about cancer prevention was not tenable if cancer prevention came at a net cost in life expectancy.

Twelve years after Cawthon, enough time had elapsed for a Danish group to compile a prospective study of the same question with a sample population that was 500 times larger [21]. Telomere length robustly predicts longevity, even after factoring out the effect of age, smoking, exercise, blood cholesterol, BMI and alcohol consumption. We now know that stress [22] and unhealthy life choices [23, 24] erode telomeres more rapidly; nevertheless, short telomeres are driving higher mortality by some mechanism over and beyond these known correlates. The 10% of people with the shortest telomeres were dying at 1.4 times the rate (adjusted for age) of the 10% with the longest telomeres, a result that was overwhelmingly statistically apparent ($p < 2 \cdot 10^{-15}$). When broken out, all individual morbidities were found to decrease with telomere length. *Cancer rates in particular were significantly higher in people with short telomeres.*

This finding vitiates the hypothesis that telomerase rationing is an evolutionary adaptation to protect against cancer. According to the hypothesis, telomere length has been optimized by natural selection for a compromise between cancer prevention (short telomeres) and adequate capacity for tissue renewal (long telomeres). It follows that, since the length is at an optimal level, there should be a smooth, flat top in the mortality curve. People with slightly longer telomeres will have greater death rates from cancer, but lower from other causes; and people with shorter telomere length will have slightly greater death rates from other causes, but lower from cancer; and the sum (all-cause mortality) should be comparable for the two groups. But what the Danish group found instead (consistent with Cawthon and other previous studies in the last 10 years, but now unassailable because of the large sample) is that all-cause mortality and even cancer mortality decreases with telomere length.

The net effect of telomerase rationing on humans is to decrease lifespan. Telomerase rationing in humans is a form of programmed death, a conserved program with a function that is closely analogous to the function in one-celled ciliates.

Limited Evidence for Cancer Prevention

Some studies in mice have found an increase in cancer incidence when telomerase was overexpressed. Female mice with extra (transgenic) copies of the telomerase gene developed breast tumors, while control mice had cancers in other organs, but not breast [25]. Transgenic telomerase targeted to thymocytes (stem cells of the thymus) resulted in an increased incidence of T-cell lymphoma [26]. Similarly, telomerase overexpression in skin stem cells increased the rate of skin cancer [27]. In a mouse model genetically engineered to be prone to endocrine cancers, disabling telomerase dramatically reduced the frequency of tumor formation [28].

All authors of the mouse studies note a puzzling aspect of their results: telomerase is already abundantly expressed in mice and telomeres are never critically short.

According to the standard hypothesis, telomerase rationing should serve the body by halting tumors when they reach a size determined by beginning telomere length. Any association of telomerase with initiation of cancer must be by a different mechanism, not yet understood.

A surprising line of research has indicated that telomerase has other functions besides maintaining telomeres. All these cases in which telomerase appears to promote cancer seem to depend not on immortalization of the cells, but on other, auxiliary functions of telomerase. As Jerry Shay and Woody Wright put it so colorfully in a 2005 editorial, telomerase appears to "moonlight" in other roles [29, 30], as a signal molecule [31] and as a kind of growth hormone [32], especially growth of new ribosomes [33]. These may be regarded as a kind of pleiotropy, but not counted as evidence for the original hypothesis of Greider and Sager which involved telomere length explicitly. For pleiotropy to be an explanation for the evolution of aging, it is necessary that the pleiotropy be essential and unavoidable—that the body is stuck with a bad effect in pursuit of a good one. These extra roles for telomerase look more like the kind of opportunistic recycling that we see so often in evolution, rather than antagonistic pleiotropy—"exaptation" is the term introduced by Gould [34].

In the large Danish epidemiological study cited above [21], one finding that could most easily be mistaken for vindication of the cancer hypothesis concerns three genetic markers of telomere length that were also tracked in these 65,000 subjects. The three genetic markers correlate with higher cancer risk and also with longer telomeres. The way in which this result is reported is confirmation-biased, a bit misleadingly, toward the standard cancer hypothesis. The authors write, "We found that genetically short telomeres were associated with low cancer mortality but not low cardiovascular mortality, death from other causes or all-cause mortality. This implies that genetically long telomeres are associated with higher cancer mortality."

The misleading thing is the use of the words "genetically short telomeres". Of course, without being able to go back in time, they had no way to know what was the subjects' telomere length at birth. They explain that what they mean by "genetically short telomeres" is the variant of these three genetic polymorphisms that is statistically associated with shorter telomeres late in life. There are three SNPs in the region around the telomerase gene that presumably help to determine when and how much telomerase is transcribed. What the study shows is that the version of these three SNPs associated with longer telomeres is also associated with higher cancer rates.

This result is expected and could hardly be otherwise. If the standard neo-Darwinian paradigm works anywhere at all, it must work for mutations at the smallest level of the SNP. Indeed, that is where the theory logically must apply and that is the only place it has been tested. I have been critical of the neo-Darwinian paradigm in this book and elsewhere [35, 87, 36-38], maintaining that the Selfish Gene cannot explain the big picture in evolution. By the big picture I mean sex, aging, cooperation, speciation, evolvability, the structure of the genome. But I would not deny that standard theory can explain the small picture. Of course, the standard neo-Darwinian analysis works well for SNPs.

Withholding telomerase, allowing cells and whole animals to senesce, is a "big picture" adaptation, built deeply into the structure of the genome. One small part of this picture is ruled by just three SNPs and this small part appears to be guided by a tradeoff between cancer and other forms of mortality.

A Comparative Study of Rodent Species

Motivated by the cancer hypothesis as a premise, Vera Gorbunova and colleagues at University of Rochester undertook a comparative study of leukocyte telomere length in various species of rodents [39]. Based on the two examples of humans and mice, their hypothesis going into the study was that telomere length should be *inversely* correlated with lifespan and with body size. The rationale is that cancer generally takes a long time to germinate and longer-lived animals tend to have a higher risk of cancer and thus they need protection that shorter-lived animals can do without. Larger animals have that many more cells in which cancer may arise, so they expected telomere length to be inversely related to body size, too.

They measured characteristic telomere lengths for 15 rodent species and looked for relationships with lifespan and also body size. What they found was that telomere length is not correlated with mass or with body size. They went on to measure telomerase expression in a sample of stem cells, since stem cells are where cancer is thought to originate. There was great variability, uncorrelated with either lifespan or size. They measured telomerase activity in a variety of different tissues and found great variability from tissue to tissue, but not correlation with lifespan. They found a negative correlation between the average somatic telomerase activity and the log of body mass ($p = 0.002$). The authors noted the puzzling result that the finding was in somatic tissue only, while cancers arise in stem cells. Nevertheless, such is the power of presumption in favor of the cancer/telomere hypothesis that the results were reported as limited vindication for the theory that telomeres are limited in length as an evolved defense against cancer.

This is an influential paper that continues to be cited as primary evidence that the evolutionary purpose of telomerase rationing is to prevent cancer. Looking beyond the headline and the abstract, we have seen that the evidence it presents is indirect, ambiguous and tentative at best. In fact, the reason that this hypothesis has persisted in the research community is almost wholly theoretical.

Further Evidence Against the Cancer
Hypothesis of Telomere Rationing

In studies with mice, it has been found that excising the telomerase gene (TERT) actually increases the cancer rate [3, 40], while adding an ectopic gene for TERT does not increase cancer rates [41].

Before the Danish study, it was argued [42-44] that short telomere length is merely a marker for accumulated damage and not an independent cause of mortality. The robust data set demonstrating a residual predictive power of telomere length after effects from so many other risk factors are removed makes this far less plausible. Further tightening the case for programmed death is an understanding of the mechanism by which short telomeres lead through cell senescence to systemic self-destruction and disease.

Senescent cells are themselves at risk of becoming malignant. Short telomeres are detected by the cell's chromosome repair machinery as a form of DNA damage. Chromosome instability creates a risk of neoplastic conversion.

Damage is multiplied greatly by hormonal signals secreted by the senescent cell. This is "SASP", Senescence-Associated Secretory Phenotype [45]. Pro-inflammatory cytokines from the senescent cell can induce senescence in neighboring cells and raise the level of inflammation system-wide. Inflammation, in turn, has been associated with all the major diseases of old age. The toxic effect of senescent cells is strong enough that simply removing senescent cells substantially improves health and increases lifespan 20 to 30% (female and male, respectively) in mice [46].

The body's signaling pathways are not easily dismissed as "damage" or "dysregulation". In many, many contexts, signal transduction has been optimized for different adaptive functions. It is natural to assume that increase in pro-inflammatory signaling with age must have an adaptive purpose and we can judge by its result that this purpose is self-destruction. The interpretation of SASP as an aspect of programmed death is also consonant with the ancient evolutionary function of cellular senescence in protists.

Short telomeres leading to senescence can cause system-wide problems another way. Stem cells are responsible for renewing body tissues that are subject to high rates of damage: the stomach lining has the highest turnover rate in the body and skin cells and blood cells also have short lifetimes and need constantly to be renewed. Satellite cells are specialized stem cells for renewing muscles. When stem cells reach their Hayflick limit, they fall down on the job and in old age there are insufficient stem cells to maintain the digestive system, skin, blood and muscles. Leukocytes are a special case, because they must be able to replicate rapidly in response to infection. When leukocytes become senescent, the whole body is more vulnerable to disease. Old people commonly die of influenza, pneumonia and other infections that rarely kill people in the prime of life. Leukocytes are also important for elimination of cancerous and pre-cancerous cells and this contributes to the increase of cancer rates with age. This is another pathway by which short telomeres contribute to *higher* cancer rates.

Of all pathologies associated with short telomeres, cardiovascular disease is statistically the strongest and best established. Short telomeres affect the health of arteries [47, 48] as well as the muscle cells of the heart [49].

Telomere length is one mode of changing epigenetic profiles with age. Telomere length affects gene expression, the "telomere position effect" or TPE [6]; and though the telomere is only a tiny percentage of the length of a full chromosome, TPE can affect up to 3% of the genome [7]. Changes in gene expression with age are a direct cause of senescence [50-52] and the role of TPE is thus an indirect cause of senescence.

A battle still rages between researchers who say that short telomeres lead to cancer [53, 54] and those who say that long telomeres lead to cancer [55, 56]. But by now, it should be abundantly apparent that short telomeres are not only a marker of damage but also an independent cause of heart disease, cancer, Alzheimer's disease, frailty and increasing vulnerability to infectious disease [57, 58]. The sequestration of telomerase is not any kind of tradeoff or compromise, but poses a large net cost, accelerating the rate of aging and all its concomitant pathologies. Telomeric senescence is a clear, well-understood and abundantly documented mode of programmed aging.

Part II: Apoptosis

Apoptosis: Cell Suicide

The head of this chapter promised two evolutionarily ancient mechanisms of programmed death, both of which continue to play a role in the aging of our own bodies. The second is *apoptosis*.

It was first observed in the 1840s that cells sometimes kill themselves. Ordinarily, cells will fight approaching death with every means at their disposal. If they are short of food, they will conserve, then begin to digest inessential molecules. If they are short of oxygen, they will move into an anaerobic mode of energy generation. If they are poisoned, they pump the poison out of their cytoplasm as fast as they can. By the time they die, they are battle-worn and show multiple signs of damage. But in cell suicide, the cell makes orderly arrangements for its own demise. It chops up its DNA into pieces that can no longer direct the cell's metabolism. It burns (oxidizes using hydrogen peroxide) the highly-refined proteins that once regulated its chemistry. Far from resisting death, the cell is working in an efficient and orderly manner to shut down its own metabolism and turn itself into food for its neighbors. Apoptosis can be triggered in a process of self-policing, as when a cell detects that it has been infected by a virus and it falls on its sword rather than give the virus more opportunity to grow and spread. Pre-cancerous cells figure out that they are pre-cancerous and eliminate themselves with apoptosis. And when the young body is forming itself, much of its shape is sculpted not with creation but with destruction, as the unwanted in-between areas are eliminated with apoptosis.

Evolutionary Origins of Apoptosis

Mitochondria are organelles that dot the inside of every eukaryotic cell and burn sugar to generate its electrochemical energy. Lynn Margulis proposed in 1967 [59] that mitochondria are derived from aerobic bacteria, parasites that invaded the first eukaryotic cells and were gradually tamed and incorporated into cell metabolism over hundreds of millions of years. This hypothesis, so radical as to be nearly un-publishable at the time, has since become a standard part of textbook biology. Though mitochondria serve at the pleasure of the cell's central command in the nucleus, they retain a small snippet of their own DNA* and they have their own

---

* Only 13 genes remain in mitochondria Through the course of evolutionary time, most of the mitochondria's original DNA has migrated to the cell nucleus. It is in this way that the locus of control is maintained in the nucleus, where it belongs, for the health of the cell. Mitochondrial behavior and reproduction is tightly controlled from the nucleus.

reproduction cycle. Mitochondria die and new mitochondria are cloned from the old, even as the cell goes about its metabolic business. They reproduce, under tight control from the cell nucleus and maintain their numbers. They burn themselves out and need to be recycled.

Mitochondria retain from their pathogen past the capacity to kill the cell. They no longer do this for selfish reasons; the signal that initiates their murder-suicide originates in the command center of the cell nucleus. But the destruction is initiated by the same simple and highly reactive chemicals that are part of the mitochondrial energy-generating cycle. Hydrogen peroxide, H_2O_2, is a mitochondrial product and in excess quantities, it becomes both signal and one means of destruction. Normally, mitochondria have efficient chemical means to mop up their peroxide as fast as it is produced*. When the signal for self-destruction is received, mitochondria respond by creating peroxide in much larger quantities. The peroxide spreads through the cell, burning (oxidizing) essential biochemicals, efficiently destroying the cell.

The evolutionary history of apoptosis and its origin with the mitochondria is known well enough to biologists, but the radical message has not been assimilated. The message is that the capacity and the regulated mechanism for self-destruction has been part of the life cycle since before the first eukaryotes. It is more than two billion years old (far older than telomeres or conjugation). Apoptosis predates multicellular life. This means that programmed death exists in single-celled eukaryotes, where the cell is the entire organism. A suicide program evolved very early in life's history. Its purpose can only have been extreme altruism and its evolution must have involved group selection that overpowered individual selection.

But historically, apoptosis was discovered in higher animals as part of the developmental process and it is understood now as creative destruction, in the interest of the whole organism. Apoptosis has many "legitimate" functions in higher organisms, in the sense that they contribute positively to the individual's fitness. The shape of our hands is formed in utero via apoptosis of webs between the fingers. Remarkably, our brains, too, are formed by a process of subtraction, as many more neurons are created during foetal development than survive at birth [60]. Through a lifetime, cells that are infected or pre-cancerous detect that they are a threat to the body and undergo apoptosis for the sake of the whole organism. This function is controlled by the well-known gene p53 and every pre-cancerous lesion on the way to becoming full-blown cancer must mutate away the p53 gene before it can become malignant. The immune system relies on B-cells that are precisely targeted to attack invaders. The way this is accomplished is that a huge variety of B cells is being generated all the time and all those that do not latch onto invaders die via apoptosis. A tadpole maturing to a frog loses its tail through apoptosis. Cells in skin, blood and liver which are constantly renewing themselves rely on apoptosis for recycling.

It is easy to understand the evolutionary benefit of these roles for apoptosis, because they sacrifice a small part of the organism for the benefit of the whole. But

---

* The catalyst that neutralizes peroxide is co-enzyme Q and our bodies make plenty of it in our youth. As we get older, the body makes less and more of the corrosive peroxide leaks out into the cell, occasionally triggering the suicide of healthy cells. You can buy co-enzyme Q as a nutritional supplement, sold as CoQ10 in pharmacies and health food stores.

the idea that single-celled yeast cells would commit suicide for *each other's* sake was considered heresy. Valter Longo discovered this phenomenon while still a grad student at UCLA in the 1990s. The discovery almost derailed his career, because so many in the community rejected his findings. He endured almost as many journal rejections as had Margulis thirty years earlier. It was through his persistence and the clarity of his experimental design that he eventually won acceptance for his research and his result [2].

After Longo's work became accepted, researchers' minds were open to look at the life cycle of yeast in a new way. Their surprising discovery was that 'normal' death of a yeast cell also looks a lot like apoptosis. Perhaps triggered by replicative senescence, old yeast cells will politely slice up their own DNA, digest their proteins and turn themselves into food for their own daughters and other microbes in the vicinity [61, 62].

Yeast have an opportunistic life cycle. They reproduce via "budding" of a mother cell when food is plentiful. In nature this is most often in a rotting piece of fruit. When food becomes scarce the yeasts form spores and live in suspended animation until they have their next opportunity. Those that fail must starve to death. What Longo discovered is that during food shortages, the cells do not wait for starvation. They detect the food scarcity and 95% of them sacrifice themselves via apoptosis. They chop themselves up, digest their proteins and turn themselves into food for their cousins, so that the remaining 5% are well-equipped to form dried spores, which can survive a long time without food or water and offer the species its next big chance. The details that make this adaptation possible are curious, because the 95% and the 5% carry the same genes. What tells each individual cell whether to live or to die? Perhaps there is some stochasticity, a roll of the dice built into this genetically-programmed behavior; or perhaps the cell colony as a whole is capable of detecting how many cells have sacrificed themselves and instructing the remaining ones accordingly.

Neo-Darwinists were naturally skeptical of Longo's results because classical analysis says that this is not an ESS; a colony with this adaptation should be handily invaded by any variant that found a way to bias its odds of hanging back and not undergoing apoptosis, thereby benefitting from the altruistic suicide of the majority. Though Longo is a thorough and meticulous experimentalist, theorists took one look at his result and imagined that they knew better.

In all, it took about a decade for the reliability of his result to be established and now, two decades on, the community has yet to assimilate its message. But for researchers who understand the evolutionary origin of apoptosis and its relationship to mitochondria, it should be no surprise that the most primitive, one-celled organisms already used this suicide mechanism. The same functions that now protect the body from infections once protected a yeast colony from starvation. A diseased cell already has a high probability of dying, so it is a small sacrifice for it to die promptly and voluntarily, for the sake of depriving the infection of its cellular goodies. It is a larger sacrifice for a hungry cell among many other hungry cells to single itself out to die for the sake of the others.

In fact, group selection in this case is not so difficult to understand or to model. Though the mechanism by which the 95% participation rate in apoptosis is enforced is unknown, surely there is one and it is robust against random mutations. Colonies in which this mutation did arrive went extinct from starvation, while other colonies survived starvation under comparable circumstances. Hence the trait stayed in place long enough that eventually, after a much longer time, the chromosomes managed to rearrange themselves in such a way as to make this backward mutation very unlikely. Colonies in which the chromosomes were thus rearranged did not have the problem of periodic reversions and so the rearrangement took hold and became the predominant type we see today. This is group selection on a grand scale, a process that neo-Darwinists claim does not ever take place in nature.

The process is not well-understood by which the wall is built that prevents backward mutations into the blind alley of selfish behavior. We see its results, but do not have an effective way to observe the dynamic processes of evolution because they are so very slow. Could it be that these processes themselves involve apoptosis? Cells are programmed to commit suicide, to bow out when something is wrong. Perhaps the 'something' may include changes in the metabolism that mark the reversion from cooperative behavior back toward selfishness. This hypothesis has been promoted by Vladimir Skulachev, a biochemist at University of Moscow who is renowned in his own country, but relatively unknown in the West. At the end of a long and distinguished career studying the chemical energetics of mitochondria, Skulachev became convinced that the phenomenon of programmed death was widespread in nature, taking multiple forms at the level of organelle, cell and entire organism. "It is better to die than to be wrong [63]." This he calls the "Samurai principle of evolutionary biology." Apoptosis purges the body of diseased cells. It is relatively easy to understand the function in controlling epidemics. Skulachev theorizes that it also blocks blind evolutionary alleys. Cells that detect they have mutated in a direction which might offer only short-term, selfish advantages eliminate themselves for the sake of evolutionary integrity. Thus apoptosis itself is an evolvability adaptation. This is a radical position—probably more radical than I am willing to embrace without direct evidence, certainly beyond the pale for anyone whose perspective is framed by neo-Darwinism.

And Older Yet!

Programmed death in the form of apoptosis arrived with the first steps toward eukaryotic protozoa, three billion years ago. But there is an example of programmed death in bacteria that may be even older.

We think of bacteria as primitive, independent cells, each one fending for itself. But in fact bacteria commonly form structures with a collective purpose, in an early step toward multicellularity. In a true multicellular organism, cells form tissues and organs that support the whole, even though they have no possibility of reproducing themselves. Bacteria do not do this, but they can form biofilms that cover liquid nutrients and efficiently channel the nourishment to all their parts. In the process, they create porous structures with embedded flow channels. And how are the hollow channels created? The cells signal to each other in a way that indicates the shape and position of each; where the blueprint calls for empty tubes, the cells that occupy that region are told to eliminate themselves with programmed death.

But apoptosis is for eukaryotes. Bacteria do not have mitochondria and they do not have the metabolic machinery they would need to kill themselves in this way. The corresponding process in bacteria is called *autolysis*, meaning that the cell lyses or splits open to dump its chemical contents into the surrounding medium.

The way in which bacteria learned to kill themselves with autolysis closely echoes the story of mitochondria being adopted into the eukaryotic cell. The mitochondria were once infectious bacteria and they retain the capacity to kill the cell, though they never do so except when called upon to provide their murderous service by a cell nucleus that issues the command for suicide. Similarly, the bacterial genome contains DNA from an infectious virus (a 'bacteriophage') that long ago insinuated itself into the bacterial DNA, but is well regulated and prevented from harming the cell most of the time. But when the cell receives the news that its neighborhood is scheduled for demolition 'for the good of the biofilm', it orders its own destruction through autolysis and calls upon the ancient viral DNA to perform the execution [64, 65].

The message is that programmed death is probably even older than eukaryotic life.

The Role of Apoptosis in Whole-Body Aging

There is broad evidence that apoptosis also plays a role in mammalian aging. This evidence comes from human pathology and also from one animal study in which mice were genetically engineered to have a slower, less sensitive trigger for apoptosis. Diseases of old age in which apoptosis is implicated include Alzheimer's, Parkinson's, ALS, sarcopoenia (muscle loss), osteoporosis (bone loss) and Huntington's Disease.

Alzheimer's Disease in milder form is so prevalent among older people that it may be considered a condition of old age as well as an acute disease. In Europe and America, one person in five suffers from measurable cognitive impairment already by age 65 [66]. By age 90, the figure is three out of five [67]. Could it be that relatively healthy neurons are simply eliminating themselves and this is the primary cause of Alzheimer's disease? There is direct biochemical evidence of this [68], but it is such a radical idea that most researchers continue to propose it cautiously as a hypothesis. There are four lines of evidence:

- Caspases are enzymes that dismember proteins and they are most active during apoptosis. Elevated levels of caspases have been detected in early stages of AD [69].
- Alzheimer's disease runs in families, suggesting that part of the cause is genetic. In the 1990s, technology became available to identify the particular genes that are associated with AD and some of these genes have a primary role in regulating apoptosis.
- AD is characterized by massive loss of brain cells. Are these cells dying through a process of necrosis or apoptosis? In other words, is something killing the cells or are they eliminating themselves? Most studies of the biochemistry and appearance of the dying cells indicate that it is apoptosis

[70]. This is the more striking, since brain neurons are not supposed to undergo apoptosis at all after the very early stage of development. They do not turn over in an ongoing process of recycling, like skin or blood cells. In fact, they are the longest-lived cell group in the body.

- Do the cells become diseased and then eliminate themselves or do they eliminate themselves while they are still healthy? This is a difficult question to answer, because researchers do not get to watch the behavior of cells inside a living human brain. There is evidence that the amyloid plaques that are observed in autopsies to accompany the disease are triggering sensors on the outside of the brain cells that tell them to initiate apoptosis. Another theory is that mitochondria are more essentially involved, damaging the cells with excess reactive oxygen and then the damaged cells recognize themselves as such and go into apoptosis. Probably both processes are occurring.

From our perspective, it does not matter too much whether perfectly healthy cells are committing suicide or whether the cells are becoming damaged and the damage triggers a suicide mechanism. The point is that there is no danger to the body from these nerve cells. They do not harbor infections and they are not cancerous. So there is no legitimate reason for apoptosis to be invoked. There is no possible benefit to the individual whose brain is (rapidly or gradually) being dismantled in old age. The facts that Alzheimer's in mild form is near-universal and that the oldest mechanism for programmed death of a cell is being invoked as the executioner are further suggestions that AD is a genetic program for death on a timetable.

One more striking feature from the epidemiology of AD is the "use it or lose it" phenomenon. There is no particular physiological reason why neurons that are firing more often should be protected from apoptosis and yet intellectual activity is well-known to offer protection from dementia. It seems almost as if nature is saying to us, "we know you're not strong enough to contribute to your community as a workhorse at this stage, but we still value your wisdom. If you're not exercising your brain, then maybe it is time to bow out." Could natural selection at the group level possibly be that smart? Certainly, within the framework of neo-Darwinism, this is inconceivable.

Sarcopoenia and Parkinson's

Sarcopoenia is the age-related loss of muscle mass, leading to frailty, fractures and sometimes death. It is universal in humans, beginning usually around age 40. Some of the reason for muscle loss is simply healthy cells eliminating themselves via apoptosis [71, 72].

Young people almost never get Parkinson's and prevalence rises sharply with age. Early-stage Parkinson's is very, very common—perhaps universal in elderly people. The cause of Parkinson's is the loss of a particular kind of nerve cell in a particular part of the brain (*dopaminergic neurons* in the *substantia nigra*). It may be that these cells are eliminating themselves via apoptosis, even though our ability to move depends on them [73, 74].

Alzheimer's disease, Parkinson's disease and sarcopoenia are all common afflictions of the elderly, almost completely absent in young people. All three are connected to programmed cell death.

Apoptosis and Menopause

Women are born with tens of thousands of eggs in their ovaries, but through the course of their fertile lives, they go through only about 500 menstrual cycles. Around age 50, they run out of eggs and menopause ensues. What happened to all the rest of those eggs?

Each month, there are dozens of eggs that ripen, but only one passes into the *ampulla* where it is eligible for fertilization. The rest succumb to a process known as *atresia*, which is intimately related to apoptosis [75, 76]. The numbers are different for other mammals, but the outline of the story holds: the vast majority of a woman's eggs die unnecessarily and then she runs out of eggs and fertility ends. This is a direct link between apoptosis and reproductive aging, which is the most relevant form of aging for evolution. In this view, a woman's evolutionary 'death' is a direct result of programmed cell suicide.

There is a link to lifespan as well. It turns out that hormones from the ovaries have a *positive* effect on a woman's (and a mouse's) lifespan, defying the expectations of pleiotropic theory. When ovaries from a young mouse are transplanted into an old mouse, not only is her fertility restored, but her lifespan is extended as well [77-79]. Experimental treatments along this line are being tried in human cancer patients. Chemotherapy and radiation typically destroy a woman's fertility or create unacceptable risk of birth defects should she want to conceive after her cancer is cleared. In the experimental procedure, a piece of the woman's ovary is removed *before* her cancer treatment and flash frozen. Then, if cancer treatment is successful, her own ovary is thawed and re-implanted [80].

An Apoptosis Gene that Shortens Lifespan in Mice

In 1999, an Italian research group headed by Enrica Migliaccio discovered that they could make mice live 30% longer by deleting a gene that promotes apoptosis. This confirms that apoptosis is important in determining lifespan and it suggests that apoptosis is on a hair trigger, destroying healthy cells and cutting the animals' lives short as a result [81, 82].

The gene named *p66^{Shc}* is found in wild mice and laboratory mice and was knocked out in a line of mice developed in Migliaccio's lab. These mice lived longer and showed better resistance to stress and toxins. Migliaccio's 'p66-knockout' mice have inspired hundreds of papers in the ensuing decade, some of which report that they have improved resistance to cardiovascular damage [83] and to diabetes [84]. The knock-out mice regenerate more readily from physical injury [85] and show improved cognitive performance. They even suffer less liver damage after binge drinking [86].

What's going on? Is p66 an 'aging gene', pure and simple? Probably not. Neo-Darwinian understanding works well for traits governed by a single gene. If it is so easy for Migliaccio to knock out the p66 gene, then some mouse somewhere would have lost this gene by a chance mutation and its progeny would have survived to have more offspring and soon p66 would have been gone from the gene pool. Hence it is probable that the story is more complicated and that there are chromosome structures and genetic mechanisms that hold the p66 gene in place and prevent its loss. It is likely that benefits of p66 will be discovered, that help keep it in the genome despite its lifespan-shortening effects.

p66 may be an example of antagonistic pleiotropy, but not the kind of "compulsory" pleiotropy that has become the dominant theory for evolution of aging. Once we realize that aging is programmed for the good of the community, it becomes clear that there must be mechanisms in place that guard against cheaters and prevent the loss of traits that are important for the community. I have proposed that antagonistic pleiotropy, where it is observed, is an adaptation that prevents the loss of altruistic traits to short-term selection [87].

Summary: Replicative Senescence and Apoptosis

Apoptosis and cellular senescence are two ancient forms of programmed death that existed long before multicellular life. Both evolved at a time when their only conceivable function must have been to sacrifice individual cells for the long-term health of a cell colony. Both have carried forward into life forms and both are implicated in the aging and death functions of animals and plants.

It is clear that apoptosis has 'legitimate' functions in the bodies of higher animals, functions that support individual fitness. This is distinguished from the case of telomerase and replicative senescence; there the evidence for a positive role is weak and mostly theoretical. In man, telomere attrition functions primarily as a mechanism of programmed death. But apoptosis, in contrast, has many vital functions. Our everyday metabolisms have come to depend on apoptosis for defense and recycling.

Compulsory death in animal communities evolved in the same way and serves some of the same functions as programmed death in *Paramecia* and *Saccharomyces*. In the case of yeast, the primary function is population homeostasis and avoiding famines. In the case of ciliates, the population is turned over, diversity is enhanced and individual organisms are sacrificed for the long-term health of the community. Both functions are important to communities of higher organisms.

References

1. Karakashian, S.J., H.N. Lanners and M.A. Rudzinska, *Cellular and clonal aging in the suctorian protozoan Tokophrya infusionum.* Mech. Ageing Dev., 1984. **26**(2-3): p. 217-29.
2. Fabrizio, P., et al., *Superoxide is a mediator of an altruistic aging program in Saccharomyces cerevisiae.* J. Cell Biol., 2004. **166**(7): p. 1055-67.
3. Shay, J.W. and W.E. Wright, *Hayflick, his limit and cellular ageing.* Nat. Rev. Mol. Cell Biol., 2000. **1**(1): p. 72-6.

4. Strehler, B.L., *Time, Cells and Aging.* 1977, New York: Academic Press.
5. Witkowski, J., *The myth of cell immortality.* Trends Biochem. Sci., 1985. **10**(July): p. 258-260.
6. Baur, J.A., et al., *Telomere position effect in human cells.* Science, 2001. **292**(5524): p. 2075-2077.
7. Robin, J.D., et al., *Telomere position effect: regulation of gene expression with progressive telomere shortening over long distances.* Genes Dev., 2014. **28**(22): p. 2464-2476.
8. Bell, G., *The Masterpiece of Nature: The Evolution and Genetics of Sexuality.* 1982, Berkeley: University of California Press. 635 p.
9. Peck, J.R., *Sex causes altruism. Altruism causes sex. Maybe.* Proc. R. Soc. Lond., Ser. B: Biol. Sci., 2004. **271**(1543): p. 993-1000.
10. Maynard Smith, J., *Evolutionary Genetics.* 1989, New York: Oxford University Press.
11. Muller, H.J., *The relation of recombination to mutational advance.* Mutat. Res., 1964. **106**: p. 2-9.
12. Ridley, M., *The Red Queen.* 1993, London: Penguin.
13. Mitteldorf, J. and J. Travis, *An evolved mechanism to enforce gene-sharing.* forthcoming, 2017.
14. Lewis, W.M., Jr., *The cost of sex, In: The Evolution of Sex and its Consequences*, S. Stearns, Editor. 1987, Birkhäuser Basel. p. 33-57.
15. Layzer, D., *Genetic variation and progressive evolution.* Am. Nat., 1980. **115**(6): p. 809-826.
16. Rode, L., B.G. Nordestgaard and S.E. Bojesen, *Peripheral blood leukocyte telomere length and mortality among 64 637 individuals from the general population, In: J NCI Suppl Mat.* 2015.
17. Greider, C.W., *Telomeres, telomerase and senescence.* Bioessays, 1990. **12**(8): p. 363-369.
18. Sager, R., *Senescence as a mode of tumor suppression.* Environ. Health Perspect., 1991. **93**: p. 59-62.
19. Campisi, J., *Aging, cellular senescence and cancer.* Annu. Rev. Physiol., 2013. **75**: p. 685.
20. Cawthon, R.M., et al., *Association between telomere length in blood and mortality in people aged 60 years or older.* Lancet, 2003. **361**(9355): p. 393-5.
21. Rode, L., B.G. Nordestgaard and S.E. Bojesen, *Peripheral blood leukocyte telomere length and mortality among 64 637 individuals from the general population.* J. Nat. Cancer Inst., 2015. **107**(6): p. djv074.
22. Epel, E.S., et al., *Accelerated telomere shortening in response to life stress.* Proc. Natl. Acad. Sci. U.S.A., 2004. **101**(49): p. 17312-5.
23. Epel, E.S., et al., *Cell aging in relation to stress arousal and cardiovascular disease risk factors.* Psychoneuroendocrinology, 2006. **31**(3): p. 277-87.
24. Puterman, E., et al., *The power of exercise: buffering the effect of chronic stress on telomere length.* PLoS One, 2010. **5**(5): p. e10837.
25. Artandi, S.E., et al., *Constitutive telomerase expression promotes mammary carcinomas in aging mice.* Proc. Natl. Acad. Sci., 2002. **99**(12): p. 8191-8196.
26. Canela, A., et al., *Constitutive expression of tert in thymocytes leads to increased incidence and dissemination of T-cell lymphoma in lck-tert mice.* Mol. Cell. Biol., 2004. **24**(10): p. 4275-4293.
27. Gonzalez-Suarez, E., et al., *Increased epidermal tumors and increased skin wound healing in transgenic mice overexpressing the catalytic subunit of telomerase, mTERT, in basal keratinocytes.* EMBO J., 2001. **20**(11): p. 2619-30.

28. Katsimpardi, L., et al., *Vascular and neurogenic rejuvenation of the aging mouse brain by young systemic factors.* Science, 2014. **344**(6184): p. 630-634.

29. Shay, J.W. and W.E. Wright, *Does telomerase moonlight?* The Scientist, 2005. **19**(4): p. 18-19.

30. Flores, G., *New function for telomerase?* Genome. Biol., 2005. **5**(8): p. spotlight-20050819-02.

31. Park, J.-I., et al., *Telomerase modulates Wnt signalling by association with target gene chromatin.* Nature, 2009. **460**(7251): p. 66-72.

32. Cong, Y. and J.W. Shay, *Actions of human telomerase beyond telomeres.* Cell Res., 2008. **18**(7): p. 725-732.

33. Lee, J., et al., *TERT promotes cellular and organismal survival independently of telomerase activity.* Oncogene, 2008. **27**(26): p. 3754-3760.

34. Gould, S.J. and E.S. Vrba, *Exaptation-a missing term in the science of form.* Paleobiology, 1982: p. 4-15.

35. Mitteldorf, J., *Evolutionary orthodoxy: how and why the evolutionary theory of aging went astray.* Current aging science, 2014. **7**(1): p. 38-47.

36. Mitteldorf, J. and J. Pepper, *Selection in ecosystems. In: Fifth International Conference on Complex Systems.* 2004. Boston, MA: NECSI.

37. Mitteldorf, J. and J. Pepper, *How can evolutionary theory accommodate recent empirical results on organismal senescence?* Theory in Biosciences, 2007. **126**(1): p. 3-8.

38. Mitteldorf, J., *Neo-Darwinism and the group selection controversy, In: Lynn Margulis: The Life and Legacy of a Scientific Rebel*, D. Sagan, Editor. 2012, White River Junction, VT: Chelsea Green Publishing. p. 86-96.

39. Seluanov, A., et al., *Telomerase activity coevolves with body mass not life span.* Aging Cell, 2007. **6**(1): p. 45-52.

40. Rudolph, K.L., et al., *Longevity, stress response and cancer in aging telomerase-deficient mice.* Cell, 1999. **96**(5): p. 701-12.

41. Bernardes de Jesus, B., et al., *Telomerase gene therapy in adult and old mice delays aging and increases longevity without increasing cancer.* EMBO Mol. Med., 2012: p. 691-704.

42. Serra, V., et al., *Telomere length as a marker of oxidative stress in primary human fibroblast cultures.* Ann. N.Y. Acad. Sci., 2000. **908**(1): p. 327-330.

43. Houben, J.M., et al., *Telomere length assessment: biomarker of chronic oxidative stress?* Free Radical Biol. Med., 2008. **44**(3): p. 235-246.

44. Zglinicki, T.v. and C. Martin-Ruiz, *Telomeres as biomarkers for ageing and age-related diseases.* Curr. Mol. Med., 2005. **5**(2): p. 197-203.

45. Davalos, A., et al., *Senescent cells as a source of inflammatory factors for tumor progression.* Cancer Metastasis Rev., 2010. **29**(2): p. 273-283.

46. Baker, D.J., et al., *Clearance of p16Ink4a-positive senescent cells delays ageing-associated disorders.* Nature, 2011. **479**(7372): p. 232-236.

47. Chang, E. and C.B. Harley, *Telomere length and replicative aging in human vascular tissues.* Proc. Natl. Acad. Sci., 1995. **92**(24): p. 11190-11194.

48. Samani, N.J., et al., *Telomere shortening in atherosclerosis.* The Lancet, 2001. **358**(9280): p. 472-473.

49. Oh, H., et al., *Telomere attrition and Chk2 activation in human heart failure.* Proc. Natl. Acad. Sci., 2003. **100**(9): p. 5378-5383.

50. Johnson, A.A., et al., *The role of DNA methylation in aging, rejuvenation and age-related disease.* Rejuvenation Research, 2012. **15**(5): p. 483-494.

51. Mitteldorf, J., *How does the body know how old it is? Introducing the epigenetic clock hypothesis.* Biochemistry (Moscow), 2013. **78**(9): p. 1048-1053.

52. Rando, T.A. and H.Y. Chang, *Aging, rejuvenation and epigenetic reprogramming: resetting the aging clock.* Cell, 2012. **148**(1): p. 46-57.

53. Donate, L.E. and M.A. Blasco, *Telomeres in cancer and ageing.* Philos. Trans. R. Soc. Lond. B Biol. Sci., 2011. **366**(1561): p. 76-84.

54. Nan, H., et al., *Genetic variants in telomere-maintaining genes and skin cancer risk.* Hum. Genet., 2011. **129**(3): p. 247-53.

55. Mehdipour, P., et al., *Evolutionary hypothesis of telomere length in primary breast cancer- and brain tumor-patients: a tracer for Genomic-tumor heterogeneity and instability.* Cell Biol. Int., 2011. **35**(9): p. 915-925.

56. Liu, J., et al., *Longer leukocyte telomere length predicts increased risk of hepatitis b virus-related hepatocellular carcinoma: a case-control analysis.* Cancer, 2011. **117**(18): p. 4247-4256.

57. Blasco, M., *Telomeres and human disease: ageing, cancer and beyond.* Nat. Rev. Genet., 2005. **6**(August): p. 611-622.

58. Fossel, M., *Cells, Aging and Human Disease.* 2004, New York: Oxford University Press. 489.

59. Sagan, L., *On the origin of mitosing cells.* J. Theor. Biol., 1967. **14**(3): p. 225-IN6.

60. Roth, K.A. and C. D'Sa, *Apoptosis and brain development.* Mental retardation and developmental disabilities research reviews, 2001. **7**(4): p. 261-266.

61. Herker, E., et al., *Chronological aging leads to apoptosis in yeast.* J. Cell Biol., 2004. **164**(4): p. 501-507.

62. Fabrizio, P. and V.D. Longo, *Chronological aging-induced apoptosis in yeast.* Biochim. Biophys. Acta, 2008. **1783**(7): p. 1280-1285.

63. Skulachev, I.V., *Phenoptosis: programmed death of an organism.* Biochemistry (Mosc.), 1999. **64**(12): p. 1418-1426.

64. Webb, J.S., et al., *Cell death in pseudomonas aeruginosa biofilm development.* J. Bacteriol., 2003. **185**(15): p. 4585-92.

65. Gordeeva, A.V., Y.A. Labas and R.A. Zvyagilskaya, *Apoptosis in unicellular organisms: mechanisms and evolution.* Biochemistry-Moscow, 2004. **69**(10): p. 1055-1066.

66. Hendrie, H.C., *Epidemiology of dementia and Alzheimer's disease.* Am. J. Geriatr. Psychiatry, 1998. **6**(2 Suppl 1): p. S3-18.

67. Launer, L.J., et al., *Rates and risk factors for dementia and Alzheimer's disease: results from EURODEM pooled analyses. EURODEM Incidence Research Group and Work Groups. European Studies of Dementia.* Neurology, 1999. **52**(1): p. 78-84.

68. Su, J.H., et al., *Immunohistochemical evidence for apoptosis in Alzheimer's disease.* Neuroreport, 1994. **5**(18): p. 2529-33.

69. D'Amelio, M., et al., *Caspase-3 triggers early synaptic dysfunction in a mouse model of Alzheimer's disease.* Nat. Neurosci., 2011. **14**(1): p. 69-76.

70. Behl, C., *Apoptosis and Alzheimer's disease.* J. Neur. Trans., 2000. **107**(11): p. 1325-1344.

71. Marzetti, E. and C. Leeuwenburgh, *Skeletal muscle apoptosis, sarcopoenia and frailty at old age.* Exp. Gerontol., 2006. **41**(12): p. 1234-8.

72. Pistilli, E.E., J.R. Jackson and S.E. Alway, *Death receptor-associated pro-apoptotic signaling in aged skeletal muscle.* Apoptosis, 2006. **11**(12): p. 2115-26.

73. Mochizuki, H., et al., *Histochemical detection of apoptosis in Parkinson's disease.* J. Neurol. Sci., 1996. **137**(2): p. 120-3.

74. Lev, N., E. Melamed and D. Offen, *Apoptosis and Parkinson's disease.* Prog. Neuropsychopharmacol. Biol. Psychiatry, 2003. **27**(2): p. 245-50.

75. Bosco, L., et al., *Apoptosis in human unfertilized oocytes after intracytoplasmic sperm injection.* Fertil. Steril., 2005. **84**(5): p. 1417-23.

76. Morita, Y. and J.L. Tilly, *Oocyte apoptosis: like sand through an hourglass.* Dev. Biol., 1999. **213**(1): p. 1-17.

77. Cargill, S.L., et al., *Age of ovary determines remaining life expectancy in old ovariectomized mice.* Aging Cell, 2003. **2**(3): p. 185-90.

78. Mason, J.B., et al., *Transplantation of young ovaries to old mice increased life span in transplant recipients.* J. Gerontol. A-Biol., 2009. **64A**(12): p. 1207-1211.

79. Mason, J.B., et al., *Transplantation of young ovaries restored cardioprotective influence in postreproductive-aged mice.* Aging Cell, 2011. **10**(3): p. 448-456.

80. Huser, M., et al., *Ovarian tissue cryopreservation in cancer patients–six years of clinical experience.* Ceska. Gynekol., 2012. **77**(2): p. 118-26.

81. Orsini, F., et al., *The life span determinant p66Shc localizes to mitochondria where it associates with mitochondrial heat shock protein 70 and regulates trans-membrane potential.* J. Biol. Chem., 2004. **279**(24): p. 25689-95.

82. Migliaccio, E., et al., *The p66shc adaptor protein controls oxidative stress response and life span in mammals.* Nature, 1999. **402**(6759): p. 309-13.

83. Napoli, C., et al., *Deletion of the p66Shc longevity gene reduces systemic and tissue oxidative stress, vascular cell apoptosis and early atherogenesis in mice fed a high-fat diet.* Proc. Natl. Acad. Sci. U.S.A., 2003. **100**(4): p. 2112-6.

84. Rota, M., et al., *Diabetes promotes cardiac stem cell aging and heart failure, which are prevented by deletion of the p66shc gene.* Circ. Res., 2006. **99**(1): p. 42-52.

85. Zaccagnini, G., et al., *p66(ShcA) and oxidative stress modulate myogenic differentiation and skeletal muscle regeneration after hind limb ischemia.* J. Biol. Chem., 2007. **282**(43): p. 31453-9.

86. Koch, O.R., et al., *Role of the life span determinant P66(shcA) in ethanol-induced liver damage.* Lab. Invest., 2008. **88**(7): p. 750-60.

87. Mitteldorf, J., *Adaptive aging in the context of evolutionary theory.* Biochemistry (Moscow), 2012. **77**(7): p. 716-725.

6
CHAPTER

Evolving Population Control

Synopsis

The key to resolving the paradox of aging in evolution is to question the persistence of ecosystems. In both neo-Darwinism and MLS theory, a static ecosystem is assumed as the background within which evolution of a single species occurs. But demographic stability is not to be taken for granted. A race among individuals to reproduce as fast as possible can lead to a tragedy of the commons. If individual organisms succeed, then they do so by grabbing the available resources more aggressively than their sisters and brothers. Then they produce offspring that are even more profligate in the next generation. This process of evolving individual super-competitors leads to collective consequences that can destroy the ecosystem on which all their lives and their children's lives depend. No species that is evolved to reproduce without restraint can expect to survive more than a few generations in its habitat. This is the dynamic we examine in this chapter.

Yes, evolutionary fitness is about efficient reproduction; but it is also about stability and sustainability. All animal populations exist in the context of an ecosystem and if they kill the tree in which they are perched, the tree brings them down with it. Hence species have evolved cooperation in order to tame the boom/bust cycles of nature: to prevent extinction.

The science of ecosystem stability—like the science of aging—has run afoul of evolutionary theory and has its own contentious history. The two stories are intertwined.

Taking Stock

We have seen abundant evidence that group selection has been far more effective than theory would lead us to believe. Even the expanded framework of multilevel selection theory fails to predict natural selection of such adaptations as dioecious sex, which have steep short-term costs and advantages that only accrue over many generations.

The previous chapters contain a diverse body of evidence that aging, like sex, has evolved based on its adaptive value to a unit of selection larger than the individual. It is easier to see that the prevailing evolutionary theories of aging are flawed than to construct a plausible theory to replace them. It is not merely that there are so many diverse forms of aging in different species, so many kinds of phenomena that demand explanation. Even the basic facts constitute a genuine scientific dilemma.

If it were only a matter of demonstrating an evolutionary advantage for aging, this would be easy. Aging helps maintain population diversity, it increases population turnover and (through these two effects) aging enhances the rate at which a population can adapt and evolve. Although these advantages are effective, they cannot compete with the immediate benefit of increased lifespan and extended fertility; the benefits of aging take a long time to manifest and they accrue to a broad community, not just to the individuals within that community whose genes cause them to die early. In any mixed community of agers and non-agers, the non-agers have all the advantages of the extra slots in the niche freed up by those others that die of old age, but none of the disadvantages of weakening and dying themselves. Why would the non-agers fail to dominate?

The neo-Darwinists are correct in saying that evolution of aging as an adaptation cannot take place within the context of the selfish gene paradigm, the only mechanism that neo-Darwinists recognize. And they are correct in demanding that an evolutionary theory should stipulate a mechanism in detail and should substantiate an evolutionary advantage for aging sufficiently strong to overcome its manifest disadvantage. The next logical step is Multilevel Selection Theory (MLS). But we shall see that the MLS paradigm confirms that aging should not be able to compete with non-aging and should be rejected by natural selection. If aging has evolved as an adaptation, it has done so via a mechanism outside the models of the selfish gene and outside the extensions to that model that have been developed in MLS.

The challenge is clear: to find the least radical extension of MLS that can support the evolution of aging as an adaptation. What assumptions of MLS theory can be relaxed? What can be added to the MLS picture that would help us understand how aging might have evolved?

If evolutionary theory is to be broadened to encompass unrecognized mechanisms, the most plausible and economical extension is to consider evolution of populations and entire ecosystems. When we ask how it came about that there are stable, persistent ecosystems, we may begin to understand that there are evolutionary forces powerful enough to compete with the Selfish Gene. In this context, a new theory of aging will take its place, but not before calling into question the postulates of neo-Darwinism.

We shall see that population dynamics provides the only selective mechanism that is rapid and potent enough to be a plausible counterweight to individual selection for higher fertility and longer life.

Sustainability is the Missing Piece of the Puzzle

How must the neo-Darwinian paradigm be extended to be broad enough to embrace adaptive aging? The short answer is: ecosystem stability. Neo-Darwinian analysis and MLS are conceived in the context of a stable population, in a stable biological environment. It is assumed that the total population and the condition of the surrounding ecosystem remain stable while some genes succeed in launching more copies of themselves at the expense of other genes. But nature does not always behave this way. The environment can change substantially from one generation to the next and—crucially—there is a feedback loop. The present behaviors of parents, in the aggregate, contribute to shaping the ecology into which their children are born. The behaviors of each generation affect the environment in which the next generation grows up.

Early in the 20th century, the science of population genetics was formulated by scientists with impressive mathematical sophistication, but little experience with wildlife. They knew that in nature, ecosystem communities often persist and remain stable over many generations. Species extinctions are rare compared to individual deaths. It was natural for them to take the fact of ecosystem stability as a simplifying assumption to make the formidable problem of genetic evolution more tractable. Hence the stability of ecosystems was taken as an implicit assumption by the inventors of neo-Darwinism, an assumption that became explicit during the "group selection" debates of 1966-1975. In the standard population genetic model, unchanging ecosystems are the assumptive background within which alternative alleles vie for prevalence.

We now ask, how it has come to be true that (most) ecosystems are stable and resilient. Is it just something that happens when you throw together a large number of diverse players, each clamoring for domination? Is it the "invisible hand" of a competitive marketplace at work? Or is stability the result of a Darwinian process, a long period of trial-and-error before organisms learned the communal traits that would allow them to coexist as predator and prey, as parasite and host, symbiont and commensal? Can it be that entire ecosystems are co-evolved for stability?

These questions have a history, a scientific story every bit as intricate and contentious as the evolution of aging. In fact, the two stories interweave and the evolutionary emergence of aging can only be understood in the context of ecosystem evolution.

The Rocky Mountain Locust: A Morality Tale

Populations can explode and overshoot their carrying capacity; whole species can crash to extinction, carrying their ecosystem with them into the dust. A stable ecosystem must not be taken for granted and no species can afford to trash its ecosystem*. Through historical examples, through studying the work of computational ecologists and through my own computer modeling, I have come to believe that it is actually quite a trick to construct a stable ecosystem out of many unrelated species, each of which is trying to grow exponentially at the expense of the others. I think the only reason that we see stable ecosystems in nature is that evolution has arranged it so, and this is the missing piece from the standard picture of how natural selection operates. Ecosystem stability is a collective adaptation, evolved in a Darwinian process on an extended scale of time and space.

---

* Exceptions includes some highly mobile predators that have evolved a hit-and-run lifestyle.

An ecosystem that is out of balance is in danger of collapsing to extinction, taking all its species out when it loses one or two that throw the populations out of balance. But a robust ecosystem is able to thrive and to expand its territorial dominion, with all its constituent species moving and growing together. A robust ecosystem resists disturbances (from within or without) and is able to restore homeostasis when it is upset. The individual life history qualities that make an ecosystem able to compete with other ecosystems can be a target of natural selection.

In the late nineteenth century, the American Midwest was plagued periodically by incursions of Rocky Mountain locusts. The appearance of this pest was devastating and unforgettable. Laura Ingalls Wilder wrote in her childhood memoir [1]:

> Huge brown grasshoppers were hitting the ground all around her, hitting her head and her face and her arms. They came thudding down like hail. The cloud was hailing grasshoppers. The cloud was grasshoppers. Their bodies hid the sun and made darkness. Their thin, large wings gleamed and glittered. The rasping, whirring of their wings filled the whole air and they hit the ground and the house with the noise of a hailstorm. Laura tried to beat them off. Their claws clung to her skin and her dress. They looked at her with bulging eyes, turning their heads this way and that. Mary ran screaming into the house. Grasshoppers covered the ground, there was not one bare bit to step on. Laura had to step on grasshoppers and they smashed squirming and slimy under her feet.

In 1874, a swarm was described as being half a million square kilometers in area (for comparison, California is 425,000 sq Km). When a cloud descended, the land was denuded of everything green for many miles in all directions. The ground was thick with egg masses, ready to renew the plague the following year.

But the last reported sighting of a Rocky Mountain locust was in 1902. There are preserved specimens in museums and laboratories today, but no living locusts. Entomologists interested in the locust's rise and fall travel to the glaciers of Wyoming, mining hundred-year-old ice for carcasses that they might study.

It appears that the Rocky Mountain Locust drove itself to extinction by overshooting its sustainable population. These locusts did not die out because they were insufficiently "fit"—in the sense of aggressive competition and prolific reproduction. They disappeared because they were *too aggressive* and *too prolific*. If this kind of event is rare in the present, it is only because natural selection has been at work for hundreds of millions of years, punishing species that were individually superperformers, but were collectively unable to restrain their numbers and avoid population crashes.

Why is the Earth Green?

Why is the sky blue? Every child asks this question eventually and pursuit of an answer can extend well into the career of a college physics major. The sun's blackbody spectrum is 5700 Kelvin, peaked in the yellow, but molecules of nitrogen and oxygen that make up our atmosphere have vibrational resonances at much higher frequencies, in the ultraviolet. Because the frequencies are mismatched, there is very little interaction between visible light and molecules of air, but higher light frequencies are closer to the UV end of the spectrum and interact more strongly with the molecules. Thus the yellow and red light from the sun tends to go right through 10 Km of air to reach our eyes, but the blue and violet light bounces around among the air molecules and comes to us from every which way. "Sky blue" represents the highest frequencies that are present in the sun's yellowish spectrum.

Why is the earth green? Another question a child may ask, this one reaching deep into ecodynamics. Though it is seldom addressed in this form, it is a story that will lead us into a major theme of this book and interesting as well in its own right.

The proximate answer, of course, is that green is the color of the molecule chlorophyl, which is the most efficient solar collector known to man. Chlorophyl turns sunlight into biologically usable chemical energy (food) better than any other substance and so important is this function that all those living things that make their living directly from the sun must use it or else lag behind and fail to compete with those that do.

But the part of the question on which I want to focus attention is this: Animals all depend on green plants for food. Animals are in competition for each other to expand and sustain their numbers. Growth and reproduction, for an animal, depends on the conversion of food biomass. Consumption is the universal bottleneck, determining the rate of growth and reproduction. Given the relentless competition for animal growth, why do we not see the level of predation rise to the point where green shoots are consumed pretty much as soon as they come out of the ground? Why does the food pyramid flourish so spectacularly at its base that (wherever there is water) the earth looks green from above?

Most of the earth's biomass is in the form of cellulose and only specialized bacteria can digest cellulose. Leaves and wood can be food only for animals that host these bacteria in their guts—termites and ruminant mammals. That is the beginning of an explanation.

Cellulose and starch are both chains of 6-carbon sugars, differing only in conformal structure that affects shape of the molecule (and steric access of digestive hormones to the most active chemical bonds).

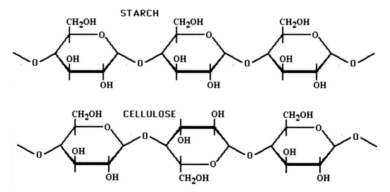

The chemical structures of cellulose and starch differ only in the directional shape of oxygen bonds that link sugars together in a chain. Starch molecules tend to coil around, making the links accessible to chemical attack from the outside, while cellulose molecules are linear, and the links are better protected from chemical attack.

We know that cellulases evolved in several different bacterial species and that a huge adaptive benefit accrues to any species that is able to tap into the most abundant food source on earth. Why have so few animals evolved to do this?

The answer, I suggest, is that the keys to this wooden chest, like Pandora's box, carry an awesome destructive potential and must be wielded with great care and restraint, on pain of wholesale destruction of ecosystems, which, of course, quickly bring about the extinction of the species that opened the box. Any species that learns to digest cellulose must find a way to limit its numbers and its rate of growth.

An ecosystem containing powerful, greedy predators is not just a barren ecosystem of rather low productivity—it is unstable and must collapse.

Stability of the Two-Species System

If the predator's (collective) success is measured by the total population that can be sustained ("K-selection" [2]), it is clear that protecting the prey species at high levels, close to the "untouched" carrying capacity, is the best strategy. This was pointed out in a classic paper of Slobodkin [3]. But this conclusion rests on an abstract notion of fitness, one step removed from the mechanics of selection.

Here we show why, quite generally, a predator *must* maintain the prey at levels close to the carrying capacity. To do otherwise leads to prompt ecosystem collapse.

Consider a toy ecosystem comprising two species, a consumer (y) and a producer (x), which I will call sheep and grass. The grass, in the absence of the sheep, grows exponentially at low density, asymptotes to a fixed carrying capacity at high density. This behavior is classically modeled with a logistic curve.

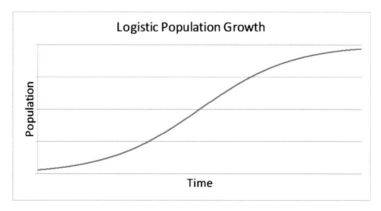

Classic logistic growth curve.

The logistic curve is solution of the differential equation

$$dx/dt = x(1 - x)$$

This equation says that the growth rate of the grass is small when the grass density is small, rises to a maximum at intermediate levels of grass coverage and falls to zero when coverage reaches its carrying capacity.

If the grass ever exceeds carrying capacity, the curve continues downward, reflecting negative growth that brings the population back to the sustainable limit. But in the simplest assumption, feedback of grass density on growth rate is instantaneous and under these circumstances, the grass approaches its carrying capacity smoothly and asymptotically, either from above or below.

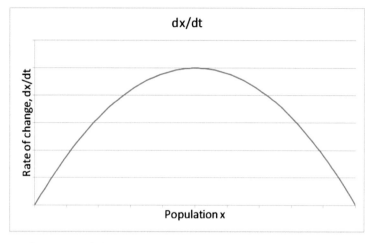

Another view of the same logistic equation. Rate of change of the population is plotted against the population itself.

Only the qualitative shape of the curve is important for the dynamic we want to examine. In reality, the shape of the curve is often skewed to the right, because onset of the damping effect of limiting resources is steep.

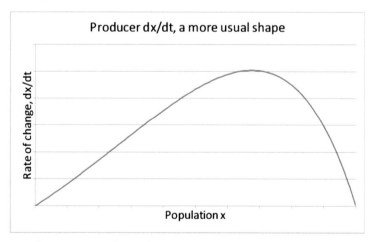

In real ecosystems, the peak rate of change tends to be skewed to the right, i.e., closer to the carrying capacity.

It is reasonable to assume that the grazing of the sheep is some function of the number of sheep and of the grass coverage and that the function increases monotonically with both arguments. The more sheep, the more they eat and the more grass is available, the more they will eat. Whatever they eat is subtracted from the growth rate of the grass:

$$dx/dt = \text{logistic growth} - \text{predation} = x(1-x) - f(x, y)$$

For a constant value of *y*, the two components of *dx/dt* might look like this:

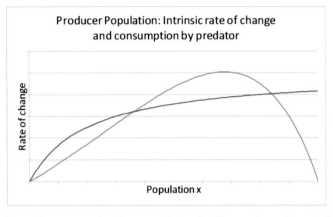

Rate of consumption by a predator (red) may be subtracted from the intrinsic logistic growth (blue) of the prey population.

Let's look now for stable, steady-state solutions. "Steady-state" means that *x* and *y* are both constant, so *dy/dt* = 0 and *dx/dt* = 0. "Stable" means that if either *x* or *y* varies slightly from their steady-state values, the dynamic is such as to restore each one toward steady-state.

Steady state can occur when the two curves cross, so that the net change in *x* is zero. This happens, very generally given the shape of the curves, at two points, one to the left and the other to the right of the peak. Both are steady state solutions. (The curves also cross where both *x* and *y* are 0. This represents extinction.)

We ask now about stability of the two solutions. It is appropriate to focus on *dx/dt* first, because grass grows more quickly than sheep. (We find rather generally in nature that predators have longer life histories with slower growth than prey. This can be interpreted as an adaptation for system stability.)

The difference between the two curves looks like this:

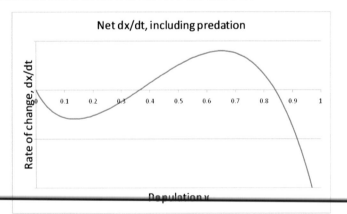

The net rate of change of the prey population is the difference between red and blue curves plotted in the above fig.

Steady states are at the zero crossings, where $dx/dt = 0$. The crossing on the right (here shown about 0.83) is stable, because a little to the left of the crossing, dx/dt is positive and a little to the right, dx/dt is negative. Thus x tends to be restored to the steady state value. Likewise, the crossing at the far left (extinction) is also stable. Small values of x lead to dx/dt that is negative, terminating in extinction. But the middle crossing (around 0.36 in our example) is unstable. If grass cover is just a bit more than 0.36, then it will continue to increase until it reaches 0.83. But if coverage falls below 0.36, dx/dt is negative and the grass will be gobbled up by increasingly desperate sheep until there is none left.

The conclusion is that the sheep must arrange their grazing intensity, life history and population dynamics in such a way as to maintain nearly full grass coverage. The "green earth" solution on the right is stable. The "brown earth" solution on the left is on a path to extinction.

The Sheep Population Must also Find a Stable Equilibrium

The sheep population grows much more slowly than the grass. The sheep have the luxury of averaging over fluctuations in the grass cycle. But in the long run, they must maintain a stable steady state as well,

$$dy/dt = 0$$

The simplest assumption about the sheep is that their population growth depends on the food they are able to forage and that depends on the grass coverage. Physiologically, we might expect that the growth rate of the sheep is a monotonically increasing function of the grass consumed per capita.

$$dy/dt \sim f(x, y)$$

where "$\sim$" is meant to indicate not strict proportionality, but any monotonically increasing function. The danger for the sheep arises because populations will tend to fluctuate stochastically. If the sheep population should rise above the steady-state value, they must not persist with the same individual consumption behavior as though they had a sustainable population. Since there is plenty of grass, the sheep as individuals will be tempted to eat just as much as they did when the population was within sustainable limits.

Suppose the sheep were individually adapted only, without willingness to adjust their consumption behavior based on danger to the community or without sensing population density at all. Here is what the curves for dx/dt would look like with 10%, 20% and 30% overpopulation, assuming the sheep's consumption (per capita) depends only on the grass coverage.

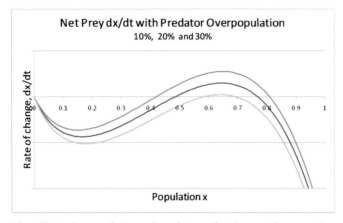

The effect of a population of predators that is over the carrying capacity on the rate of change of the prey population. The blue curve is 10% excess, red is 20% excess and green is 30% excess. The message is that even a small excess over carrying capacity is sufficient to drive the prey population (temporarily) to zero, risking extinction (permanent) of the predator.

In this example, 10% looks manageable and 20% looks dangerous. 30% overpopulation translates to no margin at all. *dx/dt* is negative everywhere and the grass coverage is collapsing to zero. In the real world, this means extinction for the sheep. The grass will eventually recover, re-seeded by a far-off wind.

Though the specific numbers in this example are arbitrary, the general finding is that there is a looming tragedy of the commons [4]. Natural populations of large animals typically range over a factor of 3 or more. A 30% margin for avoiding extinction is not viable, not even close. If predator species are not adapted in some way to sense crowding and avoid food shortages *before they occur*, then a collective tragedy is unavoidable.

The earth is green because every animal species is collectively adapted to protect the base of its food chain. No ecosystem can be stable in the long term without a large, standing producer reservoir at its base.

The present analysis is not standard ecological theory. Standard theory as quoted in textbooks is often based on a pair of differential equations due (independently) to Lotka and Volterra. Lotka-Volterra dynamics leads to less restrictive predictions about stability, as we shall see in the next section.

An Ecosystem in a Bottle

When Leo Luckinbill was a grad student in the Zoology Department at UCLA in the late 1960s, mathematical ecology was in its heyday. The field had evolved largely from pure thought, pushed forward by mathematicians and physicists. Their *modus operandi* was the most fruitful methodology of classical physics: First they would abstract from a system a differential equation* that describes the way

---

* Just as the solution to an algebraic equation is a number (or family of numbers), the solution to a differential equation is a graph (or family of graphs), showing how one some quantities change over time.

in which it changes over time, given its present status. There was already a rich theoretical literature of such equations and their solutions, but very little contact with experiment. "As a consequence, mathematical models of simple predator-prey systems have been developed to a degree of sophistication far advanced beyond the support of empirical experimentation," he noted. Luckinbill's plan for his dissertation was to compare the behavior of the simplest solutions to the simplest ecosystem he could create in the lab.

He prepared a water bottle with appropriate nutrients and seeded it with two protist species, one of which is known to eat the other [5]. In ponds the world over, *Didinia* thrive on *Paramecia* and Luckinbill thought it would be an easy matter to establish this simplest ecosystem in his lab, by providing food for the *Paramecia* and allowing the *Paramecia* to provide food for the *Didinia*. He would observe the system through a microscope and track the numbers of the two species as they changed over time.

But the result of the experiment was more interesting than he had anticipated and his careful observations and analysis helped launched a new wave of thinking in the field. No matter how he tried to set up the advantage of one species or the other, Luckinbill always found that one of two things would happen: Either the *Paramecia* would fend off the predators and all the *Didinia* would die out; or else the *Paramecia* would be wiped out entirely by the predators and then the *Didinia* would starve to death. This would happen quickly — in a matter of hours. He was unable to establish a stable community with predator and prey in balance, so long as they were freely mixed in one bottle. Remember the condition,"freely mixing in a single bottle"—we shall come back and finish this story in Chapter 8.

The differential equation that theorists had used to describe this situation is the Lotka-Volterra equation and it is "neutral stable". This means that it will cycle forever, repeating the same shape curve, without a tendency for the cycling to grow in amplitude over time or to damp out to a constant.

$$\frac{dx}{dt} = ax - bxy$$

$$\frac{dy}{dt} = cxy - dy$$

(where a, b, c and d are constants, t is time and y and x are predator and prey populations, respectively, as above).

Solutions to the Lotka-Volterra equations can be very flat, with little amplitude or they can look like periodic population blooms, with long periods of near-zero population in between. Curiously, the character of the solution is completely determined by the initial ratio of predator to prey. Theorists imagined that nature must have found ways to keep the stable solutions and standard practice among theorists was to amend the original Lotka-Volterra equation with a simple, plausible extra term that assured stability.

But in lab experiments, stability seemed to be elusive in a way the equations did not predict.

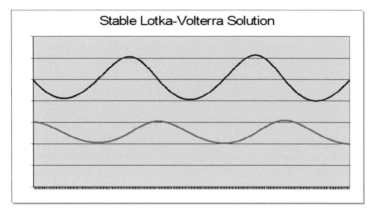

This graph shows how the number of predators (pink) and prey (blue) change over time. The curves are derived by solving a standard differential equation. The populations vary periodically, but never fall so low as to risk extinction.

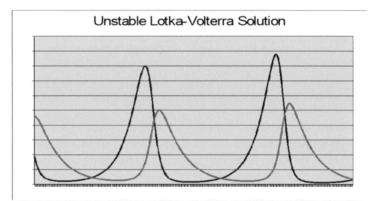

This graph shows another solution of the same equation, this one quite unstable. Population counts for predators and prey both dip very close to zero and stay there a long time. If this were reality of idealized mathematics, this would be extinction.

After 1973, a number of lab experiments were performed with different species. They all found instability, leading to rapid extinction. A few scientists looked for evidence of this kind of instability with simple ecological systems in the wild, but the wild ecologies seemed to be unaccountably stable [6]. How does nature avoid the wild population fluctuations and quick extinctions that characterize laboratory systems and also theoretical models?

It seems plausible that ecosystem stability is an evolved trait. A detective might note that nature has the means, the motive and the opportunity. Indeed, there have been a few articles in prominent ecology journals suggesting this possibility [7] but they have not taken root in the scientific community. Most evolutionary theorists prefer to see ways that more traditional modes of natural selection might lead incidentally to population stability [8, 9]. The reason why is clear: to embrace this mechanism is to abandon the Selfish Gene, foundation of neo-Darwinism. This would be a fundamental change in the way that evolutionary biology is understood.

Based on any one study or one experimental result, to abandon a good theory would not be good science. But, in fact, there is an abundance of evidence from diverse phenomena in biology, all suggesting that the Selfish Gene is not the whole story. It is long past time for a theoretical acknowledgment of these other mechanisms of natural selection. (More of this story to come in Chapter 8.)

Theorists are Surprised

What had theorists been thinking before Luckinbill? Theorists, especially in biology, like to look for reasons that the world is the way it is. Stable ecosystems are observed in nature, so stability became the "right answer" that the theorists were seeking from their equations. With hindsight, it would be unfair to judge them as naïve. There are many ways to arrange the terms of an equation and many approaches to analyzing stability.

Michael Rosenzweig today is a wise elder of the ecology community, advocating passionately for simple measures that might help humans to coexist with other species in a quasi-natural ecology. When I asked him whether it could be true that ecosystems were stable only because they were evolved to be that way, he would say only that it is a deep question. This was a remarkably open-minded answer from a man who, in his youth, laid the theoretical foundation for the thesis that ecosystem stability is a "free" byproduct of individual competition.

In 1962, Rosenzweig was a bright Ivy undergrad, when he worked with his faculty adviser on the article that was and is often quoted as the definitive analysis of ecological stability [10–12]. Erudite and abstractly mathematical, his analysis introduced a new and elegant way to visualize simultaneous changes in predator and prey populations. But at the root, the idea was very similar to economic theory of supply and demand: Rosenzweig and MacArthur identified an equilibrium and asked whether small departures from that equilibrium tend to expand over time or to drift back toward equilibrium. Part of the reason that their answer was quickly accepted was that it comports with our intuitions and with the observation that persistent ecosystems are frequently observed in nature. (And of course, it did not upset the apple cart of established neo-Darwinian theory.)

The supply/demand analogy is compelling. If there are too many birds for the available supply of worms, then the worms will be harder to find and some of the birds will die off; then, with fewer birds, on the hunt, the worm population can replenish. If too many seeds take root in one patch of ground, then they will crowd each other out and only the seedlings that catch enough sun will survive. Ecology provides many sources of negative feedback, which is the basis for all self-regulation.

I believe, despite the manifest and universal operation of negative feedback, that ecosystems are inherently unstable unless specifically evolved for stability. The reason involves not just the direction of feedback, but also the time scale for its operation and the need to overcome inertia that tends to keep populations growing (or collapsing) long after they have passed (or collapsed) through their steady state value.

There are two factors in the instability: exponential growth and delay. Delay means simply that growth takes time; a population may continue to grow and overshoot its carrying capacity. Exponential growth is growth that feeds on itself. Characteristically, it looks as though nothing is happening for a long while, then suddenly all hell breaks loose. Biological populations tend to grow (or to shrink) exponentially just because the number of children tomorrow is proportional to the number of parents today. Population growth cannot turn on a dime and neither can population collapse be quickly halted.

It's all in the Timing

We think of the self-regulating marketplace as a model of a naturally stable system based on negative feedback. The law of supply and demand operates by automatically lowering the price of goods that are in oversupply and raising the compensation for goods (or professions) when there is a shortage. But suppose this feedback operated with a delay: For example, there may be a doctor shortage driving up medical fees and salaries, but the only way to get more doctors into the system is to send them through four years of medical school and three more years of internship and residency. Worse—medical schools may already be operating at capacity. Getting each new medical school up and running might require a decade. And the doctor shortage is now! In our economic world, there is communication and planning and people operate with some amount of foresight, so this situation is less likely to arise. But as an example of how nature operates, it can offer some insights. If people built medical schools only in response to present shortages of medical personnel, we might have large numbers of people dying for lack of hospital care before a new supply of doctors arrived on the market. By the time the situation began to correct itself, there would be more medical schools than the country can support, training more doctors than the community ultimately needs. A fully trained doctor is highly motivated to continue in his profession for the full duration of his career. So the dearth of doctors might be followed by a glut of doctors for a generation to come. The profession would lose prestige and the ability to command a professional salary. People would have to have fanatical devotion to begin medical school under the circumstances—and so the stage is set for an even steeper shortage of doctors in the next generation after the doctor glut.

Without adaptations that specifically address stability, ecosystems could well behave this way. The negative feedback in ecosystems comes with an insupportable delay. Larger animals, especially, have long generation times. They cannot afford to reproduce based on the present availability of food, because the next generation is likely to starve. If the caribou living in tundra were to eat all the ground cover that was available to them, not only would their offspring die off, but the tundra might take decades to regenerate itself. The caribou in Alaska are smart enough (this intelligence is in their genes, of course, not their brains) to eat lightly and to mate only in alternate years. Their cousins (same species) that live further south can afford the luxury of reproducing every year and so they do. This is an example of cooperation to avoid ecosystem collapse—individuals behaving in a way that is good for the species but bad for their own individual fitness.

Chaos Theory: A Different Kind of Mathematics

The logistic equation, used above to derive smooth curves for population growth, was historically connected to the birth of mathematical chaos theory in the mid-twentieth century. The difference between smooth behavior and oscillating or chaotic behavior is in the delay of feedback concerning population saturation. If the feedback is instantaneous, then the population settles smoothly into its ideal, long-term sustainable level. If the feedback is slightly delayed, there will be some overshoot in the population curve and the population will go up and down, never straying too far from its steady-state value. But if the delay is any longer, then (even in these simple, purely theoretical calculations) the population jumps about wildly and cannot find its ideal, steady-state level at all.

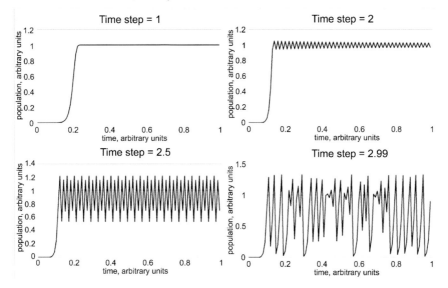

The logistic differential equation can be re-cast as a finite difference equation. This corresponds to population feedback that comes with a time delay. A short time step leads to small oscillations above and below the carrying capacity. But a time step of 3 (in units of the inverse growth rate) leads to chaotic changes in the population level.

Mathematically, chaos ensues as the delay approaches a value of 3. Is that three minutes of delay or three months or three years? The natural unit of time here is the "e-folding time" for a population. Three time units corresponds to enough time for the population to become 20 times as large, since $e^3 = 20$, approximately. This is not such a large number. A pair of mice can easily produce 40 young in their lifetime. Insects and worms can lay thousands of eggs.

The arithmetic is telling us that a single generation might be too long! If animals are reproducing apace based on abundant food supply now, then the next generation might already be too large and a catastrophic die-off will be unavoidable.

In the graphs above, you can see the effect of feedback that slows a population's growth as it approaches its steady-state level. In the first frame, the population receives feedback after one standard generation and the population grows smoothly to its equilibrium point and stays there. In the second frame, feedback comes after two standard generations and you can see some small overshoot and volatility in the result. The third frame corresponds to feedback after 2½ standard generations and now the overshoot is substantial, but long-term stability prevails. In the fourth frame, feedback requires 2.99 generations. The population dips very close to zero, but then recovers. Of course, real ecosystems cannot afford to fluctuate as wildly as this. Sooner rather than later, the last individual of a species will wink out of existence and there is no recovery ever. For feedback that is slower yet (≥ 3), the mathematical solution for population goes rapidly to negative infinity.

Delay is the first factor that distinguishes ecosystems from self-regulating markets. Exponential growth is the second. When the rate of increase of any quantity is dependent on the quantity itself, the result is exponential growth. Populations have the property that they tend to grow not by a fixed increment per unit time, but by a fixed proportion. This is the deep source of instability in biological systems. The number of offspring in the next generation depends most strongly on the number of parents in this generation. Imagine if no one could change careers and doctors could only have doctors for children. Building a stable economy out of individuals that can adapt to market conditions by changing careers may be a viable proposition; but it is far more difficult to build a stable ecosystem when the constituent species are all either growing exponentially or declining exponentially. Imbalances become the rule and populations can die out completely. There is a tendency for producer species to disappear first and to take down the entire ecosystem once they are gone.

Computer Game Ecology

Artificial Life or "ALife" is a discipline involving a small community of scientists worldwide who study life in computer simulation. They use mathematical representations of biological processes to try to capture the essence of life's behavior within a computer model. One subfield in this area is the modeling of ecosystems [13]. Equations are written down that represent the way the population of each species might change depending on the other species in the ecosystem. There are all kinds of interactions: predator/prey, competition for resources, mutualism, parasitism. Practitioners of this art have been trying for years to put together combination of virtual 'plants' and 'animals' to construct stable artificial ecosystems. And yes, they have model ecosystems to show for their efforts, but the catch is that the populations are fluctuating wildly. Typically dynamic ranges are $\sim 10^7$; in other words, population will go from one individual to 10 million individuals, before dying back to one individual some generations later. In the real world, microbes probably do experience such dramatic population blooms, followed by die-offs; but macroscopic animal populations cannot afford to have 99.99999% of the population disappear. In real ecosystems, even a 90% culling poses dangers of extinction.

Enough Reindeer

The Isle of St Matthew in the Bering Sea is barren and mountainous, with low-growing tundra in the summer and not much to eat in the winter. In 1944, the largest animals inhabiting the island were voles—rodents resembling field mice—and a few foxes that chased them. Thinking to create a hunting preserve, wildlife managers introduced 29 reindeer that year, imported from the island of Nunivak, 200 miles to the east.

The reindeer flourished, their population growing by about a third from each season to the next. That may sound like an extraordinary rate, but the ability of the population to expand rapidly is beneficially adaptive in an empty niche and may be a life-saver after a natural disaster. So the reindeer population followed a trajectory typical of an exotic species that is successfully introduced, growing on an exponential trajectory. Naturalists estimate the carrying capacity of the island at about 2,000 reindeer and the population crossed that threshold around 1960.

Such is the relentless logic of exponential growth that just four years later, the population was 6,000 reindeer.* The winter of 1964 was severe—not a dramatic

---

* $1.33*1.33*1.33*1.33 = 3.1$.

departure from what the reindeer expected, but more snow than usual. By the end of the winter, the entire population had starved to death. An expedition the following year counted 42 stragglers (and shot 10 of them in the name of sport and science). Reindeer live typically 18-22 years*, so the entire saga had unfolded within the lifetime of a single reindeer.

Scientists are privileged to witness dramatic dies-offs like this only rarely. Without exception, the cases that have been documented all involve animals that are newly-introduced into a favorable, virgin habitat. Of course, this is to be expected: in a natural habitat, the extinction event would most likely have occurred long ago, before humans were around to record it. Still, we have to wonder: when populations undergo dramatic local extinctions, do they vanish without a trace of a legacy or do some animals in some places survive. Do the survivors tend to have a different genetic make-up than those who succumbed? And does the event leave its imprint on the genome?

Yes, of course this is what we should expect. This kind of account sounds like classical Darwinian logic. The population that learns to detect the limits to growth early avoids a crash; the population that does not succumbs to extinction. Over time, those populations that carry genes that help them to moderate population growth *in advance* of food shortages persist and their legacy survives, while competing populations may vanish. The surprise is not that this kind of dynamic should occur in nature, but how vigorously this story is denied by mainstream evolutionary theorists. "There are powerful and fundamental reasons for rejecting this 'group selectionist' explanation..." [14]. How did neo-Darwinists come to think this way? And how could they cling so insistently to theory in the face of countervailing evidence? Remember that the argument against group selection amounts to a comparison of time scales: Individual lifetimes are short; extinctions are few and far between. Many individual lifetimes will take place before one extinction event, so it is expected that individual selection must be much more rapid and efficient than group selection [15]. But here we see that an entire cycle of exponential expansion into a new habitat, population overshoot and crash to extinction can unfold in one individual lifetime.

These reindeer came originally from Nunivak island. Why didn't they overgrow there? I have no certainty to offer, but I suspect it had to do with the diseases, the wolves and other predators that were part of the Nunivak ecology but missing on St Matthews. Their reproduction was attuned to a higher mortality rate and in the context of the Nunivak ecology they were (and still are) able to maintain a stable population. Freed from the predators that killed them, they grew in numbers until they starved themselves to death.

Population Regulation as an Evolutionary Force

The point of all this is that stable ecosystems cannot be taken for granted. If we see stable ecosystems in nature, this might be the result of an evolutionary process.

---

* Remember from Chapter 2 that the lifespans of Arctic animals tend to be longer than their cousins in the temperature zone.

I believe that not only do individuals compete with other individuals, but whole ecosystems compete with one another, co-evolving homeostatic systems. To many scientists, this may seem like common sense. But neo-Darwinian theory does not recognize any evolutionary mechanism that could pit one ecosystem against another in a struggle for existence. Competition is always individual vs individual and the backdrop of the competition is a stable ecosystem that is taken as a given.

This, then is a good candidate for a way to extend classical evolutionary theory beyond the selfish gene. Population stability is essentially a collective attribute; it makes no sense to talk about an individual being ecologically stable or unstable. And—crucially—population dynamics as an evolutionary force can act very fast. The essential argument that cast group selection in a bad light beginning in the 1960s was that it takes too long to work. In this way of thinking, any trait which offered a benefit to the population at the expense of the individual would be extinguished by individual selection within the group in just a few generations, long before its benefit for the group could become apparent. But I have argued theoretically that population dynamics can operate within the time scale of a single generation and cited examples from natural experiments.

George Williams [16], John Maynard Smith [15] and other astute scientists who made the argument that populations change more slowly than individual gene frequency noticed that population extinctions were relatively rare and accepted that this is the way nature works, without ever asking why. I am proposing that population extinctions must have been much more frequent in earlier evolutionary times and that ecological stability is a universal (all macroscopic animal species) evolutionary adaptation which became established so long ago that now we are tempted to take it for granted. All life is accommodated to an ecosystem and cycles of birth and death are adapted to prevent the worst kinds of abuse, that might bring an ecosystem crashing down. Williams and Maynard Smith were assuming the condition they had set out to prove.

Neo-Darwinists ask how group-level evolution can possibly compete with the quick and efficient process of natural selection for ever greater fertility and ever longer lifespan. Here is an answer for them: Population overshoots are a rapid, deadly consequence of fertility that is too high and lifespans that are too long. Ecological imbalance can generate local extinctions with the potential to be a fast-acting evolutionary force.

We may imagine many, many extinctions over a long period of time before the genes "learned" to behave less selfishly. The selfish behaviors would have evolved hundreds or thousands of times, each one leading to extinction until, by chance the right combination of genes appeared to assure moderation, preserving the prey species, fitting into a balanced ecosystem. Still, the selfish behaviors would continue to re-appear from time to time and flourish briefly. Extinctions would continue to follow until, by chance, some trait or adaptation appeared in the genome that would effectively lock moderation in place, rendering unlikely the possibility that unrestrained consumption and immoderate reproduction would re-appear. The operation of this and other long-term evolutionary forces is facilitated by the suppression of purely selfish, pro-growth behaviors based on their potential to cause prompt extinctions.

How to Stabilize an Ecosystem

If we accept the idea that natural selection has crafted stable ecosystems, the next step is to ask by what genetic traits this may be accomplished. It's all about tempering rates of population growth early, because by the time the limit to growth is felt as a deprivation, a crash is already inevitable. There are four basic principles:

- Individual selection favors ever higher reproduction rates, which lead (at a population level) to ever higher population growth rates. This is absolutely unsustainable. The first requirement is that individual reproduction rates must be tempered.
- It is best if population growth rate is flexible in responsive to the condition of the population. When the population is low, high growth rates are favored; but when crowding approaches the local carrying capacity, population growth must be halted (and reversed) as soon as possible. For this to work, individuals need to be aware of their environment and adjust their fertility and their mortality in response to perceived crowding.
- Predators must not over-exploit their prey. Ideally, the prey population should be judiciously pruned, just below its maximum sustainable level.
- Individual selection would favor a population that is uniformly strong, able to resist predators and disease. But in a population like this, either everybody dies or nobody dies. The situation is inherently unstable. In order to promote stability, the population should be diverse, with some individuals more vulnerable than others, on a smooth, graded scale. Somehow, the weaker individuals should be retained in the population, even though their individual fitness is lower. Aging provides the "somehow".

Within each of these categories, there are many strategies that may be used. Aging is not the only way to stabilize populations, but aging fits handily into each of the above. No progress can be made toward stability without compromising individual fitness and since individual selection is strong and direct, we should expect nature has found ways to stabilize populations that minimize the impact on individual fitness.

The first two strategies imply that some reproductive capacity is kept in reserve, so that individuals are not as fertile as they could be, except in times when the population is low. The most common adaptation for this purpose among higher animals and plants is territoriality.

The last strategy calls for maintenance of weaker individuals within a diverse population so that the population is sensitized to negative population feedback. If different individuals with different genetics varied in their susceptibility to starvation and disease, then the weaker genes would be promptly eliminated by natural selection. Aging serves uniquely well in maintaining diversity, because it is the same individuals who are strong and weak, at different stages in their life cycle. Numerical simulations confirm that weakening with age is a particularly effective life history adaptation in this regard and that a weak, post-reproductive period in the life cycle is most effective of all [17].

Birds Lacking Estates

In 1949, John Aldrich and Robert Stewart [18] contracted with the lumber interests that controlled timber land in northern Maine to study an infestation of budworms, a species of moth that was defoliating the fir and spruce trees and threatened productivity of the managed forest. They were ecologists of a different era and their methodology was not unusual for the time: try to understand the life cycle of the budworms by simplifying their ecology. What would happen if there were no predators eating them?

Aldrich and Stewart set about to rid an entire 40-acre plot of all songbirds, the better to study the life cycle of their prey, the budworms. A team of field biologists took a census of birds, counted 148 and set about to kill them all with small-gauge shotguns. Two weeks later, they had killed 455 birds and there were still dozens more remaining about. They must have felt like the sorcerer's apprentice.

They wrote up their results in an ornithology journal, where it continues to be cited 60 years after the fact. The story they told was of two bird populations: one nesting and mating and producing next year's crop of chicks. The males staked their territories and sang their hearts out, announcing their dominion over the little plot where they held court. The females hid unobtrusively in their nests, tending the eggs and feeding the hatchlings. But waiting in the wings were perhaps twice as many birds that did not have territories, did not have nests and did not reproduce. Crowded out of a home, they were destined to leave no offspring.

Aldrich and Stewart did not theorize on their findings—they were good field scientists, reporting their results without interpretation. But we may ask the questions for them:

This was a robust system of population stabilization, assuring that the population of breeding birds would be renewed every year, but that there would not be overpopulation or strain on the food supply. If the population was too high, the excess would hang about without breeding; if some of the birds should be lost to a famine or weather catastrophe, there was a large buffer population from which replacement breeders would instantly be drawn.

Was it just good fortune that led to this stable and durable population control system? Was it the byproduct of purely selfish selection, the "invisible hand" of the market place? Another way of asking this: what were those bench-warmer birds thinking* as they waited patiently with no offspring, forgoing their Darwinian legacy? Where were their "selfish genes", if they were willing to suffer a catastrophic fitness loss—equivalent to death—without even challenging the bird that controlled the territory? Bird fights are rare.

Of Carnivores and Cacti

Territoriality is one of the main ways that nature has been able to prevent overpopulation. It is widespread in the world of higher animals and even plants.

---

* Meaning, what were their genes thinking? How could genes for such behaviors have survived natural selection?

Birds, lizards and carnivorous mammals are famously territorial. Less well known are crabs and fish. You've seen territoriality when you bring a second cat into the house, but have you ever watched what happens when you introduce a new angelfish into your tropical fish tank?

Mountain lions in the American Midwest will patrol a territory of about 25 square miles of green forest, but in less productive land—desert or tundra—a single lion's range can be as large as 1,000 square miles. Males and females establish separate and overlapping territorial subdivisions. They will tolerate another lion of the opposite sex, but not of the same sex. (Adults hunt alone and the father does not stay with the family.)

Most surprising, perhaps, are desert plants. A mature saguaro cactus laps up the rainfall on a full acre of sand. The roots of a single plant can extend hundreds of feet in all directions and it emits chemical signals that tell other cactuses not to grow there. In fact, it's not just desert plants that are territorial: roots of forest plants rarely tangle in the competition for water and it is suspected that they have chemical means of detecting and avoiding one another. Though the chemical signals have not been isolated, the root patterns themselves tell the tale [19].

Ants are territorial, not individually but by family. Ants are exquisitely sensitive to chemical signals and one of the most powerful signals is the one established by the queen, which distinguishes her home colony. Ants cooperate famously with others from the same colony, but will avoid ants from other colonies while foraging. A solitary ant caught in foreign territory will be surrounded, attacked and killed. Different colonies that are established in close proximity lead to ant wars, with a winner and a loser. Sometimes the losers are all killed, but they may also become non-breeding slaves living within the victor colony.

Harvard Prof. E.O. Wilson, after a long career writing scientific articles and works of public advocacy, tried his hand at age 81 writing a novel. *Anthill* [20] draws a compelling analogy between the devastation wrought by ants and humans, when their respective populations grow beyond the bounds of sustainable ecology. A boy naturalist observes the unfolding story in a small tract of Georgia forest where one deviant ant colony fails to respect territoriality. A single mutation causes the ants to tolerate others from different but closely-related anthills. The result is that pioneer ants set up new colonies too close to home and a Supercolony grows to a far greater density than was possible while classical territoriality prevailed. Supercolony is able to vanquish other ant clans because of its numerical superiority, but without limits to growth, the ants begin to destroy the ecology that supports them. They become aggressive as food becomes scarce, attacking other insects that would not normally interest them. Pollination fails. Small mammals avoid the area. The ground itself becomes soft and porous underfoot, root systems suffer and the entire ecosystem crashes from overpopulation of a single species.

Private Property—No Trespassing

Everyone agrees that territorial behaviors help to stabilize population density, but classical evolutionists regard this as a lucky side-effect of behavior that is perfectly selfish. It was not always so; before the hegemony of the selfish gene, before "group selection" became a four-letter word, it was common to speak of homeostasis as an adaptation that served the community.

C.B. Moffat addressed the Dublin Naturalists' Field Club in 1903 on the subject of population regulation among birds (which he had observed extensively) and among higher animals in general (about which he frankly was speculating). Moffat counted himself as a disciple of Darwin, but recognized that his views contradicted the literal interpretation of the *Origin*: that the competition for a place in the biosphere was fierce and all-consuming, that all but a tiny minority of animals in each generation died in the struggle.

> What is the real reason why birds—and perhaps the higher vertebrate animals generally—do not increase in number from year to year? This question has, I think, always puzzled field observers, the answers commonly given being of that class which looks well on paper, but which somehow do not carry conviction so readily when we close our books and look all round us... That great tragedy, the "struggle for existence," as pictured for us by Darwin, requires such a death-rate among the young in their first year or before they are of age to mate, as could not be less than 90 percent in the case of most of our finches and other common small birds. For my part, I cannot believe that the theory of Natural Selection—for which I have the greatest respect and which I must carefully guard myself against appearing for a moment to call in question—requires this sacrifice or anything like it.... as regards birds I am altogether unable to find grounds for believing in so great a death-rate, at any rate in our own land.

Moffat goes on to elaborate his theory that bird songs are a claim to territory and that un-landed birds are silent. Coloration, he argues, is a kind of war-paint, advertising that birds of another species may stake out overlapping territories, but birds of this particular color are enjoined to respect property rights established by the bearer of the plumage. Thus the destructiveness of an all-out war for existence is avoided and a stable equilibrium is peaceably maintained.

Up through the early 1970s, this is the way that ecologists understood territoriality. Students were taught that ecologies had evolved for homeostasis because those ecologies that were unstable did not last long. V.C. Wynne-Edwards cited Moffat in the book [21] that was at once the culmination and the downfall of his long career as a naturalist. Subsequently, the quantitative *coup d'état* in evolutionary biology spilled over into ecology (and other biological fields). Today, territoriality is understood as a fiefdom maintained by the strongest, using force or implicit threat of force to assure one family's license to forage and thus to reproduce. It is assumed that the losers are all doing their best to reproduce, but have simply been overpowered. Here is how the issue is framed in a popular 2005 textbook on ecology [14]:

> Individuals from a territorial species that fail to obtain a territory often make no contribution whatever to future generations. Territoriality, then, is a "contest". There... can only be a limited number of winners...

One important consequence of territoriality, therefore, is population regulation...

Some have felt that the regulatory consequences of territoriality must themselves be the root cause underlying the evolution of territorial behavior—territoriality being favored because the population as a whole benefitted from the rationing effects which guaranteed that the population did not overexploit its resources. However, there are powerful and fundamental reasons for rejecting this "group selectionist" explanation (essentially, it stretches evolutionary theory beyond reasonable limits). The ultimate cause of territoriality must be sought within the realms of natural selection, in some advantage accruing to the individual [22].

Territoriality functions beautifully to maintain population stability, but there are "powerful and fundamental" reasons for thinking that this is just a lucky break and that it did not evolve for this purpose. The 'realms of natural selection' are explicitly assumed to be limited to "advantage accruing to the individual." Here, as elsewhere, the author does not undertake to explicate the 'powerful and fundamental' reasons or to inform the student that they are the subject of a persistent controversy within the evolutionary community. Actual tooth-and-claw battles for territory are very rare in nature and yet the theoretical presumption is that every individual is doing its utmost to establish a territory. This is no mere luxury or fitness bonus: the individual's entire Darwinian legacy depends on success in obtaining a territory. Still, the competition is carried out symbolically with vocal and visual displays, with chemical signals and physical posturing. The game's losers accede quietly to the system's judgment and rarely challenge the territory-holder directly or try to cheat.

There is an analogy here between the way ecologists changed their understanding of territoriality, based on pure theory and the way gerontologists changed their understanding of aging. Both have imposed a rigid theoretical framework on a pre-existing body of data that seemed to point in another direction entirely.

The Prudent Predator?

In addition to territorial protocols, there are other ways that individuals might alter their behavior for the sake of the ecology. All of them involve sacrifices in individual fitness for the sake of long-term sustainability; there is no way that a population can stabilize its size without imposing sacrifices in fitness upon individual members. Restrained predation is a very direct sacrifice of individual for community. Reproduction is energy-intensive for females and with less food, the body generally restrains reproduction. If a predator spares some of its prey, it not only denies its metabolism the resources needed for reproduction but also preserves the pool of food available to its intraspecific competitors. Thus a neo-Darwinian perspective would predict that predators ought to kill as many prey as physically possible, even beyond their own capacity to absorb nutrition. This is the behavior that optimizes the increase in frequency of their own genes. But in nature we rarely see predators that kill for sport when they are not hungry; quite the contrary, we observe restrained predation that maintains a prey population near the steady-state level that would be sustainable in the absence of predation. We rarely see cannibalism, though this would be an ESS, from the perspective of pure individual selection [23]. The result that we do see serves the population ideally, but at the expense of the individual. Field biologists take it as a matter of course that predator species hold back when their prey is plentiful, apparently for the purpose of modulating population overshoot; but, once again, evolutionary theorists deny that this is a possibility. Were it not for prejudice against "group selection", it would be natural to interpret restrained predation as a behavior adapted for population stability.

From Foe to Friend: The Evolution of Reduced Virulence

There is one situation which is well-accepted by neo-Darwinists as an example of "predatory restraint" or "prudent predation". It's about disease and the pathogens that cause them. You and I may not be accustomed to thinking of viruses as "predators", but they fit the formal definition used by ecologists. The dynamics of predator/prey and pathogen/host have much in common. Microbes that cause infection are subject to just the same population dilemma as are predators, with the same split between the best interest of the individual and the best interest of the group. For each individual virus, its fitness is maximized by attacking the host cells with maximum efficiency and gaining the resources of those cells which it needs to reproduce. The microbes that are better at reproducing faster will quickly take over the population at the expense of microbes that are less aggressive.

The countervailing force comes from variable contagion, which is essential for the microbes in spreading to a new host. If the microbes attack too hard, too fast, then their victim will become sick and despondent and have less social contact, less opportunities to spread. The worst case is if the microbes attack with such force that they quickly kill the host. Then they're really stuck in a body that's dead and buried, with no opportunity to infect someone new. So clearly, for the best interest of the microbes as a community, they should hang back, multiply slowly, allow the host to thrive and to function normally (and socially) while slowly infiltrating his mucus or the droplets in his sneeze spray, allowing contagion to the next host before this one either dies or develops an immune response that knocks out the microbes.

Everyone agrees this process actually happens and that it is a process of group selection. The neo-Darwinists call it an exception to the rule, based on unique circumstances: First, the "group" is clearly defined: all the microbes within a given individual form a trait group. Second, the group members are closely related, strengthening the force of kin selection. Usually infections begin with a few invading microbes and the entire population in the body is descended from these. And third, the pathogen's lifestyle makes it absolutely essential to jump from one host to another. What about cheaters? Presumably, mutations arise that give rise to a more virulent strain. Perhaps they take over and kill the host quickly and then it is likely that their progeny have no future and so the progressively less virulent strain is the one that continues to propagate.

Spumaviruses are retroviruses, closely related to HIV: their core is an RNA molecule that copies itself into the host's DNA. Unlike HIV, they have been around for a long time—so long that they have learned to live with humans and humans have learned to live with them. In the human body, they are harmless. They attack cells viciously, create lots and lots of copies of themselves and kill the cell. Harmless? Yes! The way they stay harmless is that they only attack cells that the body is about to slough off, cells that were about to die. There are a lot of cells in this category: skin cells, blood cells and the lining of the stomach, all of which are recycled and replaced every few days. You could say that the spumavirus helps our bodies get rid of those cells that were ready to be recycled.

Of course, the absolute classic story of an infection evolving into an essential helper is the case of mitochondria, related in Chapter 5.

Do Animals "Hold Back" their Reproduction?

V.C. Wynne-Edwards was an old-school naturalist, a broadly-educated scholar and eloquent writer, who collected evidence from nature in a book [21] on population control as a group-level adaptation. It is a fat compendium of examples drawn from lab experiment and diverse natural populations. No one piece of evidence can be expected to provide a slam-dunk proof, but the breadth of the examples looks only the more impressive 50 years on.

Wynne-Edwards begins by telling us that animal communications are much more extensive than we might expect, from pheromonal signals in ants up to clicks and whistles and ultra-low-frequency broadcasts by elephants and whales. Many animals coordinate their reproduction at special places and times of year. This is widely interpreted as having a protective benefit for each individual, but Wynne-Edwards argues that it limits total population size and that individuals would have more reproductive success if they avoided the intense competition of collective breeding.

He describes pecking orders and dominance hierarchies in many different species of birds. These are behavioral norms that limit access to food and opportunities for reproduction and yet to which individuals submit, for the most part, without raising a defense. He makes a case that territorial behaviors are not optimized for individual success, but for preservation of communal food resources. He documents the existence of large buffer populations of non-breeding birds that represent a reserve reproductive capacity to compensate for population declines for any reasons. These birds are content to serve as bench warmers, sacrificing their reproductive capacity in order to preserve demographic homeostasis. Elephants and other large herbivores delay their maturity in times of draught, forgoing their opportunity to compete in order to conserve scarce communal resources. Lion mothers space their offspring. Many mammals have evolved longer gestation periods and smaller clutch sizes than physiology permits. Remarkable birth control adaptations in turtles include species that have sex ratios favoring females, 3:1 and yet the males limit population growth by remaining monogamous.

Whales and elephants have very low mortality rates and so they reproduce much less frequently than their physiology permits. Lions and tigers spend much less energy on reproduction than smaller cats and Wynne-Edwards says that is because they live so much longer that they would overpopulate if they reproduced more frequently. Flies bred in jars will reach a limited density before they cease to lay eggs, even if plenty of food is provided. Beetles eat their young, but only in conditions of crowding. Mice and other rodents respond to crowded cages by refusing to reproduce, even when they have plenty of food. Game fish can be bred in tanks and the number of fish remains remarkably constant if a proportion of the fish are periodically harvested. Long-lived birds—penguins, auks, condors, vultures, eagles, albatrosses—lay only one egg at a time, even when the physiological burden of producing an egg is trivial. In fact, if the one egg is lost or broken, the bird will replace it. You have to wonder: if the birds can lay two eggs so easily, what stops them from doubling up in Darwin's lottery? (All the above examples are drawn from *Animal Dispersion in Relation to Social Behavior* [21].)

Concerning primitive human populations, Wynne-Edwards cites his predecessor, Alexander Carr-Saunders who compiled his own book a generation earlier, limited to anthropological examples [25]. Hunter-gatherer populations were stable for hundreds of thousands of years before agriculture and Carr-Saunders lists the ways that overpopulation was avoided: fertility limits and abortion, warfare and even infanticide had its place.

Near the end of the book, Wynne-Edwards includes a chapter on lifespan, which he assumes, naturally enough, has evolved as part of a population regulation program, anticipating the thesis of my own work by half a century.

Wynne-Edwards offered a compelling barrage of evidence for natural population control. Still, the book ultimately failed in its mission for lack of mathematical and deductive structure. As a naturalist, he had no peer, but as a theoretician, Wynne-Edwards was naïve and his arguments were fuzzy. His book was slammed on theoretical grounds [16] and even though the field evidence in Wynne-Edwards's book was never refuted, it became highly unfashionable to talk about evolution of population control. The naturalists had met the theorists head-on and the theorists had won. This is not how science is supposed to work.

Taken individually, the claims of Wynne-Edwards can each be diluted by a broader view of the data or explained by suitable adaptation of accepted theory. But collectively, as a volume, they tell a story of a world of social adaptations in stark contrast to expectations based on inclusive fitness of the Selfish Gene. By what perversion of the scientific method was this encyclopedic collection of observational evidence dismissed on theoretical grounds?

Less is More: David Lack's Perspective, Based on Individual Selection

Eight years before Wynne-Edwards, David Lack [26] had tackled the same subject of population regulation. He thought and wrote from a perspective consonant with the framework of standard evolutionary theory. If he is correct, then there is no real conflict between the individual's interest in maximizing reproductive success and the collective interest in avoiding overshoot and extinction. Is it plausible that populations can regulate themselves via an "invisible hand," a free benefit that accrues even as each individual maximizes its own reproduction? Or was Lack's thesis accepted uncritically because it fit so conveniently with prevailing theoretical ideas?

When conditions are crowded, birds lay fewer eggs. Wynne-Edwards claimed that this was a collective adaptation to preserve population homeostasis. Lack offered an explanation that fit better within the framework of standard evolutionary theory: Crowded conditions make the parents' task more difficult. Birds are evolved to lay as many eggs as they can successfully rear to maturity, given the resources currently available to the parents. In support of this idea, Lack performed field studies in which he determined that those birds laying more eggs than average could not feed them and in the end they fledged fewer offspring. Similarly, those that laid fewer eggs than average fledged fewer offspring. Thus Lack showed that the evolved average was optimal from the perspective of the parents' individual fitness.

This is a compelling finding and offered assurances for adequacy of prevailing theory. But when follow-up field studies failed to replicate Lack's findings, these results never reached the mainstream and it is Lack's work that continues to be cited today. In 1989, Ydenberg and Bertram [27] revisited Lack's thesis and reviewed the results of studies of clutch size in the intervening years.

> We review studies reporting experiments in which the broods of sea-birds were enlarged. In more than half of the 25 studies (on 21 species) seabird parents successfully reared the extra chick(s) added to their broods. This large proportion of successes contrasts with the way that the outcome of these studies has often been reported in the literature.… The studies clearly do not support Lack's clutch size hypothesis, but in spite of their inconsistency with Lack's outlook, the results on seabird brood enlargement studies were not used to weaken Lack's argument, but were often used as support for it!… We discuss how Lack's hypothesis came to be widely accepted in spite of all the contradictory data.

A debate between Lack and Wynne-Edwards continued until Lack's death in 1973. History records that Lack won the debate, but in a review of the content they exchanged, it is not clear that the evidence he cited was more compelling. Rather, the abundant exceptions to Lack's thesis have come to be regarded as anomalies or as problems that smart theorists will someday incorporate into the accepted canon of individual selection. For a detailed account of the debate and a general rehabilitation of Wynne-Edwards's work, I recommend Mark Borrello's book, *Evolutionary Restraints* [28].

Michael Gilpin: A lone Mathematician Supports the Theory of Cooperative Evolution

The direction of evolutionary biology in the twentieth century was centrally influenced by interlopers from mathematics and physics. Alfred Lotka and R.A.

Fisher were mathematicians. Max Delbrück and Leó Szilárd were physicists. George Price and J.B.S. Haldane were physical chemists. Even Erwin Schrödinger, famous as a father of quantum mechanics, wrote a seminal book about the origin of life.

All of these embraced the neo-Darwinian model of gene frequency in a static population as their primary model of how evolution works and together they did much to establish this paradigm as the standard way to view natural selection.* Standing alone is the mathematician turned ecologist, Michael Gilpin.

During the 1960s and 1970s, quantitative methods were taking a primary place in the study of evolution and an agreement was forming among the luminaries of the field that group selection is very generally much weaker than individual selection. This thesis was advanced from pure thought, often by people who had little experience studying animals and plants in the field.

Gilpin had just received his PhD in mathematics from Stanford and around the time of the first Earth Day, developed a keen interest in ecology. He determined to set Wynne-Edwards's thesis on a firm mathematical foundation. Computer resources were cumbersome and expensive at the time, requiring great patience and significant expertise specific to the computing platform in order to perform complex calculations. But in this area Gilpin was right at home. He had the mathematical chops to argue his point with great clarity and precision.

Gilpin wrote a closely-argued monograph [29] on the subject of predator restraint. He assumed that predators who ate more would be able to support a higher fertility rate and would thus come to dominate their local population. However, if they became too greedy in the aggregate, he showed that their offspring (and the offspring of those around them) would all starve in short order. He demonstrated with computational models that famine and extinction could be powerful evolutionary forces at the group level. Interspersed with his computer calculations, he included logical and mathematical arguments to show that the assumptions behind his calculations were reasonable and that the real world was likely to be, in every way, more conducive to the evolution of predator restraint than his model.

Gilpin showed that the balance of evolutionary forces could be expected to create predators that were restrained and conservative, holding back to protect their prey for future generations. But the scientific currents of the times were flowing against him and few biologists took his work to heart.

Predator populations limit their growth rate to match the availability of prey. Of course, individual selection working on the predators would tend to raise reproduction rates to unsustainable levels. The results of this are catastrophic for the population as a whole. Famines are quick and effective means to eliminate populations that have evolved to be too aggressive. Evolutionary theorists in the 1960s and 70s wondered what possible group selection mechanism could be efficient enough to counterbalance the directness and efficiency of individual selection for higher rates of reproduction. Famines are the answer to this question! Populations

---

Price was the only one of these who considered the mathematics of group selection and derived an equation which predicts the circumstances under which cooperative behaviors can be selected over selfish behavior. See Chapter 7.

can wink out of existence in a single generation when their food supplies become exhausted. Predators must 'learn' to limit their reproduction in response to the availability of food*. What is more, halting the growth of a predator population is like stopping the course of an ocean liner: there is considerable momentum implicit in the exponential expansion so retreat must begin well in advance of a famine. Predators cannot afford to wait until food is scarce to limit reproduction, because the next generation of predators will always be larger and the prey species scarcer yet. Food may be stored in the larger bodies of the adults, but the young are always most vulnerable and will be the famine's first victims.

Gilpin's work is badly out-of-fashion today and the man himself has moved from a career in mathematical ecology to the more urgent business of conservation advocacy in his adopted state of Montana. When the pendulum swings back and the importance of evolved eco-dynamics is recognized, Gilpin's theoretical contribution will be honored as an insight ahead of his time.

Time Scales of Ecology and Evolution

There has been recognition in recent years that ecological time scales and evolutionary time scales are not necessarily different [30, 31]. Already in 1998, Thompson [32] listed dozens of diverse examples, based on Endler's volume a decade earlier [33]. These include co-evolution of insects with their host plants; collective evolutionary response of snails in response to novel predators; and rapid adaptation of guppy populations to environments with and without predation. A few years later, alewives in different ecological niches became a popular model system for studying rapid evolution [34, 35].

> Metapopulation structure can rapidly shape and reshape the genetic structure of species at different geographical scales and interspecific interactions have now been shown to coevolve over the timescale of decades. Nevertheless, much ecological research continues to be carried out without considering—as one of a group of working hypotheses— whether some of the observed patterns and ecological dynamics are the result of rapid evolutionary change within and among populations [32].

It follows that evolution and ecology are not separate processes; that evolutionary theory that operates under the assumption of a fixed ecology is suspect; and that the great majority of experimental studies in laboratory evolution are inapplicable to the real world. The implications are profound; they negate face-on the argument by which "group selection" was rendered an irrelevant folly a generation earlier. The inertia of the neo-Darwinian paradigm and the primacy of individual selection continue, but their theoretical foundation has long since crumbled away. There is a scientific revolution waiting to happen.

---

* Of course, it is not the brains but the genes that are doing the 'learning' and the word 'learning' is just a useful metaphor. Predators with no capacity for awareness at all, such as worms or even protists, can "learn" in this sense.

Summary

To the extent that we see persistent and stable ecosystems in nature, this reflects broad (group-selected) adaptation for stability and not an "invisible hand" of homeostasis. Yes, starvation is a homeostatic force that can correct population overshoot, but it operates after too long a delay. If starvation were the only thing enforcing population limits, population dynamics would be violently volatile, threatening extinction at every turn.

An assumption at the foundation of standard evolutionary theory is that individual gene frequencies change on a time scale of a few generations within an ecology that remains stable over much longer periods. Fisher [36] argued for this assumption based on general observations of natural ecosystems and Maynard Smith [15] evoked it explicitly in arguing against group selection. Only recently has this assumption been questioned and it has not borne up well against field observation. Typically, populations are changing just as rapidly as the gene frequencies within those populations [37]. Evolutionary changes feed back to affect the ecology and of course the ecology sets the context for evolution. The rate of ecological change is such that evolution and ecology must be considered as a single dynamic.

The logic of this situation is a wholesale negation of standard individual-level evolutionary theory, with its gene-centered dynamic. This is a theoretical vindication of Wynne-Edwards's observations and the mother of all group selection mechanisms. The evolutionary community has been slow to acknowledge the need for a re-thinking of what has been the predominant strain of evolutionary theory since 1970, based on the fact that genetics and ecologies are changing on the same time scale.

The evolution of population regulation has a long and contentious history. Thought and fashion on the subject closely parallel the corresponding history for evolution of aging. At one time, biology was a field science. Naturalists noticed many examples where populations seemed to be self-limiting in the wild and they had every reason to believe that this was the result of evolved traits. But once the rigor of neo-Darwinian theory was imposed, observation yielded to reason and experiment to theory. This is not a recipe for healthy science.

The naturalists were silenced by the theorists, but all along it was the naturalists who had observation on their side, even if they could not articulate a theory to explain their observations. The theorists understood that the implications of evolved population regulation would be deep and broad and they were understandably reluctant to re-think the foundations of their science. They could not have known that the key to a new understanding was already seeded with the concurrent dawn of a computer age. Quantitative science before computers was rooted in the ability to abstract simple rules about average behavior, and long habit had made a virtue of necessity. After computers became commonplace, theorists were able to model the complex and to highlight those situations in which the predictions of individual-based models differed markedly from calculations based on averages alone. Gilpin's model was not difficult or sophisticated, but it already demonstrated a new kind of evolutionary dynamic.

In the chapter that follows, I put forth my own theory of aging, based on the contribution that aging makes toward stability of ecosystems.

References

1. Wilder, L.I., *On the Banks of Plum Creek*. Little House. Vol. 4. 1937, New York: Harper & Bros.
2. Benton, T. and A. Grant, *Evolutionary fitness in ecology: comparing measures of fitness in stochastic, density-dependent environments*. Evol. Ecol. Res., 2000. **2**: p. 769-789.
3. Slobodkin, L.B., *How to be a predator*. Am. Zool., 1968. **8**(1): p. 43-51.
4. Hardin, G., *The tragedy of the commons*. Science, 1968. **162**: p. 1243-1248.
5. Luckinbill, L., *Coexistence in laboratory populations of paramecium aurelia and its predator Didinium*. Ecology, 1973. **54**(66): p. 1320-1327.
6. Vos, M., et al., *Inducible defences and the paradox of enrichment*. Oikos, 2004. **105**(3): p. 471-480.
7. Turelli, M. and D. Petry, *Density-dependent selection in a random environment: an evolutionary process that can maintain stable population dynamics*. Proc. Natl. Acad. Sci. U.S.A., 1980. **77**(12): p. 7501-5.
8. Mueller, L.D., A. Joshi and D.J. Borash, *Does population stability evolve?* Ecology, 2000. **81**(5): p. 1273-1285.
9. Prasad, N.G., et al., *The evolution of population stability as a by-product of life-history evolution*. Proc. Biol. Sci., 2003. **270 Suppl 1**: p. S84-6.
10. Rosenzweig, M.L. and R.H. MacArthur, *Graphical representation and stability conditions of predator-prey interactions*. Am. Nat., 1963: p. 209-223.
11. Gilpin, M.E. and M.L. Rosenzweig, *Enriched predator-prey systems: theoretical stability science*, 1972. **177**: p. 902-904.
12. Rosenzweig, M.L., *Exploitation in three trophic levels*. Am. Nat., 1973. **107**(954): p. 275-294.
13. Mauno, R. *An artificial ecosystem: emergent dynamics and lifelike properties*. Artif. Life, 2007. **13**(2): p. 159-187.
14. Begon, M., C.R. Townsend and J.L. Harper, *Ecology: From Individuals to Ecosystems*. 2005, New York: Wiley-Blackwell. 752 p.
15. Maynard Smith, J., *Group selection*. Q. Rev. Biol, 1976. **51**: p. 277-283.
16. Williams, G., *Adaptation and Natural Selection*. 1966, Princeton: Princeton University Press.
17. Mitteldorf, J. and C. Goodnight, *Post-reproductive life span and demographic stability*. Oikos, 2012. **121**(9): p. 1370-1378.
18. Stewart, R.E. and J.W. Aldrich, *Removal and repopulation of breeding birds in a spruce-fir forest community*. The Auk, 1951. **68**(4): p. 471-482.
19. Schenk, H.J., R.M. Callaway and B.E. Mahall, *Spatial root segregation: are plants territorial?*, In: *Adv. Ecol. Res.*, A. Fitter, Editor. 1999, Academic Press: London. p. 145-180.
20. Wilson, E.O., *Anthill*. 2010, New York: W. W. Norton. 381 p.
21. Wynne-Edwards, V., *Animal Dispersion in Relation to Social Behavior*. 1962, Edinburgh: Oliver & Boyd.
22. Moffat, C.B., *The spring rivalry of birds. Some views on the limits to multiplication*. The Irish Naturalist, 1903. **12**(6): p. 152-166.
23. Stenseth, N.C., *On the evolution of cannibalism*. J. Theor. Biol., 1985. **115**(2): p. 161-177.
24. Sage, L., *Bad Blood*. 2000, New York: Harper Collins.
25. Carr-Saunders, A.M., *The Population Problem*. 1922, Oxford UK: Clarendon Press. 516 p.
26. Lack, D., *The natural regulation of animal numbers*. The Natural Regulation of Animal Numbers., 1954.

27. Ydenberg, R. and D. Bertram, *Lack's clutch size hypothesis and brood enlargement studies on colonial seabirds.* Colonial Waterbirds, 1989: p. 134-137.

28. Borrello, M., *Evolutionary Restraints: The Contentious History of Group Selection.* 2010, Chicago: University of Chicago Press.

29. Gilpin, M.E., *Group Selection in Predator-Prey Communities.* 1975, Princeton: Princeton University Press.

30. Hairston, N.G., et al., *Rapid evolution and the convergence of ecological and evolutionary time.* Ecol. Lett., 2005. **8**(10): p. 1114-1127.

31. Turcotte, M.M., D.N. Reznick and J.D. Hare, *The impact of rapid evolution on population dynamics in the wild: experimental test of eco-evolutionary dynamics.* Ecol. Lett., 2011. **14**(11): p. 1084-92.

32. Thompson, J.N., *Rapid evolution as an ecological process.* Trends in Ecology & amp; Evolution, 1998. **13**(8): p. 329-332.

33. Endler, J.A., *Natural Selection in the Wild.* Monogr. Popul. Biol. 1985, Princeton, NJ: Princeton University Press. 354 p.

34. Palkovacs, E.P., et al., *Independent evolutionary origins of landlocked alewife populations and rapid parallel evolution of phenotypic traits.* Mol. Ecol., 2008. **17**(2): p. 582-597.

35. Post, D.M. and E.P. Palkovacs, *Eco-evolutionary feedbacks in community and ecosystem ecology: interactions between the ecological theatre and the evolutionary play.* Philosophical Transactions of the Royal Society B: Biological Sciences, 2009. **364**(1523): p. 1629-1640.

36. Fisher, R.A., *The Genetical Theory of Natural Selection.* 1930, Oxford,: The Clarendon Press. xiv, 272 p.

37. Schoener, T.W., *The newest synthesis: understanding the interplay of evolutionary and ecological dynamics.* Science, 2011. **331**(6016): p. 426-429.

7

How Might Aging Have Evolved as an Adaptation?

We admit possibility only after we grant necessity.
— Harold Pinter

This book began with a statement of paradox: Natural selection in favor of aging for its own sake is impossible within the framework of classical neo-Darwinian evolutionary theory. In the first five chapters, I have arrayed the evidence that aging has all the characteristics of an evolutionary adaptation in its own right, not an artifact lurking in a selection shadow, as Medawar supposed, nor a pleiotropic side-effect of selection for fertility, as theorized by Williams.

Only now that we have been compelled to grant the necessity for a mechanism of selection that can have the perverse effect of preferring death to life do we ask, "how can this be possible?" In strict accord with neo-Darwinian theory, it is not possible. The challenge, as I take it, is to specify the least-radical extension of neo-Darwinism that is capable of supporting affirmative natural selection for aging.

This chapter explores three mechanisms that might fit the bill.

I am a computer modeler and I approach this question through the discipline I know best. I have too much experience with models to suppose that the existence of a successful computational model for a mechanism compels a presumption that the model embodies anything of the natural world. Rather, I take the models as existence proofs, counter-examples to the common belief that evolutionary theory categorically rules out programmed aging. This should give us confidence in taking the evidence of the first five chapters at face value, granting the necessity once we have been convinced of the possibility.

Among the three, the most important and most robust is the Demographic Theory of Aging. Fixed lifespans evolved for the purpose of stabilizing population dynamic fluctuations. Death is brought under the control of the genome so that it can be meted out a little at a time and the result is to avoid deaths occurring all at once. I credit Wynne-Edwards [1] with the insight that animal species are broadly adapted for demographic homeostasis and Gilpin [2] with having explained why we should expect that local famines are a powerful agent of natural selection, opposite in direction and comparable in magnitude to the force of competition for ever higher reproductive output. Population dynamics are inherently volatile, subject to crashes that risk extinction. Limited lifespan has evolved, first and foremost, to address this existential danger.

I do not consider this a full and final answer to the question, however, because the problem of overpopulation can be solved by limiting fertility as effectively as by limiting lifespan. It remains to be explained why nature sometimes chooses one or the other tact and frequently both in tandem.

In fact, the insight that Gilpin bequeathed us explains an essential omission in the foundation of standard population genetic theory and it opens the door for all theories of aging and beyond this, provides the basis for understanding all the diverse phenomena of cooperation that have hitherto been squeezed into the implausibly tight container of kin selection theory. The second mechanism that I proffer depends explicitly on the high cost of allowing populations to rise to a density that tempts fate (though this is not the focus of the model). The third lacks this explicit connection, but also requires the logic of a fixed population limit, with the implicit assumption that Gilpin's mechanism has already taken its toll.

Mechanism number two has been dubbed by Dorion Sagan the "Black Queen," by close analogy to the Red Queen hypothesis, a leading candidate for explaining the evolution of sex. A population that becomes too dense and homogeneous risks epidemics and limited lifespan helps to reduce both density and homogeneity, just as the mixing of genes, which many evolutionists believe to be well-explained by this mechanism.

Mechanism number three is the optimization of evolvability, which has been a second-order target of natural selection for fitness since the dawn of life. Darwin overstated the case for evolution as an inevitable property of self-reproducing systems; only since 1996 has the community of evolutionary scientists begun to come to terms with the fact that a system needs special properties in order to support the process of variation and natural selection that Darwin described. Without adaptations specifically to support evolvability, the pace of evolution would be many orders of magnitude too slow to matter in a world only a few billion years old. Where does evolvability come from? We must assume that it has evolved in parallel to fitness in a bootstrapping process, as first described by Layzer [3]. Many deep aspects of living metabolisms, development and its governance, gene sharing, the structure of the genome, the genotype-phenotype map, all give the appearance of having been optimized for evolvability. Aging takes its place among these deeper properties of life as contributing to a rapid and efficient evolutionary process. Population turnover is limited by recruitment rate, which, assuming fixed carrying capacity, is controlled by the death rate. Hence programmed lifespan can enhance diversity and reduce the effective generation time, supporting evolvability by both means.

That Others Might Live

Preliminaries

Before proceeding to present three mechanisms that I believe to be good candidates for explaining the evolution of aging, I should like to clarify why some popular ideas are not adequate.

I

First is a variation on the selection shadow. Once an individual has finished reproducing, evolution does not care if she dies. For mammals and birds, it is useful for the parent to live on for a time after the last reproduction in order to rear her young; but most animals do not care for their young, so even that short period of post-reproductive life becomes an extravagance. If an insect has laid all the eggs she has to lay, then her fitness is not affected whether she lives or dies. Can this be the evolutionary explanation for aging that we have been seeking?

Yes, but only in a very limited sense; the idea comes from a correct understanding of evolutionary theory, but based on a restricted definition of aging. We can understand why an animal dies once its fertility has ended, but then we must ask: why does it lose its fertility? For many animals, loss of fertility is integrated into the life cycle [4, 5]. The deep question about evolution of aging is not why animals die after they become infertile, but why they should grow infertile in the first place.

II

Second is the mechanism proposed by Weismann [6] at the end of the 19th century. With wear and environmental exposure, the soma inevitably becomes damaged over a lifetime and aging has evolved to get older, damaged individuals out of the way and make room for younger individuals. This hypothesis has many problems; Weismann himself realized them and never pursued the idea further. For an organism that is capable of molecular-level repairs from the inside out, why should it ever be more economical to throw away a damaged soma and begin building another from sperm and egg? There is no mechanical or metabolic necessity for damage to accumulate over time, no inherent limit to the efficiency of repair. This argument was made in detail in Chapter 3. We may wonder, along with Williams, why "after a seemingly miraculous feat of morphogenesis a complex metazoan should be unable to perform the much simpler task of merely maintaining what is already formed [7]."

III

Evolution of aging as an adaptation, a thesis for which so much evidence has been adduced in this volume, really does present a dilemma for evolutionary theory that is not easily resolved. Obviously, no individual selection mechanism can do because the impact of senescence on the individual is wholly detrimental, depleting its ability to survive and to reproduce. A simple application of Hamilton's rule shows that no kin selection mechanism can work, either. If we consider the individual giving up its place in the niche as an act of altruism, then that one death makes room in the niche for just one replacement and even if that individual has relationship coefficient of 100%, as a clone or identical twin, then the transaction is only neutral and not beneficial; in reality, there is no assurance that the individual's replacement is related at all. And even if we embrace the logic of multilevel selection (MLS) based on the Price equation [8, 9]—an extension to neo-Darwinism that has been grudgingly incorporated into the canon in recent years—aging does not look like a viable adaptation. The individual cost of aging is too steep, the benefit is too small and not focused on those that share the trait of aging, but accrues quite generally to any rogue who takes up the slack. So we expect something more radical than MLS will be required.

All three mechanisms described below depend upon group selection, as they must, since aging offers no individual benefit. In the first, the groups are explicit and discrete. The other two use limited mobility, "population viscosity" [10-12] to simulate an amorphous, constantly shifting geometry of group associations. The difference between population viscosity and explicit group selection is superficial and generally the same evolutionary dynamic can be modeled in either way [10, 12].

What MLS Adds to Classical Population Genetics and What Remains to be Added

Fisher

In the original 1930 formulation [13] of population genetics, fitness is a property of the individual allele. The fitness of an allele is equated to its generational increase in frequency in a population, in comparison to competing alleles. Fitness of an allele is conceived as deriving from its contribution to either the survival or the fecundity of the bearer.

Fisher explicitly assumed that the genetic background, the physical environment and the ecology could all be regarded as constant during this process. He argued that variations in all these could be subsumed in a grand average and thus change in the frequency of individual genetic alleles was the primary process at the heart of evolutionary change.

Fisher's fundamental theorem says that the increase in the frequency of an allele over one generation is proportional to the covariance of that allele with fitness of the individuals carrying the allele.

$$\Delta \bar{z} = Cov(w, z)/\bar{w}$$

Haldane/Hamilton

Haldane [14] realized that an allele could be selected because it promotes identical copies of itself that appeared in family members. This is "kin selection" and it is how we understand the care of a mother bird for its hatchlings and the reason that worker bees, all descended from a common queen, can cooperate so effectively. An allele may be selected even if it detracts from the fitness of the individual who carries it, so long as the allele promotes behaviors that sufficiently increase fitness of related individuals carrying copies of the same allele.

Hamilton [15, 16] summarized this principle in a simple equation that bears his name. An allele can be positively selected so long as the aggregate benefit it provides to related individuals, weighted by their relatedness r, outweighs the cost to the individual carrying the allele.

$$\sum br = c$$

This idea was popularized by Dawkins as The Selfish Gene [17] and it is one mechanism for evolution of altruism that everyone agrees on.

Price/Wilson

Price [8, 9] generalized the idea of relatedness in Hamilton's Rule (above). An allele for an altruistic behavior may be selected if the behavior increases the fitness of others bearing copies of that gene. These others need not be close relatives or their exact relationship may not necessarily be traceable, as siblings or parent/offspring.

The Price Equation is a basis for understanding group selection. What matters is an individual's contribution to a group's increase in numbers relative to other groups and how that depends on the frequency of the altruistic allele within each group.

Price's paradigm relaxes in part the classical limitation of Fisher's model, which is that it assumes a static demographic background. In Price's model, there is a metapopulation of fixed size, while subpopulation groups may increase or decrease their relative proportion within the whole. Thus selection is taking place simultaneously at two level: groups are advancing or receding in size within the metapopulation, while individuals are competing against one another within each group.

The Price Equation partitions the aggregate change in frequency of an altruistic trait as the sum of within-group and between-group selection. Within each group, the altruistic trait is losing ground, while groups that contain more altruists are growing at the expense of groups with fewer altruists.

One way to write the Price Equation is identical to Hamilton's Rule, but with the symbol r reinterpreted to mean the probability that any beneficiary of an altruistic behavior carries the altruistic allele. In its most abstract form, the Price Equation can be written as Fisher's Fundamental Theorem with one additional term for between-group selection.

$$\Delta \bar{z} = \frac{Cov(w, z) + E(w\Delta \bar{z})}{\bar{w}}$$

Through the last decades of the 20th century, Wilson [18] applied the Price Equation to diverse situations in nature. He popularized the term *multilevel selection* (MLS) to capture the idea that selection is simultaneously occurring between groups and within groups and that groups might be hierarchically structured. He introduced the idea of a *trait group*, which is the set of individuals that benefit from a particular altruistic behavior. A trait group may or may not be localized in space and different altruistic traits are associated with different, possibly overlapping groupings in a population.

Gilpin

Gilpin [2] realized that population dynamics could be the basis of a potent selective force. He worked not with a single equation but with a computer simulation that could model more complex behaviors, including interaction of ecology with evolution. Since Darwin, the idea of gradual change had been a staple assumption of evolutionary theory. But Gilpin showed using simulation that population sizes could expand exponentially or collapse precipitously on a time scale much shorter than the time scale on which gene frequencies were changing.

Gilpin's monograph was based on predator/prey interactions, but it carries implications that affect our understanding of the nature of evolutionary competition for any consumer species. Gilpin provided the basis for understanding why plants evolve to maximize seed production, but animals cannot afford to reproduce too rapidly, vitiating a central assumption of population genetic theory.

This story with mathematical detail, up to but not including Gilpin, is concisely presented by Steven Frank in the journal *Evolution* [19].

The Demographic Theory of Aging—Model #1

It must be considered well within the framework of Darwinian thinking that surviving species are those that have adaptations making extinction less probable. It must be considered an omission in the foundation of standard population genetic theory that there is no explicit consideration of existential threats to a species.

If predation is the most serious threat to individuals in nature, starvation is the most dangerous to the species as a whole, because by its nature famine tends to affect an entire population at once. I believe that avoidance of famine is a major driving force in evolutionary selection. Against this proposition is the fact that it implies cooperation on a broad scale and that it requires a major sacrifice of individual fitness to achieve it. In favor of the proposition is the theory (from simulations [2, 20, 21]) demonstrating that this is a form of group selection that can easily compete with individual selection. Also in favor is a huge body of observations [1] of ways in which populations seem to be cooperatively adapted for the sake of ecological stability. The CR response and other forms of hormesis may be understood as adaptations for the purpose of stabilizing population dynamics.

Starvation is not an effective means of maintaining population homeostasis because hunger does not become lethal until there is a crisis, and then it is too late. Starvation cannot gently trim the population back to a more appropriate level; rather, no one dies until there is a famine and then everyone dies at once. By the time hunger first appears, the prey population is devastated and will require a long while to recover, at a time when any remaining predators are desperate and vulnerable.

Aging provides an alternative, steady and predictable mode of death. What is more, the Caloric Restriction adaptation assures that death from old age does not add to starvation deaths and aging will take its largest toll when food is plentiful and deaths from starvation rare. In this way, the CR adaptation enhances the effectiveness of aging as an adaptation for population homeostasis.

Predator species are dependent on a living community of prey and in the long run, the fate of the predator population is intimately tied to the prosperity of the prey community. Some predator species operate on a hit-and-run basis. They nab their prey and quickly move on, seldom re-visiting the area they left behind. But many more are territorial. They have a vested long-term interest in maintaining a thriving community of prey among which they may freely roam and strike at will (generally selecting the old, the weak and the sick and thus contributing to the health of the prey community by their mode of pruning it). This strategy requires territorial protection and also reproductive restraint—adaptations touched upon in Chapter 5. For most predators, remaining in a sustainable relationship with their prey is sufficiently important to their (collective) fitness that it justifies multiple accommodations, including aging on schedule.

In 1968, Larry Slobodkin [22] wrote an influential article with the cute title, 'How to be a Predator'. His prescription was not sharp claws and quick reflexes, stealthy approach or ruthless attack. His focus was on the long-term advantage of husbanding a thriving community of prey. (1968 was probably the last point in the history of evolutionary ecology in which such a paper could have been so prominently published, as soon afterward the backlash against Wynne-Edwards and the study of population homeostasis set in with full force.) Slobodkin emphasized that an ideal predator population should sit as lightly as possible on the prey population. "The optimal system for a predator wishing to insure the continued availability of its prey is to take animals which are about to die anyway, i.e., to alter the natural pattern of mortality as little as possible. It is concluded, with some reservations, that predators in nature generally act in this manner." The larger the herd of prey, the greater the harvest that can be sustainably extracted. The ideal predator, he theorized, would take prey when they are done reproducing, at a time in life when they were near to death from some other cause. (We note, in retrospect, that he took for granted the cooperation of the prey population, in aging on a predictable schedule. Thus aging in a prey population may be considered a product of coevolution.)

I developed the Demographic Theory based on chaotic logistic population dynamics beginning in 2002 [23] and (after protracted back-and-forth with journal editors skeptical of adaptive aging in any form) it was published formally in 2006 [20]. A similar model was developed independently and published in Russian by Trubitsyn [24]. The model was updated and expanded in 2012 [21] to compare and optimize the effectiveness of a broad array of life history profiles in stabilizing population dynamics.

Dynamics of the Time-Delayed Logistic Equation

The time-delayed logistic model was introduced in the last chapter. It is at once the canonical example of a simple equation that displays chaotic behavior and also a natural and plausible model for the behavior of animal populations, where the future population growth depends on the past availability of resources. Crowding inhibits population growth, but does so with a time lag. The time-delayed logistic equation can be written

$$\frac{1}{x}\frac{dx}{dt} = r(1 - x_d/K)$$

The left side is the logarithmic growth rate of population x; r is the maximal growth rate in the absence of intraspecific competition; and K is the steady state population level. The x/K term represents crowding that limits growth and the subscript d indicates that it is not the present x but the population at some time in the past, a time-delayed population measure, that comes into the calculation.

Let Δt be the time delay implicit in the subscript d. (Crowding how far in the past determines population growth inhibition today?). Then $r\Delta t$ is the dimensionless parameter that determines the behavior of the population x over time, described and illustrated in the last chapter. If $r\Delta t < 2$, then the behavior is smooth. The population responds to feedback promptly enough that it finds its steady state level and remains there, with small fluctuations. But for $r\Delta t > 2$, the behavior changes drastically, in a manner very sensitively to $r\Delta t$. As $r\Delta t$ approaches 3, the population fluctuates chaotically and for $r\Delta t \geq 3$, the formal solution heads to negative infinity, indicating extinction. Hence $r\Delta t$ can be called the "chaos parameter" (See graph on page 147).

Evolution with Delayed Logistic Dynamics

Consider a model population, whose life history parameters are allowed to evolve. (Life history parameters may include fertility, maturation time and lifespan.) The ecological background is not modeled explicitly, but is subsumed in the parameter Δt, which is the characteristic time for the ecosystem to respond to disturbance by population x. Think of Δt as the time necessary for the modeled species x to deplete the reservoir of living foodstock or as the time necessary for the foodstock to regrow after it has been depleted. (Though these two times need not be the same in general, the qualitative behavior of the model is not sensitive to this detail.)

When population is sparse and resources plentiful, the population x is able to grow at its maximal rate r. r is a function of the life history traits of the species, as determined by its genes. Considered from an individual perspective, r is also the Malthusian parameter, which is a target of individual selection. As we expect, genetic components of fertility and lifespan increase, while maturation age evolves lower in the model. All these have the effect of increasing r. In this model of exclusively individual selection, r evolves ever higher. The population, meanwhile, remains close to $x \sim K$, because of logistic feedback. r evolves ever higher, while Δt remains fixed and x holds steady close to the value K. The dynamic changes rapidly when r exceeds the threshold $2/\Delta t$. Then the chaos parameter enters its critical range and x begins to oscillate with higher amplitude and then to fluctuate chaotically. Soon after r has evolved in excess of $2/\Delta t$, we observe the population fluctuate to extinction.

This behavior, described heuristically, was observed in numerical models [20] and an example is plotted in below figure.

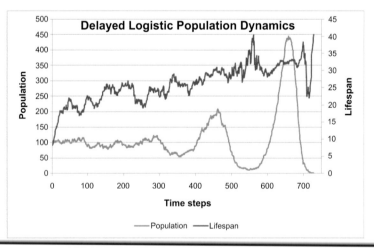

As lifespans evolve ever longer, the population's growth rate becomes too rapid relative to the inverse delay time Δt and the population gradually loses its logistic homeostasis.

A Subdivided Population Model with Delayed Logistic Dynamics

Consider now a metapopulation model, with many subpopulations arrayed on a map, each responsive (after delay Δt) to its own local population density and each evolving as above. Assume that there is weak interaction among the subpopulations, such that there is occasional migration among nearby subpopulation sites.

What we might expect (what I actually found) is that individual subpopulations are constantly evolving longer lifespans and greater fertility, until they become dynamically unstable and fluctuate to extinction. Then the site is vacant and it is re-seeded by migration from a nearby site. The founder population migrating in derives from a subpopulation that has not yet fluctuated to extinction, so it is likely to have a lower r than the subpopulation that it is replacing. So long as all subpopulation sites do not fluctuate to extinction at the same time, migration keeps the metapopulation viable indefinitely (long compared to the lifespan of any individual subpopulation).

The metapopulation evolves to a dynamic steady state, dependent on the rate of migration and the rate of individual selection within the subpopulations. Predictably, the steady state is characterized by a value in the neighborhood of $r = 2/\Delta t$, just below the threshold of chaos.

In below figure, this model has been run in a version where fertility is held fixed (value on the x axis) and lifespan is permitted to evolve to a steady state value.

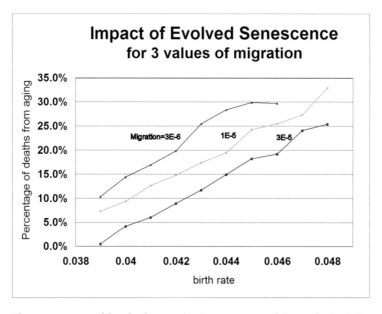

The percentage of deaths from aging is a measure of the ecological significance of senescence. Values in the chart are long-term population averages for three different values of migration rate and 10 different values of fertility.

This is a simple, clean model that arguably applies quite generally to animal species. It demonstrates that individual selection pressure for ever longer lifespans can be held in check by group selection for population homeostasis. Results indicate more senescence evolves when the migration rate is lower, illustrating that highly mobile populations can afford longer lifespans, while for those that stay close to home it is more prudent to keep growth in check and protect the producer species. I chose to measure senescence on the y axis by the dimensionless quantity, percentage of all deaths attributed to senescence. This is a convenient and appropriate choice especially because it is commonly reported for field studies of senescence in the wild.

One thing that stands in the way of this being a fully satisfactory explanation for the evolution of aging is the assumption of fixed fertility. In reality, we expect fertility to be evolving under selection pressure in parallel with lifespan. Any combination of shorter lifespan or lower fertility can keep the population safely out of the chaotic regime. Is there a reason to expect that nature might prefer to curtail lifespan in preference to birth rate or *vice versa*? Yes, shorter lifespan and higher reproductive rate are conducive to population diversity and evolvability. These are long-term values to a population that could not evolve on their own without some powerful constraint being placed on individual selection. We have seen the power of demographic homeostasis in this regard. The imperative to keep the population out of the chaotic regime handily holds down individual selection for ever higher r. This allows play for the longer-term values of diversity and evolvability to have their effects. These results will be seen in the following two models.

In an extension to the above model created in cooperation with Charles Goodnight [21], we found that differences are small so that many combinations of limited lifespan and limited fertility are almost equally viable. Interestingly, we also noted that post-reproductive lifespan has an extra stabilizing effect. These results handily explain some observations of nature that defy classical predictions of population genetic theory:

- that senescence is *de rigeur* in populations of animals (predators) but optional in populations of plants (producers).
- that a variety of different life history strategies are almost equally viable, so long as fertility and lifespan are matched appropriately.
- The model also handily explains the otherwise puzzling observation that nature seems to have a preference for continued lifespan after fertility has ended [5, 25].

The Black Queen—Model #2

The evolution and maintenance of sexual reproduction is recognized as a substantial challenge to evolutionary theory. Like aging, sex cannot evolve via traditionally-recognized population genetic mechanisms [26-28]. In its common dioecious form, sexual reproduction carries a fitness cost of a full factor of two; on the other side of the equation, the benefits of sex accrue many generations downstream in a diverse lineage. If costs and benefits are weighed using standard kin selection or MLS criteria, sex appears to be a losing proposition.

One of the best-accepted candidates for a mechanism by which sex may have evolved is the Red Queen* hypothesis [29-31]. Multicellular organisms with long life cycles and corresponding low rates of evolutionary change must maintain population diversity in order to protect against pathogens, which evolve much more rapidly. Pathogens that are narrowly adapted to infect a particular genotype can spread rapidly through homogeneous populations, causing local extinctions. Thus they provide a powerful incentive at the group level to maintain immunologic diversity. Sexual reproduction contributes to this end by recombining genomes, providing unique and diverse genomes for each member of a community.

The same Red Queen mechanism that provides a powerful selective force for the evolution of sex also favors the evolution of senescence. This has been dubbed by Sagan [32] the *Black Queen*. Senescence contributes to epidemic resistance in two separate ways:

- Population density promotes the transmission of disease. Senescence lowers population density by increasing the death rate; moreover, it does so in a way independent of stochastic causes of mortality in the environment. Senescence at the population level can contribute to leveling the death rate in fluctuating environments.
- Senescence contributes to a shorter effective generation time, thereby increasing population turnover and enhancing genetic diversity.

The fitness cost of senescence is high [33-35], but not so high as the cost of sex. Application of the Red Queen logic to evolution of senescence is at least as plausible as for evolution of sex.

In 2008, John Pepper and I published a Black Queen model for the evolution of aging, descended from an elegant mathematical model of Josh Socolar et al. [36]. Agents live on a Cartesian grid and reproduce to vacant neighbor sites, at a rate controlled by an evolving fertility gene. Similarly, an evolving gene for mortality controls the rate of random events removing the occupant of a site. With low probability ($\sim10^{-6}$ to 10^{-4}) an epidemic can begin at a selected site, from which it spreads through *every available contiguous pathway* of occupied sites, killing all agents in its path. Socolar explored the evolution of a constant, age-independent mortality rate under genetic control. Pepper and I extended his analysis to evolution of a programmed lifespan.

We also added to the model the concept of immunological diversity. In some variations, we allowed for different immune phenotypes, with pathogens presumably adapted to be able to bring down just one host type. Population turnover, facilitated by senescence, could maintain a diversity in the population that protected against spread of epidemics, adding to the protection from limiting overall population density.

---

* The name derives from a line in Lewis Carroll's fantasy, *Through the Looking Glass.* The Red Queen says to Alice, "Here, you see, it takes all the running you can do, to keep in the same place. If you want to get somewhere else, you must run at least twice as fast as that!"

The principal result of our study was the finding that the Black Queen mechanism works handily to evolve a fixed lifespan and that the lifespan that emerged depended little on the frequency of epidemic over a broad range. In common with other models for evolution of senescence as an adaptation, we found that senescent mortality evolved in a way that complemented background mortality (please see below figure). This is a prediction that distinguishes programmed aging theories from most traditional theories based on pleiotropy or the "selection shadow". In non-programmed aging theories, senescent deaths are predicted to rise in parallel with the background death rate, while in programmed aging theories, senescent deaths tend to complement the background death rate. Both relationships are observed in nature [5, 37-39]. I interpret this to mean that both effects are real and important. It is true that bats have a lower rate of aging than mice because bats are less subject to predation and can afford to evolve a life history that evolves at a slower pace. It is also true that guppies in an environment protected from predators evolve a lower fertility and shorter lifespan in order to avoid the hazard of overpopulation. Local ecology determines which relationship between background death and senescent death prevails.

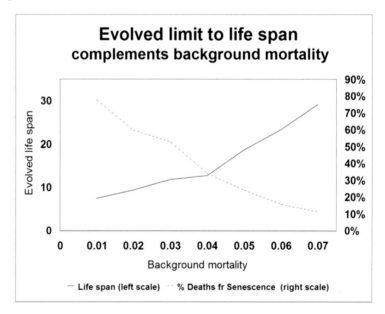

A background mortality rate is assumed and lifespan is permitted to evolve. The lifespan that is selected tends to complement background mortality so that the total is sufficient to limit population density on the grid as a firewall against epidemics.

The Black Queen mechanism is based on avoidance of epidemics and the Demographic Theory is based on avoidance of famine. The two models have this in common: total population density is limited by the imperative to avoid existential calamities that become probable with crowding.

Le Rouge et le Noir

Diversity in a population offers powerful advantages, but these advantages accrue to the population as a whole and only over long time spans. It is not easy to understand how long-term advantages for the population can outweigh short-term disadvantages that accrue to the individual bearing these genes. The devastating rapidity of epidemics in a population that has grown too homogeneous suggest a process by which diversity may offer a powerful advantage that does not require thousands of generations. The Red Queen has been embraced by the theoretical community as an explanation for the evolution of sex because it gets them out of a great pickle. But the evolution of aging has not yet been recognized as a pickle. So the same selective mechanism is considered a leading hypothesis in the case of sex, but unnecessary baggage in the case of aging. Instead the three standard theories (of Chapter 4) are endlessly embroidered as each new experiment comes forward with data that doesn't seem to fit.

Sauce for the goose is sauce for the gander.

Population Turnover and Evolvability—Model #3

The need to limit population density can be satisfied either with lower birth rates or with higher death rates. The choice is biased by the long-term need of the population to evolve, to keep pace with changing environmental conditions and to compete with other species that are evolving. The two population dynamic models presented above invoke a rapid, efficient mode of selection. The evolvability imperative, in contrast, is slow and diffuse as a selective modality. Group selection for evolvability would not be able to compete with individual selection for long life and high fertility were it not for the fact that individual selection is blunted by the population dynamic mechanisms.

The theme of evolvability harkens back to Weismann's 19th century hypothesis about the evolutionary provenance of aging. Weismann's hypothesis has been widely caricatured as a need for the old generation to get out of the way and allow room for the young generation to grow up. Within the neo-Darwinian picture of the world, this mechanism appears to be highly implausible. But suppose the message of the population dynamic models is taken to heart, in the form of an imperative that population density is absolutely capped. With selfish competition for higher resource consumption and faster reproduction effectively stifled, the long-term advantage of evolvability may prove a decisive selective force.

This was the starting place for a computational model contributed by Martins [40]. Before describing the Martins model, we fill in some background on the concept of evolvability in evolutionary theory.

Evolvability

Darwin took much of the machinery of biological reproduction for granted when he formulated his evolutionary theory. To this day, it is widely misstated (e.g. [41]) that a Darwinian process requires only three things: imperfect reproduction, an excess population and competition such that only a fraction of entities are viable. But in practice, the great majority of systems that meet these criteria cannot evolve. The crux of the problem is in the kinds of variation that are available during imperfect reproduction and the genotype/phenotype map.

Imagine you have a crude, working automobile engine and you want to evolve a better one by trial and error. If you try varying the cylinder size, larger and smaller, you will soon find a size that is optimal. But this requires changing the sizes of the piston, the rings, the cylinder housing and the crankshaft all in a coordinated way. If each of these parts were varied independently—say a larger piston without changing the bore of the engine block—then the result would *always* be nonfunctional—all point mutations would be lethal.

Similarly computer scientists experimenting with evolvable systems find that standard computer languages, designed for human readability and efficiency, are not capable of supporting evolutionary algorithms [42]. For a computer program written in Java or Visual Basic, changing one letter at a time will always produce uninterpretable nonsense. Special computer languages have been designed for "genetic algorithms" [43] that seek to evolve, rather than design, more efficient algorithms.

Hence, eukaryotic genomes are structured hierarchically, with hox genes at the apex of a genetic bureaucracy and transcription factors deploying hundreds of genes at a time to get a job done in coordinated, systematic fashion. A structure like this at the seat of evolutionary change, the core of genetic information, goes far toward explaining how evolution can take place efficiently. But it also raises the question: where did this structure come from? How was an evolvable system installed in the first place? This subject is the evolution of evolvability.

Ahead of his time and outside his field (astrophysics), David Layzer [3] first proposed that natural selection might favor the rate of increase of fitness over evolutionary time, apart from selection for fitness itself. He cited hierarchical genetic architecture as a powerful indication that evolvability has been a target of selection. He described a mechanism by which natural selection might occur not just for fitness but also for the rate of change of fitness. The mechanism was closely analogous to what is called in evolutionary theory "hitchhiking", [44] (though Layzer did not use the word). Over time, genes that manifest as increased rate of change become associated with individuals that have both higher and lower fitness compared to ambient means. The ones with lower fitness tend to die out, while those with higher fitness tend to survive. Thus genes for change become linked to genes for greater fitness and selection for the latter indirectly selects for the former. This was the Layzer hypothesis for evolution of evolvability.

In part because Layzer's ideas were out of tune with the times and in part because his language was that of a physicist, not a biologist, his work had little impact. Similar ideas developed without reference to Layzer by computer scientist Michael Conrad [45] met a similar fate. It was sixteen years later that Wagner and Altenberg [46], unaware of the precedents of Layzer and Conrad, independently proposed some of the same ideas and biochemical advances in the interim helped them to make their case more convincingly, using genetic examples. Evolvability became a new area of evolutionary study.

Adaptations that promote evolvability at a direct and immediate cost to individual fitness include, famously, sexual reproduction. There is broad agreement that the evolutionary basis for sexual reproduction is related to its contribution to evolvability, but there is yet no agreement about how sex might have evolved [26, 28, 47-49]. The mapping of genotype to phenotype is another crucial evolvability adaptation, because it affects the way in which the feedback of selection works on the raw material of variation [50, 51]. The simplest mappings that we might devise in the abstract would not provide a viable basis for a Darwinian process. Yet the mapping ultimately adopted by biology cannot have evolved by incremental mutations in nuclear DNA; rather, it reflects the holistic system of gene transcription, developmental timing, self-organizing cell structures and other processes that are yet poorly understood. Though the evolution of such holistic attributes does not fit easily within models, the genotype/phenotype map has nevertheless evolved in such a way as to make evolution possible and even efficient.

Similarly, other recognized adaptations that have been interpreted as promoting evolvability include different mutation rates for core metabolism and peripheral traits [52], adaptive mutation rates that depend on environmental cues [53] and hierarchical organization of genes (with hox genes on top and layers of subordinate instructions under them) [54]. Selective mechanisms for each of these fundamental features of life remain unexplained, though there is little doubt that their adaptive purpose is connected to evolvability. These precedents make plausible the acceptance of aging as another evolvability feature, even though standard theoretical frameworks suggest no selective mechanism.

The idea that evolvability could be the basis for evolution of aging was implicit in the early ideas of Weismann [6], first revived in the modern era by Libertini [55] and similar ideas with greater physiological detail were expounded by Skulachev [56] and Bowles [57, 58]. Goldsmith [59] has self-published and continually updated a volume on the subject. All these were qualitative descriptions of the mechanism. It was only in 2011 that a general numerical model for evolution of aging based on evolvability was proposed by Martins [40].

The Martins Model

Like the first two models of this chapter, the Martins model [40] tracks individuals with different genomes, competing and reproducing on a two-dimensional grid. All three models are simple and general for illustrative purposes, with an enormous amount of biological detail deliberately subsumed in as few parameters as possible. In the Martins model, total population density is fixed, with a Cartesian grid of sites that are densely filled. Each individual, in order to reproduce, must displace an existing occupant of a neighboring site. By assumption, the incumbent can only be replaced by an individual of strictly higher *fitness**, so fitness in the model must

---

* "Fitness" here has a completely abstract and limited meaning within the context of the model. It is a genetic trait of each individual, subject to mutation upon reproduction and its function within the model is as a criterion in competition for real estate. It is not claimed that this variable is isomorphic to Darwinian fitness in the actual biosphere, from which the word is borrowed.

evolve ever higher. A crucial feature of the model is that even when the offspring/ challenger has higher fitness than the incumbent at the target site, recruitment only succeeds with a probability $p < 1$. Senescence is modeled as a fixed lifespan, controlled by a single gene, such that each individual dies when its age attains the genetically determined lifespan. At that point, its site is available for occupancy by the next comer, without having to exceed a fitness threshold determined by an incumbent. Hence, senescence promotes more recruitment, faster population turnover and fitness progresses at a higher rate. Shorter lifespans are selected on this basis, despite the individual cost. The model robustly evolves shorter lifespans, defying intuition that enhanced reproductive potential of individuals with longer lifespans ought to trump the long-term advantage of greater population turnover.

In a 2014 sequel to this study [60], I worked with Martins to ask the question, how realistic is this model? We stripped the model to its essence, then varied it with different parameters, with gradual senescence instead of fixed lifespan, with a high burden of detrimental mutations, overwhelming a much smaller proportion of mutations that increased fitness. We conclude that, though the model is an abstraction, all its essential features have broad applicability in the biosphere. One of the factors that makes the model plausible (omitted in the original version) is the biased competition between mature adult and young offspring that limits recruitment in many species. Mature individuals are often able to out-compete younger challengers, even if the challenger has higher intrinsic (age-independent) fitness and this is an important effect limiting recruitment, slowing population turnover, cutting off potentially fruitful evolutionary pathways. Without senescence, the youngest group would always be the smallest, the weakest, the least experienced, the most vulnerable and the least able to compete. Senescence creates job opportunities for aspiring young offspring and the most prodigious among these carry the future of the species in their genes.

Aging in Prey Species

It is a common observation of field biologists that predators live longer than their prey. Foxes live 10 to 15 years in the wild, while rabbits live three to eight years. Lions live 30 years and gazelles 12. Wolves are smaller than the deer they hunt, but live longer [61]. Perhaps this is because the predator-prey ecosystem is more stable that way. The logistic model presented earlier in this chapter demonstrates that when the consumer species has a faster life cycle compared to the producer species, this relationship leads to demographic instability. Also, the longer life cycle of the predators gives them every motivation to protect their prey from population crashes, even for their own future, let alone their progeny.

We have seen how difficult it is for predators and prey to establish a stable demography. Both species have a common interest in assuring that the prey are not hunted to extinction. This is a classic setup for co-evolution: the predators evolve toward moderation, so they only capture the weaker prey; the prey evolve aging so as to assure that the weakest prey are not the youngest but the oldest.

Co-evolution is common in the biosphere, if challenging to understand (Darwin's "abominable mystery", [62]). Species that are entirely separate from each other evolve in parallel to tighten their ecological relationship. The mystery is that the traits of each species may benefit the other species, without providing any benefit to the individual which actually bears the trait. The neo-Darwinian paradigm has difficulty with many forms of co-evolution. Some dramatic examples involve wasp species that are exquisitely adapted to pollinate a single species of orchid. Birds get nourishment from eating berries and in return they spread the seeds within the berries far and wide. Most forms of co-evolution are difficult to explain within the vantage of pure individual selection, as illustrated by the problem of cheaters. For example, providing nectar in a flower is not an evolutionarily stable strategy, because any individual flower is tempted to attract the bee with smell and appearance and then skimp on actually providing the nectar. A mutation that led the flower to invest more in pollen and less in nectar would succeed in spreading, so long as it was rare. It would continue to spread even when not rare, because it might take many generations for the bees to evolve a system for detecting which flowers actually contain pollen. The prediction of classical evolutionary theory is that this mutation should evolve to fixation, undermining the symbiosis, before selection pressure at a higher level could reward the benefits of cooperation. The general conclusion is that most forms of co-evolution require group selection on a scale which mainstream evolutionists regard with extreme prejudice.

We usually think of co-evolution as applying to cooperative, symbiotic relationships, in which each species benefits from the other. But there is no reason why a predator and prey species cannot co-evolve a relationship that mitigates the ecological conflict between them and helps stabilize both populations. The principal danger to the predator/prey ecology comes from over-exploitation. Individually, the predators are evolving to be better at their 'job' and able to capture the prey more efficiently. But to the extent that they succeed, there is a tragedy of the commons: if the predators capture the prey too efficiently, there is no food left for the next generation. So predators as a group want to be fast, but not too fast.

Prey evolution may also be subject to a tragedy of the commons. Individually, prey are evolving to be better and better at evading the predator. But if the levels of reproduction are already evolved for stable replacement in the presence of predators, then the prey may collectively get into trouble with overpopulation if they evolve to be too slippery. This situation was illustrated with the story of the reindeer of St Matthews Island in Chapter 6.

Both predator and prey species have an interest in stabilizing population levels so that they can co-exist in a robust ecosystem, less liable to extinctions when the environment varies.

Predators may chase a herd of prey and take down the lagging member. In the absence of aging, the youngest members of the prey species would be the laggards. They are small, weak and vulnerable. But aging assures that the older members gradually reduce their speed and agility over time, until they reach the point where the oldest members of a herd are even more vulnerable than the youngest. Without aging, the weakest members would be the youngest and they would be the preferred targets of the predators. Not only is the number of young attaining to reproductive age drastically curtailed; the feedstock for population growth becomes extremely sensitive to the intensity of predation. For example, suppose that two species attain a balance in which 90% of the young prey, on average, are eaten by the predators, so that only 10% are growing to maturity. 10% may be just what is needed to replace the dying adults, so the population would appear to be stable. But this is an extremely precarious situation, because it may be that the next generation of predators is just slightly larger and they eat 100% of the young prey instead of 90%—so that now *none of the prey* are able to grow up and the population of prey disappears.

The instability of this situation is largely due to the fact that it is the youngest that are being preyed upon. Aging can overturn this dynamic. Suppose the prey grow progressively weaker with age, so that at any given time, the slowest and weakest members are not the youngest but the oldest. If the oldest members are taken down after they have already reproduced, then this poses little threat to the viability of the herd. Whether the predators take a few more or less from year to year has little effect on the size of the following year's harvest. Better yet, if the oldest members are post-reproductive, then they are (demographically) completely irrelevant and therefore expendable. It does not matter if the predators are out in force or if their numbers are very thin—the effect on reproduction rate of the prey herd is negligible [21].

In order for this to work, the predators must co-evolve moderation in the intensity of their hunt. Ideally, they should be just fast and agile enough to capture the aged prey, but they should be unable to capture the young ones. The reward is that this system provides a large and steady herd for the predators' dining pleasure. Over time, not only is their food reservoir maximized, they also get to harvest every prey animal, fully grown.

Theory based on pure individual selection would have a hard time with this mechanism. Selfish evolution favors cheaters in both species: predators that go after the young and prey that do not age. However, this is the best possible configuration for both the predator and prey species, if it can be attained and sustained. The most robust measure of fitness is the population density that can be supported; and by this standard, the arrangement with senescence on the part of the prey and restraint on the part of the predator maximizes productivity and population density for both species.

Why the Gazelle Doesn't Live Forever A Just-So Story of Co-Evolution

Once there was a race of gazelles that were all above average. In fact, they had attained the pinnacle of Darwinian fitness and were just as strong and as fast as the laws of physics would allow. And every one of them was at this peak, all proud and fit Survivors in the race that goes to the swift.

Of course, they were immortal. Not only were they uniformly in top form, but they could stay that way indefinitely. They never got old and they never lost their speed.

They shared the plain with a pride of lions. The lions were the very reason that the gazelles had evolved to be so fast. Every one of them could outrun the lions, except...

Except that the very young gazelles were small and new and shaky on their feet and slower than their perfectly fit mothers and fathers. The lions could catch the babies and they did.

So this race of immortal gazelles had no children. They went on living forever, almost, but whenever one of them died, by chance, it was a devastating tragedy, because there was no one to replace him. The herd got a little smaller each year.

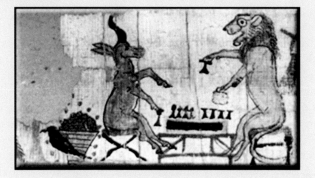

The population dwindled. Rumors flew. Elsewhere, there were other herds of immortal gazelles in even worse straits. Many had already been lost. Extinct. They couldn't get their babies to grow up. The situation was desperate.

An assembly was convened of the wisest elders. (Luckily, there was no shortage of wise elders.) They had to stop the lions from eating their children. But how?

The eldest and wisest of the group put forward his idea. There was no help for the situation without the cooperation of the lions. They must meet with the lions and ask the lions to stop eating their children. But what could they offer the lions in return?

There's only one thing that lions understand and that's red meat. We have to offer them more meat than they had before.

But where is this meat going to come from? The old, wise gazelles looked around the room and they knew the answer. To save their children, they would sacrifice themselves.

The gazelles made a pact. They would still be the fastest and the fittest, the most graceful denizens of the Serengeti, but only for a time. Each gazelle would have his chance to grow up, to live, to have children and raise them up. But at the end of the day, they would give themselves up, turn themselves in to the lions for meat.

"We'll allow the lions to eat us, every one, not when we are small and scrawny, but when we are fully grown and have much more meat to offer.

"And here's how we'll do it. We'll give up our immortality. We'll loosen our hold on perfection and we'll suffer aging over time. We'll get slower as we age, after we've enjoyed our lives and had our children.

"We give our elder selves up to the lions on one condition: the lions must stop eating our children. They'll continue to take the slowest of us, but the slowest won't be the youngest. The slowest will be the oldest."

They took their pact to the lion king and the lion king licked his lips and he signed eagerly on the dotted line. The lions would curb their appetite for speed, while indulging their appetite for meat. They'd have more to eat than ever before.

And so it was that the gazelles agreed, one and all, to give up their immortality. And the lions, too, kept to their bargain. They held back their speed, grew to be very fast, but not so fast as a gazelle at his peak. And never again did the lions eat the children of the gazelles, but always preyed upon the oldest.

The Serengeti blossomed with more lions and more gazelles than it had ever known and they all lived together in bliss and concord and demographic homeostasis.

Blunting the Blade of Selection

Over the æons, not only has the genome learned how to survive and reproduce; the genome has learned how to learn. Evolution can experiment, for example, with placement and geometry of appendages without risk of destroying the structures that have been highly optimized.

A great deal of the genome in higher animals and plants codes for basic metabolic chemistry. It has been crafted by natural selection and optimized over such an extended time that the genome knows not to monkey with it any more. Mutation rates in these areas are extremely low and one has to assume that is by design. Other areas of the genome are more recently acquired and the processes for which they code are more contingent and peripheral; mutation rates here are much higher [53, 63-65].

It is undeniable—it is a fact of logical causality—that the variation on which selection acts must always be blind to the future. But the process of evolution has been around a long while and has watched the history of many, many mistakes. So many times, selection has jumped too quickly to discard a trait that would later prove useful. Like a fortune-teller with Tarot cards and a crystal ball, somehow evolution has acquired an ability to feign foresight convincingly and to give the appearance of farsighted wisdom. The fortune-teller doesn't really know what will happen to you, but she is wise and experienced and good at reading clues in your dress, your affect, your demeanor. She makes educated guesses about the future based on her experience and sometimes she gives the appearance of being uncannily prescient.

Watson and Szathmary [66] combine learning theory with evolutionary theory with computer science to break conceptual ground in the evolution of evolvability.

The evolutionary process has itself evolved. Aging and sex were able to evolve on the basis of their contribution to evolvability; and their evolution was also made possible by earlier evolvability adaptations that softened the action of natural selection so that the short-term costs of aging and sex did not immediately blow them out of the water.

Locking the Door Against Temptation: An Alternative Explanation for Antagonistic Pleiotropy

The alcoholic who has ruined his career and his relationships once too often learns to bar temptation from his life, putting a lock on the liquor cabinet door. The short-term temptation of maximizing individual reproduction is a kind of temptation that has derailed natural selection so many times in the past, leading to so many dead ends, that eventually the genome has learned that some wide open roads turn predictably into blind alleys. Adaptations that block evolutionary pathways that provide short-term benefit at the expense of conspecifics have been incorporated into the structure of life at a deep level. This negative function is an important piece of evolvability, because it clears the way for selection of what is broadly adaptive in the long term.

The most efficient kind of natural selection is the selfish-gene variety that neo-Darwinists have studied so intensively. This is the open road to higher individual fitness. But some of these open roads lead to the blind alley of extinction. After many, many bouts with catastrophe, eventually some chance rearrangement of the genome comes along that tends to bar that road from future exploration, even as the organism continues to evolve in other ways. Then the temptation of maximizing individual reproduction in a way that does not work for the community can be avoided and thereafter the wholesale violence of group selection is experienced much less frequently.

The clearest example of a door that has been locked by natural selection is the prevalence of dioecious sex. Sharing genes across a community has huge advantages for evolution in the long run, but the temptation in the short run is for any individual to revert to cloning itself. Instantly it would be twice as fit as all its neighbors and its offspring would soon overrun the population. Only after many, many more generations would the genome begin to be polluted with mutations [67] and the population lose nature's race to keep up with changing environments. Remember that sex (gene sharing) was entirely separate from reproduction in the first protists. Cellular aging via telomere shortening was invented in order to enforce the imperative that protists must share their genes (Chapter 5).

The lock on the gene-sharing door for higher animals takes the form of tying sex to reproduction. The essential act of reproduction for higher organisms demands that genes be shared as a precondition. A double dead-bolt was provided by separation of sexual function in different individuals. Separation of the sexes minimizes the chance that any one individual can mutate to enable clonal reproduction, because each individual has only half the machinery needed to reproduce. Even self-fertilization in hermaphroditic plants and animals has been effectively barred by detailed structures of the anatomy. The extravagant adaptation of separate sexes exists for one purpose only: to bar the path of asexual reproduction as off-limits to evolving future generations. And for this lock, evolution has been willing to pay with a full factor of two in fitness (as fitness is measured by the narrow criteria of neo-Darwinism).

The defeat of aging is another very tempting target for individual selection—offering an individual advantage in the short run, but leading to trouble for the population down the road. Natural selection at the individual level is constantly pulling toward longer lifespan, trying to dismantle the machinery of death. It has been necessary to block the evolutionary road to immortality in order to guard against the temptation of individual selection and preserve the long-term advantages of aging for the population. To this end, aging has been implemented through multiple, redundant pathways, so that it is more difficult to defeat aging with a single mutation. Antagonistic Pleiotropy can be understood as one more adaptation that has grown up to guard against the loss of aging. Aging genes have sometimes been tied to essential life functions in order to lower the risk that they might be lost to selfish, short-term selection.

In Chapter 4, we described Antagonistic Pleiotropy as currently the best-accepted theory of aging among evolutionary biologists. Pleiotropy has been proffered as the root cause of the evolution of aging. The classical theory is that pleiotropy is essential and unavoidable and hence natural selection has been forced to accept aging in order to promote other aspects of individual fitness. Experimenters have searched for pleiotropy, sometimes found it and sometimes not: Pleiotropy is real, but it is not so essential or ubiquitous as the classical theory requires.

My hypothesis is that pleiotropy has been installed after-the-fact of aging. We may understand pleiotropy as a lock on the door, making it more difficult for mutations to just do away with aging—a short-term temptation that would likely lead to competitive disaster for any evolving species, over the long haul.

The Big Picture

It is easy to model natural selection for aging as an adaptation to preserve population homeostasis and prevent extinctions. It is more difficult to model the selection of aging as an evolvability adaptation. But this is not necessarily a reason to discount the importance of evolvability. The fact is that evolvability is an essential feature of life. Sex, the structure of the genome, differential mutation rates, the genotype-phenotype mapping and many aspects of the basic structure of biology are optimized for evolvability. Evolvability clearly *has* evolved, whether or not we understand how. We can see how selection for stable population dynamics has blunted the force of individual selection for ever higher growth rates and this opens the door to adaptations that may offer longer term benefits, at a short-term cost to individual fitness.

In the changing, self-modifying game of evolution, a crucial first step was the emergence of ecological webs of dependency. It became unprofitable (and sometimes disastrous) to reproduce more rapidly than the producers at the base of the ecosystem could sustain. Thus the first group-level adaptations were about cooperation to moderate growth and conserve renewable resources, as described by Wynne-Edwards [1]. But once the straitjacket of competition for ever-faster reproduction was removed, the nature of the game changed forever. The door was open for more sophisticated strategies that would bear fruit only over longer periods of time. Programmed lifespans were among the first cooperative strategies to emerge, because aging offers immediate benefits for demographic homeostasis and stabilization of ecosystems.

But as the necessity for unthrottled reproduction was tempered, the most important strategies to emerge were those that affected evolvability and the pace of evolutionary change, because such adaptations act recursively in an exponentially-accelerating progression.

The remarkable thing about aging is that it has evolved despite substantial individual cost and despite the fact that its advantage (for evolvability, for diversity and for stability of population dynamics) is very diffuse, indirect and weak. If the target of natural selection is evolvability, then aging must be considered part of the fine-tuning. Still, aging has been fiercely defended in the face of substantial selection pressure for longer lifespan; and aging has become sophisticated and plastic in its implementation. Aging must be understood in the context of an evolutionary process that is itself efficient, complex and highly evolved.

Summary

The first five chapters of this volume make a case that natural selection has included a death program in the genomes of most animals and plants. I judge that evidence to be compelling and indisputable. But the ideas in the present chapter about how that happened are more speculative. Neo-Darwinian theory about how natural selection operates will have to stretch to accommodate any aging program and the evolutionary processes described in this chapter are perhaps the most conservative, requiring the minimal extension of neo-Darwinism. All depends on the evolution of ecosystem stability, as described in Chapter 6. The need for homeostasis is easy to understand and when ecosystems are unstable, they are punished with swift extinction. This provides a plausible mechanism and a basis for understanding the evolution of aging.

Aging works very generally to level the death rate in good times and hard times. The proof of this is that animals only die of old age if they have not died of something else first. So the death toll from aging is logically bound to be higher when the death rate from all other causes is lower.

This provides a plausible rationale for aging. The changed picture of how natural selection works that is implied by these population dynamic processes is quite radical. Personally, I suspect that the truth may be even more radical and we will eventually come to realize that the ways of evolution are far more strange and wondrous than we can presently imagine. My mind is open to Lamarckian mechanisms, some currently recognized [68] and some yet to be discovered [52].

All life forms are interdependent. No species can exist without an ecosystem, and yet ecosystems are demographically very fragile, unstable and subject to destruction by any one wayward species. Species have had to adapt their ecological footprints in order to make stable ecosystems possible at all. This has been done by adjusting life cycle characteristics and aging is one of the ways that individual species are adapted to be 'good citizens' within the ecosystems upon which they depend.

Programmed death is not the strangest creation of natural selection. That title would go to sex, the "masterpiece of nature" [28]. Separation of the sexes cuts the individual organism's reproductive capacity by half. Aging is costly, but not so costly as that [69]. And compared to sexual dimorphism, aging was easier to arrange, since all that aging requires is to slow down some of the mechanisms of growth and repair, whereas sexual reproduction entails creation of new organs and new morphologies.

Neo-Darwinian theorists have had to accept sex because there are no other alternatives than to say that it evolved as an adaptation. But the same theorists have been reluctant to acknowledge that aging might have evolved by some of the same means as sex. In particular, the advantage of genetic diversity, which protects a population against epidemics, is a recognized force in the natural selection of sex; but aging also contributes to diversity and so evolution of aging might be understood in the same way.

All ecosystems include species that prey on other species. Aging of predators and aging of prey species both contribute to stable ecosystems in different ways. For prey, aging assures that it is the oldest members that are the weak ones and the most vulnerable to predation. Without aging, predators would always take the biggest bite out of the youngest age group, because they are small and vulnerable. This would be an unstable situation, indeed. Aging in predators helps to level the death rate: increasing the death rate when prey are abundant and lots of predator individuals live to a ripe old age; and also decreasing the death rate when prey are scarce, the predators are starving and therefore aging more slowly.

Aging also contributes to evolvability, though it is not so important in this regard as deeper adaptations such as the structure of the genome and gene sharing. The evolvability benefits of aging probably could not have been sufficient to account for its evolution as a group adaptation, but for the fact that strong, short-term selection for stable population dynamics had blunted the force of individual selection and opened the door to selection for features that matter more in the long term.

Natural selection acting over vast stretches of time has managed to lock some features into the genome when short-term selection might be tempted to abandon them. It appears that aging has been locked into the genome in this way, via antagonistic pleiotropy among other means.

References

1. Wynne-Edwards, V., *Animal Dispersion in Relation to Social Behavior*. 1962, Edinburgh: Oliver & Boyd.
2. Gilpin, M.E., *Group Selection in Predator-Prey Communities*. 1975, Princeton: Princeton University Press.
3. Layzer, D., *Genetic variation and progressive evolution*. Am. Nat., 1980. **115**(6): p. 809-826.
4. Finch, C.E., *Longevity, Senescence and the Genome*. 1990, Chicago: University of Chicago Press.
5. Jones, O.R., et al., *Diversity of ageing across the tree of life*. Nature, 2014. **505**(7482): p. 169-173.
6. Weismann, A., et al., *Essays upon Heredity and Kindred Biological Problems*, 2d ed. 1891, Oxford. Clarendon Press. 2 v.
7. Williams, G., *Pleiotropy, natural selection and the evolution of senescence*. Evolution, 1957. **11**: p. 398-411.
8. Price, G.R., *Selection and covariance*. Nature, 1970. **227**(5257): p. 520-1.
9. Price, G.R., *Extension of covariance selection mathematics*. Ann. Hum. Genet., 1972. **35**(4): p. 485-90.
10. Pollock, G.B., *Population viscosity and kin selection*. Am. Nat., 1983. **122**(6): p. 817-829.
11. Gadgil, M., N. Joshi and S. Gadgil, *On the moulding of population viscosity by natural selection*. J. Theor. Biol., 1983. **104**(1): p. 21-42.
12. Mitteldorf, J. and D.S. Wilson, *Population viscosity and the evolution of altruism*. J. Theor. Biol., 2000. **204**(4): p. 481-96.
13. Fisher, R.A., *The Genetical Theory of Natural Selection*. 1930, Oxford: The Clarendon Press. xiv, 272 p.
14. Haldane, J.B.C., *The Causes of Evolution*. 1932, Princeton. reprinted Princeton University Press (1990).

15. Hamilton, W.D., *The genetical evolution of social behaviour. I.* J. Theor. Biol., 1964. **7**(1): p. 1-16.

16. Hamilton, W.D., *The genetical evolution of social behaviour. II.* J. Theor. Biol., 1964. **7**(1): p. 17-52.

17. Dawkins, R., *The Selfish Gene.* 1976, Oxford: Oxford University Press.

18. Sober, E. and D.S. Wilson, *Unto Others: The Evolution and Psychology of Unselfish Behavior.* 1998, Cambridge, MA: Harvard University Press.

19. Frank, S.A., *The price equation, Fisher's fundamental theorem, kin selection and causal analysis.* Evolution, 1997. **51**(6): p. 1712-1729.

20. Mitteldorf, J., *Chaotic population dynamics and the evolution of aging: proposing a demographic theory of senescence.* Evol. Ecol. Res., 2006. **8**: p. 561-574.

21. Mitteldorf, J. and C. Goodnight, *Post-reproductive life span and demographic stability.* Oikos, 2012. **121**(9): p. 1370-1378.

22. Slobodkin, L.B., *How to be a predator.* Am. Zool., 1968. **8**(1): p. 43-51.

23. Mitteldorf, J. *Demographic homeostasis and the evolution of senescence. In: Fourth International Conference on Complex Systems.* 2002. Nashua, NH: NECSI.

24. Trubitsyn, A., *Evolutionary mechanisms of species-specific life span.* Advances in Gerontology (Russia), 2006. **19**: p. 13-24.

25. Roach, D.A. and J.R. Carey., *Population biology of aging in the wild.* Annual Review of Ecology, Evolution, and Systematics, 2014. **45**(1): p. 421-443.

26. Williams, G., *Sex and Evolution.* 1975, Princeton NJ: Princeton University Press.

27. Maynard Smith, J., *The Evolution of Sex.* 1978, Cambridge, UK: Cambridge University Press.

28. Bell, G., *The Masterpiece of Nature: The Evolution and Genetics of Sexuality.* 1982, Berkeley: University of California Press. 635 p.

29. van Valen, L., *A new evolutionary law.* Evol. Theor., 1973. **1**: p. 1-30.

30. Ridley, M., *The Red Queen.* 1993, London: Penguin.

31. Benton, M.J., *The Red Queen and the Court Jester: species diversity and the role of biotic and abiotic factors through time.* Science, 2009. **323**(5915): p. 728-732.

32. Sagan, D., *Cosmic Apprentice: Dispatches from the Edges of Science.* 2013: University of Minnesota Press.

33. Ricklefs, R., *Evolutionary theories of aging: confirmation of a fundamental prediction, with implications for the genetic basis and evolution of life span.* Am. Nat., 1998. **152**: p. 24-44.

34. Bonduriansky, R. and C.E. Brassil, *Senescence: rapid and costly ageing in wild male flies.* Nature, 2002. **420**(6914): p. 377.

35. Moorad, J.A. and D.E.L. Promislow, *Evolution: aging up a tree?* Current biology: CB, 2010. **20**(9): p. R406-R408.

36. Socolar, J., S. Richards and W.G. Wilson, *Evolution in a spatially structured population subject to rare epidemics.* Phys. Rev. E 2001. **63**(041908): p. 1-8.

37. Austad, S., *Retarded senescence in an insular population of Virginia opossums.* J. Zool. London, 1993. **229**: p. 695-708.

38. Reznick, D.N., et al., *Effect of extrinsic mortality on the evolution of senescence in guppies.* Nature, 2004. **431**(7012): p. 1095-9.

39. Ricklefs, R.E., *Life-history connections to rates of aging in terrestrial vertebrates.* Proc. Natl. Acad. Sci., 2010. **107**(22): p. 10314-10319.

40. Martins, A.C., *Change and aging senescence as an adaptation.* PLoS One, 2011. **6**(9): p. e24328.

41. Dennett, D.C., *Darwin's dangerous idea.* The Sciences, 1995. **35**(3): p. 34-40.

42. Hornby, G.S. and J.B. Pollack, *Creating high-level components with a generative representation for body-brain evolution.* Artif. Life, 2002. **8**(3): p. 223-246.
43. Ofria, C., C. Adami and T.C. Collier, *Design of evolvable computer languages.* Evolutionary Computation, IEEE Transactions on, 2002. **6**(4): p. 420-424.
44. Barton, N.H., *Genetic hitchhiking.* Philos. Trans. R. Soc. Lond. B Biol. Sci., 2000. **355**(1403): p. 1553-1562.
45. Conrad, M., *The geometry of evolution.* BioSyst., 1990. **24**(1): p. 61-81.
46. Wagner, G.P. and L. Altenberg, *Complex adaptations and the evolution of evolvability.* Evolution, 1996. **50**(3): p. 967-976.
47. Peck, J.R., *Sex causes altruism. Altruism causes sex. Maybe.* Proc. R. Soc. Lond., Ser. B: Biol. Sci., 2004. **271**(1543): p. 993-1000.
48. Hartfield, M. and P.D. Keightley, *Current hypotheses for the evolution of sex and recombination.* Integrative zoology, 2012. **7**(2): p. 192-209.
49. Margulis, L. and D. Sagan, *The Origins of Sex: Three Billion Years of Genetic Recombination.* 1990, New Haven: Yale University Press. 259 p.
50. Altenberg, L., *Genome growth and the evolution of the genotype-phenotype map*, In: *Evolution and biocomputation.* 1995, Springer. p. 205-259.
51. Wagner, G.P. and J. Zhang, *The pleiotropic structure of the genotype–phenotype map: the evolvability of complex organisms.* Nature Reviews Genetics, 2011. **12**(3): p. 204-213.
52. Shapiro, J.A., *Evolution: A View from the 21st Century.* 2011, Saddle River, NJ: FT Press.
53. Sniegowski, P.D., P.J. Gerrish and R.E. Lenski, *Evolution of high mutation rates in experimental populations of E. coli.* Nature, 1997. **387**(6634): p. 703-705.
54. Ruddle, F.H., et al., *Evolution of hox genes.* Annu. Rev. Genet., 1994. **28**(1): p. 423-442.
55. Libertini, G., *An adaptive theory of the increasing mortality with increasing chronological age in populations in the wild.* J. Theor. Biol., 1988. **132**: p. 145-162.
56. Skulachev, V.P., *Aging is a specific biological function rather than the result of a disorder in complex living systems: biochemical evidence in support of Weismann's hypothesis.* Biochemistry (Mosc.), 1997. **62**(11): p. 1191-5.
57. Bowles, J.T., *The evolution of aging: a new approach to an old problem of biology.* Med. Hypotheses, 1998. **51**(3): p. 179-221.
58. Bowles, J.T., *Shattered: Medawar's test tubes and their enduring legacy of chaos.* Med. Hypotheses, 2000. **54**(2): p. 326-39.
59. Goldsmith, T.C., *The Evolution of Aging.* 3rd Edition ed. 2013, Annapolis, MD: Azinet. 187 p.
60. Mitteldorf, J. and A.C. Martins, *Programmed life span in the context of evolvability.* The American Naturalist, 2014. **184**(3): p. 289-302.
61. Carey, J. and D. Judge, *Longevity Records: Life Spans of Mammals, Birds, Amphibians, Reptiles, and Fish.* 2002: Odense University Press.
62. Friedman, W.E., *The meaning of Darwin's "abominable mystery".* Am. J. Bot., 2009. **96**(1): p. 5-21.
63. Bejerano, G., et al., *Ultraconserved elements in the human genome.* Science, 2004. **304**(5675): p. 1321-5.
64. Sun, H., et al., *Structural relationships between highly conserved elements and genes in vertebrate genomes.* PLoS One, 2008. **3**(11): p. e3727.
65. Wolfe, K.H., P.M. Sharp and W.H. Li, *Mutation rates differ among regions of the mammalian genome.* Nature, 1989. **337**(3): p. 283-285.
66. Watson, R.A. and E. Szathmary, *How can evolution learn?* Trends Ecol. Evol., 2015.
67. Muller, H.J., *The relation of recombination to mutational advance.* Mutat. Res., 1964. **106**: p. 2-9.

68. Jablonka, E., *Epigenetic Inheritance and Evolution: the Lamarckian Dimension.* 1999: Oxford University Press.
69. Turcotte, M.M., D.N. Reznick and J.D. Hare, *The impact of rapid evolution on population dynamics in the wild: experimental test of eco-evolutionary dynamics.* Ecol. Lett., 2011. **14**(11): p. 1084-92.

8
CHAPTER

Reforming
Evolutionary Theory

I have argued for amending the current evolutionary theory of aging and expanding the recognized mechanisms of natural selection to accommodate the evidence that aging has been selected as an adaptation [1-3]. (For the opposite perspective requiring less accommodation from theory, I recommend a thoughtful discussion including commentary by several leading aging scientists, led by George Martin [4].)

Why should we overhaul the theory and not simply patch it minimally to accommodate certain facts about aging? The latter would be a proper application of Occam's Razor if aging were the only area in which neo-Darwinian theory faced difficulty. But in fact, neo-Darwinism is under siege from empirical science in many quarters. The entire neo-Darwinian paradigm is top-heavy with theory and lacking in field support. Experimental confirmation there is aplenty, but this demonstrates only that artificial selection can be designed to select individual traits in the laboratory; it says nothing about natural selection in the wild, knowledge of which is far more difficult and tentative.

What is the nature of natural selection? Does it operate exclusively at an individual level or is a communal measure of fitness commonly its target? An empirical approach to these questions draws inference from observations of what has been selected; but we have too often applied an abstract approach, attempting to derive an answer from first principles [5]. Science is served best when theory is in service of the empirical, but in evolutionary science we have persisted with experiments conducted in the service of theory. The difficulties that aging presents to evolutionary theory are not an isolated anomaly, but part of a broad pattern. I am not the first, nor the best-qualified person to press the point that the foundation of evolutionary theory is in need of fundamental reform.

Standard evolutionary theory may be uniquely vulnerable, because there are many broad features of the biosphere that do not sit comfortably in its realm. Neo-Darwinism cannot accommodate the ubiquity of sexual reproduction (especially when the twofold cost of carrying males is considered) [6, 7]; neo-Darwinism cannot explain the hierarchical structure of the eukaryotic genome, with command-and-control functions that dictate the expression of many lower-level genes [8];

neo-Darwinism takes genetic diversity as a given, but cannot account for the persistence of diversity [9]; neo-Darwinism explicitly rules out horizontal gene transfer and genome-merging phenomena that have been important at crucial turning points in evolutionary history [10, 11]; even some common examples of co-evolution between species are poorly-treated by neo-Darwinism [12]. In Chapter 6, I have proffered a quite general argument that neo-Darwinism cannot explain the observed persistence of ecosystems.

The neo-Darwinian paradigm has done well in framing the results of experiments in laboratory evolution; but this may be because lab experiments are designed around accumulation of genes that already exist as polymorphisms within the lab's breeding population. In other words, lab experiments rarely depend on creation of evolutionary novelty and never require the multiple independent new structures that are most difficult for evolutionary theory to account for. Furthermore, artificial selection in lab models is frequently designed with intention to replicate the neo-Darwinian assumption about how natural selection is supposed to work. Hence laboratory evolution offers no independent test of whether these assumptions are applicable in nature [13].

Evolution of Sex

This is the best recognized and most outrageous contradiction to standard evolutionary theory. Sex was discussed sufficiently in the previous chapter that I include here just a brief reminder.

Sharing of genes is costly and makes no contribution to the standard neo-Darwinian notion of fitness, which refers only to individual reproductive success. Sex is the most widely-recognized challenge to evolutionary theory, but it has been treated as an exception, an isolated anomaly, a mystery to be pondered by some elite and philosophically-inclined subset of the scientific community, while the rank and file goon with the quotidian business of applying standard theory, taking dioecious implementation as given. The fact that sexual reproduction has evolved as an adaptation should be a flashing neon sign advertising the inadequacy of the neo-Darwinian paradigm; but rarely have theorists taken the warnings seriously.

Hierarchical Structure of the Eukaryotic Genome

The most striking feature of the genotype/phenotype map is its hierarchical structure with hox genes controlling the development of entire organs and systems. From hox genes to chromosomes, down to the individual exons that are cut and spliced in various combinations to make genes, the entire genome has been organized in modules. This is a global adaptation that must have taken æons to develop and yet it yields no fitness benefit, only a second order benefit in the rate of change of fitness. Hence, it is difficult to reconcile with neo-Darwinian models.

Consider an analogy with computer programs: If genomes were built one mutation at a time, you might expect that they would look like what used to be called "spaghetti code" in the archaic world of Fortran programming. The genome would be full of quirks and kluges and things that happen to work in this particular case, though not in general. There is some of this; but remarkably, we find that the genome is hierarchically ordered. There are master switches—hox genes—that can turn on whole genetic programs, with many hundreds of genes, all ordered in just the right way.

The benefits of this kind of structuring of the genome are wholly long-term. Unlike the case of sex, it is difficult to estimate the cost of a structured genome. But, like sex, the benefits of the structured genome with hox genes do not accrue to the individual in the current generation or even in a small number of generations. The benefit manifests as evolvability and is realized only over evolutionary time, after thousands or tens of thousands of generations.

Phenotypic Plasticity

In adapting to any particular environment, it is enormously easier to come up with a targeted solution that narrowly addresses the particular situation. And yet, living things are plastic, adapting on the fly to individual variations in their microenvironments. To the extent that the range of microenvironments could never have been experienced in the lifetime of one individual, phenotypic plasticity represents a multi-generational adaptation. Phenotypic plasticity must have evolved as a long-term response to unpredictable change in the environment. This is 'lineage selection' on a grand scale.

Remarkably, it has been discovered in recent years that phenotypic plasticity can have a trans-generational component. This has been called "epigenetic inheritance" and its mechanism falls outside the model of neo-Darwinism.

Epigenetic Inheritance

Can traits that are acquired during an individual's life experience be passed to offspring? In the eighteenth century, this was the primary mechanism of evolution as proposed by Jean-Baptiste Lamarck. Darwin expounded a limited role for Lamarckian inheritance, which he referred to as "use and disuse" of body functions. In the generation following Darwin, August Weismann [14] reported results from one careful but limited experiment that discredited the idea of Lamarckian inheritance for generations to come. What he measured was not Darwin's "use and disuse", but the effect of cutting off a mouse's tail on the tail length of its offspring. (Weismann found there was none.) With the staged, politically-motivated experiments of Lysenko in Soviet Russia [15], Lamarckism lost all respect.

Today, Lamarckian inheritance has no place in neo-Darwinian evolutionary theory. However, experiments in recent years have uncovered intriguing examples in which the life experience of an individual affect its offsprings' phenotype for two and three generations to come [16]. This has been named "epigenetic inheritance", but its mechanisms are not well-understood. Adaptations can be passed epigenetically from the father [17] as well as the mother. The best available hypothesis is that biochemical signaling can affect the methylation patterns that control gene expression and that the chromosome's methylation fingerprint is replicated along with the DNA [18, 19].

There is a substantial literature of Lamarckian inheritance in bacteria that affects genome sequence and not just gene expression [10]. It has been argued that heritable chromatin modifications are just the beginning, that Lamarckian inheritance is a much broader phenomenon still [10, 16].

Co-Evolution

Some instances of co-evolution find a natural explanation within the framework of neo-Darwinism. For example, the symbiosis within the components of a lichen is easy to understand, because lichens comprise two individual organisms that are dependent upon one another. What each one does to benefit its partner reflects back in a direct effect on the self. But there are other examples of co-evolution that do not fit well within the neo-Darwinian paradigm [20, 21]. Consider, for example, the nectar which flowers provide to bees in exchange for pollination. In the short term, bees are attracted to flowers by their sweet smell and bright colors; but in the long term, bees continue to visit flowers because the flowers provide nectar, which is carried back to the hive for food. Neo-Darwinian logic predicts an opportunity for "cheater" flowers to undermine this system: A mutant plant may invest more in scent and appearance, but less in nectar itself. Then bees would be more likely to visit the flower and carry its pollen, though they might find out too late that there was no nectar to be harvested [22]. Another classic example of mutualism is the "farming" of aphids by ants [23]. Individuals to whom the benefit (the aphids' sweet excretion) accrues are not the same individuals that provide the reciprocal benefit (protection from predators); therefore this kind of mutualism cannot evolve via purely individual selection. The cost of the co-evolved trait is borne by the individual, but the benefit passes to many of the commensal partners and by the time it is reflected back, the benefit falls broadly on those that carry the trait and those that do not.

Diversity

When I first took up evolutionary modeling in the 1990s, I quickly discovered that, unless density-dependent selection is explicitly implemented, diversity quickly collapses. Other modelers have made the same observation [24, 25]. In simple models based on standard population genetics, a single genotype evolves quickly to fixation. Evolution proceeds to a fitness maximum and stops. The models are telling us something about the way biological evolution works: it cannot be a straightforward race to produce the most replicates. Such a simple contest produces permanent winners and eliminates losers far too quickly and a great deal of information is thereby lost.

Darwin already recognized the maintenance of diversity as a puzzle. He had no knowledge of Mendelian inheritance and believed that the attributes of an offspring were blended or averaged from the attributes of the parents. With this mode of inheritance, diversity would rapidly collapse. With the neo-Darwinian synthesis, combining Mendelian inheritance with Darwinian selection, the problem of diversity became less severe and attracted less attention. Still, it remains a weakness of neo-Darwinian theory that neutral mutation rates are inadequate and theory acknowledges no selective force capable of maintaining diversity.

In fact, diversity in itself has been a major target of natural selection, a component of fitness at the group level. Some selection for diversity can be explained by conventional models of frequency-dependent selection [26]; but such mechanisms only apply to the maintenance of diversity itself and not to the creation of second-order mechanisms (like sex and aging) that seem to exist for the purpose of enhancing diversity. In practice, one of the greatest advantages of maintaining diversity is that a trait that was useful in the evolutionary past may be useful again in the future, as environments continue to change and sometimes cycle back to features reminiscent of the past. There is a long-term evolutionary advantage to be had by silently preserving traits that were useful in the past, so they do not have to be evolved anew should they become useful again in the future.

Maintenance of diversity, sexual genetic exchange, aging and a hierarchical genome are all examples of evolvability adaptations. There is now no opposition in the scientific community to the signal importance of evolvability or to the idea that evolvability is an evolved trait. Many evolutionists who accept evolvability nevertheless reject the idea that aging might have evolved on this basis.

Reversion or *Evolutionary Capacitance*

Darwin noted that traits may be lost from the phenotype but not the genotype in the course of evolution. What he observed was that it is much easier to re-evolve a trait that was recently lost than it would be to create the same trait for the first time. But in the transition to neo-Darwinism, the idea that a trait might be stored in the genome for later use seemed untenable. This principle was formalized by Louis Dollo [27] and for many decades, it was widely quoted as Dollo's Law: "An organism is unable to return, even partially, to a previous stage already realized in the ranks of its ancestors."

But in our present understanding of molecular genetics, we say that genes remain hidden in the genome, with their expression suppressed, so that they may easily be recovered. This phenomenon has been re-discovered in the last decade and named "evolutionary capacitance", by analogy with the ability of an electric capacitor to store charge within [28, 29]. Evolutionary capacitance represents another way in which variation is not blind, suppressing random destruction and favoring adaptive change. This in itself is an exception to neo-Darwinian orthodoxy; but the larger challenge is this: How did the phenomenon of evolutionary capacitance come to be? Like aging and sex and hox genes, it is an adaptation which has value only for the *pace* of evolution and not for the fitness of the individual or its immediate progeny [30].

Horizontal Gene Transfer

Bacteria freely exchange genetic information in the form of plasmids. They are promiscuous, picking up DNA that derived from others very different from themselves. HGT in higher organisms is mediated by viruses and is far less common, but perhaps crucially important at critical junctures. HGT seems to have been responsible for some of the great transitions in evolutionary history. Every organism alive today can trace different parts of its genome to diverse lineages, very different from its direct ancestors. Carl Woese [31] has noted that Darwin's tree of life is, in fact, better characterized as a web of life.

Too Much Theory with Too Little Field Support

In fact, the science of neo-Darwinism is uniquely top-heavy with theory and lacks a solid foundation of observational support. From its origins in the 1920s, the theory was derived from axioms by mathematical scientists and not pieced together from the bottom up by field biologists [32]. Many evolutionary biologists have been educated to believe that the neo-Darwinian paradigm is "how evolution works". It is the framework within which they think and no conceivable observation could falsify that belief. New findings in genetics and even medicine are interpreted within the context of neo-Darwinian theory. For the science of aging in particular, this has been a consistent distortion of the underlying data, thwarting understanding.

The evolutionary community has been slow to embrace the modest reforms spearheaded through the distinguished career of David Sloan Wilson [33, 34]. Meanwhile, a chorus of equally distinguished voices have called for more radical changes, though there is as yet no consensus on direction and it may yet turn out that the processes of evolution are simply far more diverse than can be encompassed in an axiomatic theory like neo-Darwinism. Evolution of evolvability is one theme of the insurgent literature [30, 35-37], though there is as yet no spokesperson for the deeply subversive implications of this concept. Some broad features of the biosphere are explainable not from the imperative to survive and reproduce, but rather from the imperative to adapt in a changing world [9, 10]. Nowak [38, 39] is the most prominent voice promoting new approaches based on computational evolution. E.O. Wilson, whose career was built on classical applications of neo-Darwinism, came later in life to a realization of the radical importance of collective adaptations [40, 41]. The well-read works of Gould [42] have implications that are far-reaching and subversive. Margulis emphasized the importance of horizontal gene transfer [43] and the merging of lineages [11].

I find the wisest and broadest vision in the writings of Carl Woese.

The Legacy of Carl Woese

The late Carl Woese [44] bequeathed to us a vision of the "Path Not Taken" in 20th century biology and his plea for a more holistic approach in the 21st. I quote from Woese at length, as but a poor substitute for your reading the essay in its entirety.

[T]he colorless, reductionist world of 19th century classical physics [has] strongly affected the outlook of western society in general. The living world did not exist in any fundamental sense for classical physics: reality lay only in atoms, their interactions and certain forces that acted at a distance. The living world, in all its complexity and beauty, was merely a secondary, highly derived and complicated manifestation of atomic reality and like everything else in our direct experience, could (in principle) be completely explained (away) in terms of the ever-jostling sea of tiny atomic particles (53). The intuitive disparity between atomic reality and the "biological reality" inherent in direct experience became the dialectic that underlay the development of 20th century biology.

...molecular biology would prove a mixed blessing. On the positive side, those problems (or portions thereof) that were amenable to a reductionist approach would benefit from the fresh, no-nonsense outlook and experimental power of molecular biology. In addition, biology as a whole would benefit from the physicist's general modus operandi, i.e., from the well-honed understanding of what science is and how it should be done: the crisp framing of problems, the clear understanding of what is and what is not established truth, the importance of hypothesis testing and the physicist's disinterested approach in general. On the negative side, biology's holistic problems, which were not commensurate with the new molecular perspective, would remain relatively or completely undeveloped. The result was a distorted growth of biology in the 20th century. The most pernicious aspect of the new molecular biology was it reductionist perspective, which came to permeate biology, completely changing its concept of living systems and leading then to a change in society's concept thereof...

Fundamentalist reductionism (the reductionism of 19th century classical physics)... is *ipso facto* a statement about the nature of the world: living systems (like all else) can be completely understood in terms of the properties of their constituent parts. This is a view that flies in the face of what classically trained biologists tended to take for granted, the notion of emergent properties. Whereas emergence seems to be required to explain numerous biological phenomena, fundamentalist reductionism flatly denies its existence: in all cases the whole is no more than the sum of its parts. Thus, biology of the 20th century was in the strange position of having to contort itself to conform to a world view (fundamentalist reductionism) that 20th century physics was simultaneously in the process of rejecting...

The most transformative message of quantum mechanics is not uncertainty or wave/particle duality or discrete quanta of energy; the deepest and most revolutionary change inherent in 20th century physics is precisely the repudiation of reductionism. This is "quantum entanglement" and it is pervasive, universal. We know now that the single-particle wave function is only an approximation, that an electron is not a particle unto itself but a piece of "electron stuff" that pervades the universe. Proper treatment of the dynamics of any one electron takes explicit account of the exchange symmetry that connects this electron to all electrons everywhere.

Woese is fascinated with the irony that 20th century biology set out to emulate physics, but the physics it chose to emulate was the reductionist physics of the 19th century. While 20th century biology busied itself understanding the biological machine by studying its parts, 20th century physics was trying to understand and assimilate the message of holism thrust upon it by quantum mechanics and by the remarkable coincidences in the "six numbers" that make possible the rich complexity of the universe we know [45, 46].

I think the 20th century molecular era will come to be seen as a necessary and unavoidable transition stage in the overall course of biology: necessary because only by adopting a heavily reductionist orientation and the technology of classical physics could certain biological problems be brought to fruition and transitional because a biology viewed through the eyes of fundamentalist reductionism is an incomplete biology. Knowing the parts of isolated entities is not enough. A musical metaphor expresses it best: molecular biology could read notes in the score, but it couldn't hear the music. The molecular cup is now empty. The time has come to replace the purely reductionist "eyes-down" molecular perspective with a new and genuinely holistic, "eyes-up," view of the living world, one whose primary focus is on evolution, emergence and biology's innate complexity...

A heavy price was paid for molecular biology's obsession with metaphysical reductionism. It stripped the organism from its environment; separated it from its history, from the evolutionary flow; and shredded it into parts to the extent that a sense of the whole—the whole cell, the whole multicellular organism, the biosphere—was effectively gone. Darwin saw biology as a "tangled bank", with all its aspects interconnected. Our task now is to resynthesize biology; put the organism back into its environment; connect it again to its evolutionary past; and let us feel that complex flow that is organism, evolution and environment united. The time has come for biology to enter the nonlinear world...

[T]he entry of chemistry and physics into biology was inevitable. The technology that these sciences would introduce was not only welcome but very much needed... But the physics... was a Trojan horse, something that would ultimately conquer biology from within and remake it in its own image. Biology would be totally fissioned and its holistic side would be quashed. Biology would quickly become a science of lesser importance, for it had nothing fundamental to tell us about the world. Physics provided the ultimate explanations. Biology, as no more than complicated chemistry, was at the end of the line, merely providing baroque ornamentation on the great edifice of understanding that was physics—the hierarchy physics $\Rightarrow$ chemistry $\Rightarrow$ biology is burned into the thinking of all scientists, a pecking order that has done much to foster in society the (mistaken) notion that biology is only an applied science...

Thus, biology... must choose [to] break free of reductionist hegemony, reintegrate itself and press forward once more as a fundamental science. The latter course means an emphasis on holistic, "nonlinear," emergent biology—with understanding evolution and the nature of biological form as the primary, defining goals of a new biology...

"One would be hard put to explain evolution and the problem of biological form in reductionist terms alone." [emphasis added].

References

1. Mitteldorf, J., *Chaotic population dynamics and the evolution of aging: proposing a demographic theory of senescence.* Evol. Ecol. Res., 2006. **8**: p. 561-574.
2. Mitteldorf, J. and J. Pepper, *Senescence as an adaptation to limit the spread of disease.* J. Theor. Biol., 2009. **260**(2): p. 186-195.
3. Mitteldorf, J., *Evolutionary origins of aging, In: Approaches to the Control of Aging: Building a Pathway to Human Life Extension*, G.M. Fahy, et al., Editors. 2010, Springer: New York. p. 87-126.
4. Martin, G.M., *How is the evolutionary biological theory of aging holding up against mounting attacks?* American Aging Assoc Newsletter, 2005(May, 2005): p. 1-15.
5. Sober, E. and D.S. Wilson, *A critical review of philosophical work on the units of selection problem.* Philosophy of Science, 1994: p. 534-555.
6. Bell, G., *The Masterpiece of Nature: The Evolution and Genetics of Sexuality.* 1982, Berkeley: University of California Press. 635 p.
7. Burt, A., *Perspective: sex, recombination and the efficacy of selection–was Weismann right?* Evolution Int. J. Org. Evolution, 2000. **54**(2): p. 337-51.
8. Ruddle, F.H., et al., *Evolution of hox genes.* Annu. Rev. Genet., 1994. **28**(1): p. 423-442.
9. Kirschner, M. and J. Gerhart, *The Plausibility of Life.* 2006, New Haven, CT: Yale University Press. 336.
10. Shapiro, J.A., *Evolution: A View from the 21st Century.* 2011, Saddle River, NJ: FT Press.
11. Margulis, L. and D. Sagan, *Acquiring Genomes.* 2002, Basic Books: New York. 240 p.
12. Thompson, J.N., *The Coevolutionary Process.* 1994, Chicago: University of Chicago Press. 383 p.
13. Endler, J.A., *Natural Selection in the Wild.* Monogr. Popul. Biol. 1985, Princeton, NJ: Princeton University Press. 354 p.
14. Weismann, A., et al., *Essays upon heredity and kindred biological problems.* 2d ed. 1891, Oxford: Clarendon press. 2 v.
15. Roll-Hansen, N., *The Lysenko effect: undermining the autonomy of science.* Endeavour, 2005. **29**(4): p. 143-147.
16. Cabej, N.R., *Epigenetic Principles of Evolution.* 2012, Boston, MA: Elsevier.
17. Pembrey, M.E., *Time to take epigenetic inheritance seriously.* Eur. J. Hum. Genet., 2002. **10**(11): p. 669-71.
18. Bird, A., *DNA methylation patterns and epigenetic memory.* Genes Dev. 2002. **16**(1): p. 6-21.

19. Jones, P.A. and G. Liang, *Rethinking how DNA methylation patterns are maintained.* Nature Reviews Genetics, 2009. **10**(11): p. 805-811.

20. Goodnight, C.J., *Experimental studies of community evolution I: The response to selection at the community level.* Evolution, 1990. **44**(6): p. 1614-1624.

21. Goodnight, C.J., *Experimental studies of community evolution II: The ecological basis of the response to community selection.* Evolution, 1990. **44**(6): p. 1625-1636.

22. Wright, G.A., A.F. Choudhary and M.A. Bentley, *Reward quality influences the development of learned olfactory biases in honeybees.* Proc. Biol. Sci., 2009. **276**(1667): p. 2597-604.

23. Shingleton, A.W., D.L. Stern and W.A. Foster, *The origin of a mutualism: a morphological trait promoting the evolution of ant-aphid mutualisms.* Evolution, 2005. **59**(4): p. 921-926.

24. Rosenzweig, M.L., *Species Diversity in Space and Time.* 1995, Cambridge University Press.

25. Chesson, P., *Mechanisms of maintenance of species diversity.* Annu. Rev. Ecol. Syst., 2000: p. 343-366.

26. Takahata, N. and M. Nei, *Allelic genealogy under overdominant and frequency-dependent selection and polymorphism of major histocompatibility complex loci.* Genetics, 1990. **124**(4): p. 967-78.

27. Dollo, L., *Les lois de l'evolution.* Bull. Soc. Belge Geol. Pal. Hydr., 1893. **VII**: p. 164-166.

28. Masel, J., *Evolutionary capacitance may be favored by natural selection.* Genetics, 2005. **170**(3): p. 1359-71.

29. Bergman, A. and M.L. Siegal, *Evolutionary capacitance as a general feature of complex gene networks.* Nature, 2003. **424**(6948): p. 549-52.

30. Layzer, D., *Genetic variation and progressive evolution.* Am. Nat., 1980. **115**(6): p. 809-826.

31. Woese, C.R., *Interpreting the universal phylogenetic tree.* Proc. Natl. Acad. Sci., 2000. **97**(15): p. 8392-8396.

32. Sober, E., *Evolution, population thinking and essentialism.* Philosophy of Science, 1980. **47**(3): p. 350-380.

33. Sober, E. and D.S. Wilson, *Unto Others: The Evolution and Psychology of Unselfish Behavior.* 1998, Cambridge, MA: Harvard University Press.

34. Wilson, D.S., *Introduction: multilevel selection theory comes of age.* The American Naturalist, 1997. **150**(s1): p. S1-S21.

35. Wagner, G.P. and L. Altenberg, *Complex adaptations and the evolution of evolvability.* Evolution, 1996. **50**(3): p. 967-976.

36. Kirschner, M. and J. Gerhart, *Evolvability.* Proc. Natl. Acad. Sci., 1998. **95**(15): p. 8420-8427.

37. Masel, J. and M.V. Trotter, *Robustness and evolvability.* Trends Genet., 2010. **26**(9): p. 406-414.

38. Nowak, M.A., *Five rules for the evolution of cooperation.* Science, 2006. **314**(5805): p. 1560-1563.

39. Nowak, M.A., *Why we help.* Sci. Am., 2012. **22**: p. 92-97.

40. Wilson, D.S. and E.O. Wilson, *Evolution" for the Good of the Group": The process known as group selection was once accepted unthinkingly, then was widely discredited; it's time for a more discriminating assessment.* Am. Sci., 2008. **96**(5): p. 380-389.

41. Wilson, E.O., *The Social Conquest of Earth.* 2012, WW Norton & Company: New York.

42. Gould, S.J., *The Structure of Evolutionary Theory.* 2002, Harvard University Press.

43. Margulis, L., *Genome acquisition in horizontal gene transfer: symbiogenesis and macromolecular sequence analysis*, In: *Horizontal Gene Transfer*. 2009, Springer. p. 181-191.
44. Woese, C.R., *A new biology for a new century.* Microbiol. Mol. Biol. Rev., 2004. **68**(2): p. 173-186.
45. Rees, M., *Just Six Numbers*. 2000, New York: Basic Books. 189 p.
46. Davies, P.C.W., *Cosmic Jackpot: Why our Universe is Just Right for Life*. 2007, New York: Houghton Mifflin, 336 p.

9

A New Paradigm for Medical Research

I have long admired the parsimony and the pregnancy in the last sentence of Watson and Crick's seminal paper on the structure of DNA [1]:

> *It has not escaped our notice that the specific pairing we have postulated immediately suggests a possible copying mechanism for the genetic material.*

Emulating their concision, I should say only:

> *It has not escaped my notice that the adaptive provenance of aging suggests possible approaches to geriatric medicine and the remediation of senescence.*

But having neither the brash self-assurance of James Watson nor the prodigious vision of a Francis Crick, I risk overstepping my commission by attempting an outline of the directions in which I believe medical science should and will be propelled by a realization that aging is programmed into our genes.

Some researchers in gerontology [2, 3] have embraced the idea that the diseases of old age are best addressed not individually, but by going to the root of the problem, slowing or reversing the deterioration of the body's various defense functions that cause an exponential acceleration of vulnerability to these diseases. I support this view. Research funding, particularly in the US, has been held captive by the institutions and the historic beneficiaries of a system that separately and massively supports research into cancer, heart disease and Alzheimer's Disease. This is not just a great waste of funds, but a great waste of our best research talents and ultimately, a great waste of the lives and health of those who continue to be denied effective treatments for these diseases. Even a modest success in identifying interventions to influence the physiological mechanisms of aging would provide an outsized social benefit, whether the return be calculated in lives saved or in quality of life or in future medical costs avoided. The only argument against this research direction is the presumption that progress is impossible. Recent experience suggests that progress is more than possible, it is a present reality; but scientific attitudes and government bureaucracies have been slow to accommodate to the new reality and funding priorities are particularly slow to change, due to the inertia of entrenchment.

It is my hope that the perspective on aging provided in this volume may contribute to the new optimism in aging research and perhaps to suggest specific directions.

Programmed Aging Presents a Great Opportunity

If aging were the residue of problems that evolution has tried for æons to solve but come up short, then we would have to be very smart indeed to defeat Orgel's Second Law* [4]. If aging were the result of inevitable deterioration of a thousand bodily systems in a thousand different ways, then we would have to engineer a thousand solutions (or at least seven [5]) to forestall death. But since aging is a program of self-destruction proceeding under genetic control, there is the possibility that it can be addressed straightforwardly and efficiently by modulating gene expression. It is possible that aging may be modulated at its root by changing the gene expression of an old person to a youthful profile. This is an approach suggested by the paradigm of programmed and it may be possible to try if the young science of epigenetics advances over the next few years.

Affirmative Modes of Self-Destruction

Geriatric medicine has already discovered and begun to address several of the means by which the body attacks itself late in life. There are four modes of self-destruction that are already subjects of substantial research and though the most common approaches are not generally framed as diverting the body from its suicidal path, this is indeed the effect of at least some of the early remedies.

- Cellular senescence through telomere loss
- Inflammation
- Derangements of the immune system, including both auto-immunity and weakened ability to subdue invading pathogens
- Apoptosis, which again becomes mis-programmed in both directions, killing healthy cells while failing to halt neoplasias.

The recognition that these are not systems gone awry but part of a suicide program should only help to clarify research paths in these areas.

Cellular Senescence Through Telomere Loss

There is diverse evidence that cellular senescence is a potent mode of aging in humans, with major impact on mortality. This makes telomeres and telomerase an attractive target for anti-aging therapy. There is reason to think that longer telomeres will be an unqualified benefit to the body. Some claim that telomere length might be the body's primary aging clock [6-10].

Telomere length has been linked to life expectancy in humans [11, 12], in birds [13, 14] and in mammals [15-18]. Even in mice, which have prodigiously long

---

* "Evolution is cleverer than you are."–Leslie Orgel

telomeres and which express telomerase through their lifetimes, the rate of telomere loss has been correlated to mortality [19].

Using a large statistical sample, a Danish group [12] has been able to verify that short telomeres are robustly correlated with mortality, even after correction for age and for all the standard markers of mortality risk. This implies that short telomeres are an independent cause of mortality and also of cancer, which was separated for analysis. People with short telomeres were found to be dying at a rate 1.5 times higher than people of the same age with long telomeres. This ratio (1.5) is the actuarial equivalent of five years (my own calculation, based on Social Security Administration life tables [20]). On the one hand, five years is an eye-popping promise compared to results from traditional biomedical research; on the other hand, five years is too small to support the hypothesis that telomeres are the body's primary aging clock.

The toxicity of cells with short telomeres is well-understood [21-23] and as proof-of-principle, lifespan has been extended by removal of senescent cells [24]. Activation of telomerase has been demonstrated to extend lifespan and health span in mice with no increase in cancer rates [25] and dramatic rejuvenation has been observed in experiments with mice deprived of telomerase and then re-supplied with telomerase [26].

These results are so promising that telomerase activation should be a major research priority, but investment in this research is being held back by irrational fears that activating telomerase must increase cancer risk. There is no empirical basis for this fear [27] and the root of the fear is the evolutionary theory that says aging cannot be programmed, hence nothing as simple as expression of one gene could possibly have an unmitigated benefit for lifespan.

In the meantime, it may be that considerable life extension can be achieved simply by tagging and eliminating cells that have become senescent. Campisi has described SASP, a "senescence-associated secretory phenotype" that poisons surrounding tissue and exacerbates inflammation when a cell becomes senescent. Van Deursen [24] has demonstrated life extension in mice from removing senescent cells and (in 2015) several companies around the globe are racing to translate this concept into a pharmaceutical product.

Inflammation

Inflammation is widely recognized to increase with age in humans and the consequences have been linked to risk of cardiovascular disease [28], cancer [29] and Alzheimer's Disease [30, 31] as well as arthritis [32].

Inflammation is the body's first line of defense against invading microbes and it also plays an important role in eliminating diseased cells and damaged tissue in wounds and bruises. In old age, inflammation turns against the body and destroys healthy tissue. The standard description is that inflammation becomes subject to dysregulation with age. From the perspective of this volume, inflammation is a healthy response in youth that is co-opted into a death program at older ages. Epigenetic promotion of inflammation increases sharply with age in humans [33,

34], as you would expect if inflammation is regarded as a programmed mode of self-destruction. Pro-inflammatory cytokines include NFκB, TGF-β, COX2, IL-1β and IL-6, all of which increase with age.

Simple anti-inflammatory agents like aspirin and ibuprofen are the best-documented and best-accepted life extension pills available now, reducing all-cause mortality an estimated 13% [35]. They work because after age 50, inflammation is doing more harm than good and generally dialing it down with a "dumb" drug has a substantial benefit. But to make further progress with inflammation, we will need "smart" drugs that can reduce the harmful effects of inflammation without hampering the action of inflammation where it is needed. There is evidence that *Nigella sativa* (black cumin seed or chernushka) and *Ganoderma lucidum* (Lingzhi or reishi mushroom) have some potential in this area [36]. Among many anti-inflammatory herbs, it stands out because it simultaneously enhances immune function.

Immune Derangement

Closely related to inflammation is the problem of immune derangement. The aging human body is prone to auto-immune diseases and also to failures of the immune system to adequately defend against invading pathogens. Some of the problem can be traced to cellular senescence in leukocytes, whose telomeres shorten with age. Another factor is the loss of T-cell specificity. T-cells are named for the thymus gland, where they are "trained" to distinguish self from foreign cells. But the thymus shrinks over a life time, from a maximum size in pre-adolescence. The thymus loses half its mass by age 50 and continues its involution into old age. Thymic involution has been viewed as benign, again based on blind faith that the body cannot simply be destroying itself [37]. But old mice have shown signs of rejuvenation upon transplantation of a young thymus [38] and extracts of thymus have been applied successfully to increase lifespan in mice and in humans [39]. It may be that strategies to halt thymic involution have major potential for life extension in humans [40]. Promising trials have identified a single transcription factor capable of stimulating thymus regrowth [41]. As I write in 2015, a new clinical trial has been announced seeking to regrow the thymus in subjects age 50-65 using growth hormone.

Rapamycin is a powerful immune suppressant; that it is a life extension drug [42, 43] attests to the damage done by auto-immunity in old age. Fear of infectious disease from immune suppression has held back experimentation with rapamycin as a general-purpose tonic for humans, but Blagosklonny [44] claims it is safe, based on biochemistry and self-experimentation.

Apoptosis

Apoptosis is vitally important both in development and as protection against viral infections and cancer. But with age, apoptosis develops a "hair trigger" and healthy cells eliminate themselves. Overactive apoptosis is linked to sarcopoenia [45, 46] and also to the loss of brain cells characteristic of dementia [47]. Lifespan of a strain of mice with accelerated aging has been extended by knocking out p66^{shc}, an apoptosis signal [48].

It should not be difficult to develop drugs that simply down-regulate apoptosis and there is cause for optimism that this will offer a net benefit. One hint is that animals that live longer because of caloric restriction are found to have lower levels of apoptosis in muscles and in nerve cells. But CR animals also show higher levels of apoptosis in organs that are prone to cancer. For a major benefit to lifespan, it will be necessary to understand apoptosis and restore its proper regulation in old age.

"Natural Medicine"

A sweeping cultural change in medical research took place after the middle of the 20th century, as researchers learned to work with the body's natural defenses rather than to manipulate the metabolism with brute force. Doctors were learning a respect for the product of evolution. This is "natural medicine" and the cultural shift has resulted in a reduction of harm and brought multiple benefits.

Natural medicine is rooted in a respect for evolution's legacy (Orgel's Second Law, cited above). But the realization that aging is an evolved mode of self-destruction changes the landscape. It should be clear that natural medicine is an inapt model for the diseases of old age. We will make no progress "working with the body" so long as the body is hell-bent on destroying itself.

This is a fundamental shift in thinking and in medical culture. It affects strategy and analysis at a foundational level and disrupts habits of thought that today's professionals have formed through the entire course of their careers. Cultural shifts are never comfortable or easy, but this one will bear copious fruits for health and longevity, whenever we can manage it.

Is There a Biological Clock?

The concept of programmed aging logically implies that the body tracks its own age and at any given time has a reference clock or more likely, a small number of semi-independent clocks, that govern its metabolic characteristics. The body's age is stored as biochemical information and not simply a state of relative disrepair in various tissues. If all aspects of aging were governed by a single clock, that clock would be vulnerable to hijacking by individual selection. (This is Williams's [49] argument that no one trait subject to individual selection could have a substantial impact on lifespan.) So we might suspect that aging is governed by multiple, redundant clocks.

It may be that two such aging clocks are realized in telomere attrition and thymic involution, described above. Yet there is good reason to suppose that these two are not the whole story. Some animals suffer senescence even though their telomeres do not shorten with age. And some modes of aging in humans seem unlikely to be related to telomeres and immune function. For example, the brain ages, though neuronal growth is not directly limited by short telomere or the state of the thymus.

A broader reason for suspecting the existence of a third clock based on epigenetics comes from thinking about developmental biology. In growth, development and puberty, timing is exquisitely sensitive. It is widely believed that development is under control of gene expression, i.e., epigenetic programming. What clock tells the body when to secrete growth factors and when to stop or when to initiate puberty with gonadotropic hormones? This remains an unanswered question in developmental biology [50]. In recent years, it has become clear that gene expression is a strong function of age [51, 52]. The fact that a separate clock has never been identified suggests that gene expression itself might be a clock. Time can be measured using a feedback loop and gene expression provides such a loop:

- Epigenetic state of individual cells controls gene expression (including circulating hormones).
- Circulating hormones feedback to continually reprogram the epigenetic state of individual cells.

The existence of an epigenetic aging clock was independently suggested by Rando [53] and de Magalhães [54].

Parabiosis and Factors in the Blood

Parabiosis is the surgical joining of two bodies so that they share a common circulatory flow. Heterochronic parabiosis is the joining of a young and old animal. Experiments were done with mice beginning in the 19th century and in the 1950s, the field was renewed by the same Clive McCay [55] who discovered the life extension potential of caloric restriction in the 1930s.

The current wave of parabiosis experiments with mice grew from Tom Rando's Stanford University laboratory and several of his students in the early 2000s. The Conboys, Villeda, Wagers and Wyss-Coray today conduct parabiosis experiments in their own labs.

The first promising experiment in this new wave was published in 2005 [56], in which it was reported that impaired muscle and skin healing in an old mouse was rescued by exposure to blood from a young mouse. It was not the red or white blood cells that offered the benefit, but protein and RNA factors dissolved in the plasma. Intriguingly, gene expression was found to be broadly impacted, reverting to a more youthful profile.

These experiments established the possibility that old tissue could be rejuvenated by a young signaling environment. The next steps were to transfuse blood plasma from young to old mice and to identify specific factors in the blood that are responsible for rejuvenation. Wagers [57] found that haematopoietic stem cells could be rejuvenated by a youthful profile of blood factors.

This work is very much in progress. As I write in 2015, a number of results have been published that make the epigenetic clock model [53] look more plausible. Villeda [58] reports that infusion of young blood plasma reverses nerve damage, improves cognitive function in a mouse model of Alzheimer's Disease. It has already become clear that there are both anti-aging factors that are underexpressed and also pro-aging factors that are overexpressed in old mice. Among the anti-aging factors identified are GDF11*, which promotes nerve and muscle growth [60] and oxytocin, which is necessary for muscle maintenance [61]. Among the pro-aging factors identified are TGFβ and NFκB, which promote inflammation [56], ALK5 [62] and FSH which is associated with weight gain, osteoporosis and some cancers [63, 64].

Methylation of CpG islands in DNA is best-studied of several means by which gene expression is monitored epigenetically. Mazin [65, 66] noted loss of methylation with age in rats and associated the loss with cell senescence. Using algorithmic searches based on statistics alone, Horvath [67] has found combinations of DNA methylation sites that change so consistently with age that an accurate measure of functional age (in humans) can be constructed. There is a great deal of consistency among different tissues and different donors.

Heterochromatin refers to stretches of DNA that are tightly-spooled, suppressing transcription. With age, the proportion of heterochromatin is diminished, genes are unmasked that were repressed in youth and some of the unmasked genes are associated with pathology [68]. This also resonates with the story of sirtuins, a class of anti-aging factors that derive their name from being <u>S</u>ilent <u>I</u>nformation <u>R</u>egulators [69]. General maintenance of methylation (through overexpression of methyltransferases) has been linked to increased lifespan in flies [70] and worms [71]; but it is likely that for substantial increments of life extension in human, a finely detailed approach to epigenetic reprogramming will be necessary [72, 73].

Control from the Brain

The body's circadian rhythm is controlled by the suprachiasmatic nucleus, located within the hypothalamus in the brain's endocrine region [74]. Circadian cycles can be effected with a small number of circulating hormones, whereas development and aging probably require timing and integration of an epigenetic network that is both complex and plastic in response to signaling from the metabolic and external environments. All the more reason to expect that the locus of a clock for aging and development might be in the neuroendocrine regions of the brain.

Cavadas [75, 76] has investigated the effects of neuropeptide Y (NPY), a short peptide deriving from the hypothalamus. She has collected evidence for a role of NPY in regulating aging at a systemic level [77]. Levels of NPY decline with age and in mice, NPY seems to be necessary for the life extension effects of CR [78]. Cavadas links six modes of aging to NPY levels:

- loss of proteostasis
- stem cell exhaustion
- altered intercellular communication
- deregulated nutrient sensing

---

* GDF11 is something of a surprise since its biochemical role is closely related to catabolic hormones and the pro-aging factor TGFβ. David Glass of Novartis has reported inability to replicate Wagers's positive results 59. Egerman, Marc A., et al., *GDF11 Increases with age and Inhibits Skeletal Muscle Regeneration.* Cell Metabolism. **22**(1): p. 164-174.

- cellular senescence and
- mitochondrial dysfunction

Though NPY may be a promising target for anti-aging therapies, it is probably not an upstream determinant of age because it is a neurotransmitter and not a transcription factor. FOXO and SIRT1 are transcription factors strongly linked to aging, but are not centrally sourced in the brain. Orexin and oxytocin derive from the hypothalamus and both have been linked to effects on aging [79]. Age-dependent increase in the pro-inflammatory signal NFκB, mentioned above, seems to emanate directly from the hypothalamus [80].

Study of the nanogram secretions of neuroendocrine signals from the brain presents technical challenges for experimenters, but it may be a most promising area for high-level metabolic control of aging.

Future Directions

It is a fact that gene expression changes with age and a reasonable hypothesis that gene expression controls some aging phenotypes. There is reason to hope that restoring the body to a youthful state of gene expression will rejuvenate the repair and growth faculties, stimulating the body to repair years of accumulated damage. We have seen that a few powerful transcription factors are capable of reprogramming the epigenetic state of chromatin and this suggests a promising path for aging research.

For future medical applications, the existence of an epigenetic aging clock will do us little good if it is essentially complex and must be re-programmed, one site at a time, with the epigenetic markers characteristic of youth. But if we are fortunate, then some manageable number of circulating hormones and other blood factors will be discovered that can signal the body to return epigenetic programming to a more youthful state. If only because the prize is potentially so large, this possibility is a worthy focus for intensive research in the near future.

Epilog: Social Consequences of Increased Longevity

We have journeyed from aging as an evolved mechanism to avoid population overshoot to a derived lesson for medical interventions to increase (individual) human longevity. Increase in the human lifespan has been the driving force behind an explosion of the human population over the past 150 years [81]. The question would be obvious, were it not too terrible to ask: Are humans subject to the ecological principles of population dynamics?

Close on the heel of falling death rates, birth rates have plummeted in compensation. But there has been a generation gap between falling death rates and falling birth rates and rising human population has been a consequence. Currently, Africa is the last continent where technology is finally moving in to increase life expectancy and the African birth rate is coming down, but not fast enough to avoid devastating population increases. Over the next 30 years, the population of Africa is expected to double from 1.1 billion to 2.4 billion, a larger absolute increase than the aggregate growth in the rest of the world.

In 1850, world population was just over one billion and it is now over seven, with projections to peak somewhere north of 10 billion. A factor of seven or ten is not large in the context of local population booms. It is routine for population collapses to rebound or to be reseeded from nearby populations that have not suffered ecological collapse. One thing unique to humans is our global reach. Never before has a single species adapted to habitats over so much of the earth's land area. Wherever he has ventured, *Homo techniologicus* has displaced indigenous species, including indigenous humans. The biomass of humans is trivial compared to the biomass of insects or bacteria, but technology has swollen the human footprint. Human activity has triggered the sixth mass extinction in the half-billion year history of multicellular life [82]. Estimates of present extinction rates vary widely, with consensus estimates between 0.1% and 1% per century, numbers which are already 100 times higher than background extinction rates (before man). (The time resolution for assessing previous extinctions in archaeological time is too coarse to compare with the anthropocene extinction.) In the near future, extinction rates are expected to rise rapidly as the latent effects of habitat fragmentation and global climate change come into play [83]. Rate projections vary even more widely [84] with the highest predicting that half of all species could succumb in less than 100 years. In the oceans, the principal causes of extinction are drift net fishing, dumping of plastic waste and ocean acidification (from CO_2 emissions). 25% of all ocean species are presently listed as endangered or near-endangered. (The academic science in this and related areas has been tainted by industrial funding of researchers committed to downplaying the threat and independent scientists publishing "conservative" numbers because they anticipate being attacked as alarmist [85].)

Warnings that humans could extinguish life on earth are not worthy of consideration. It is inconceivable that human folly could destroy all of life. There are bacteria and macroscopic extremophile species that thrive in boiling and freezing conditions, extreme aridity, high levels of ionizing radiation, huge pressures under the sea and underground. Life can survive on diverse energy sources besides the well-studied standards (sunlight and food derived from sunlight). Even the realization of humanity's ultimate destructive potential in a nuclear war and speculated nuclear winter [86] could not put life in jeopardy. But it is quite possible that human activity could destroy the ecological basis that supports human life. This threat becomes the more pressing as humans are integrated into a single global economy. The few remaining pockets of hunter-gatherer tribes are considered fragile and endangered, but paradoxically they could be the only survivors after a collapse of the global production and transportation systems on which most of humanity depends.

It has been demonstrated five times in the past that the Biosphere roars back from major extinctions, with new species, greater complexity of integration and biodiversity increased each time. But speciation to fill the emptied niches is a process that extends over tens of millions of years. Our grandchildren may consider this a long time to wait.

It is an unstated and often unexamined assumption that the ecological ascent of humankind at the expense of biodiversity is "only" a crime against nature, permitting human desire for growth to take precedence over every other value.

Subconsciously, we may imagine a "farm earth" [87] that has been re-engineered to support 20 or 30 billion humans. But it is not at all clear that an artificial biosphere is possible or viable. Human knowledge of biology is strongest in the small, molecules and genetics; metabolic and systems biology are not nearly so well-developed and our understanding of ecologies and complex systems remains rudimentary. There has been exactly one attempt to engineer a fully artificial ecosystem to support a few humans in a two-acre greenhouse in Arizona in 1991 [88]. The experiment failed spectacularly.

Our species's two most ambitious attempts at bioengineering to date have been in the areas of antibiotics and factory farming. Antibiotics have neutered the threat of dozens of infectious diseases that just a century ago were life-threatening. The Green Revolution [89, 90] has increased grain yields per acre by five- or ten-fold since the 19th century. Both have played essential roles in supporting growing human populations and both are undermined by long-term consequences for which sustainable solutions remain elusive. Antibiotic resistance is now widely recognized as an impending crisis for global health [91]. Industrial farming methods are mining fossil reserves of water and topsoil that nature can replenish only over tens of thousands of years [92]. Industry-funded science and public relations campaigns can no longer keep the lid on health and environmental concerns from genetically modified organisms [93, 94].

I believe that medical progress will continue and that advances in understanding of aging will lead to lifespan extension on a global scale, perhaps more rapidly than in the past. The worst case would be if life extended only at the very end, with disabled people being cared for in a dependent, unhappy and unproductive state for additional years. I think this outcome is unlikely, because the most effective anti-aging strategies will attack the core mechanisms of aging long before its consequences are disabling. So human individuals may look forward to longer and healthier lives. The larger challenges in humanity's near future concern ecology, sustainability and overpopulation, together with the political institutions that prevent us from addressing the collective consequences of individual success.

References

1. Watson, J.D. and F.H. Crick, *Molecular structure of nucleic acids.* Nature, 1953. **171**(4356): p. 737-738.
2. Hall, S.S., *A trial for the ages.* Science, 2015. **349**(6254): p. 1274-1278.
3. de Grey, A.D. and M. Rae, *Ending Aging.* 2007, Cambridge, UK: St Martin's Press. 400 p.
4. Duntz, J. and G. Joyce, *Leslie E. Orgel, A Biographical Memoir.* Nat. Acad. of Sciences, Editor. 2013.
5. De Grey, A., *A Reimagined Research Strategy for Aging.* Sens Research Foundation 2016 [cited 2016 16 May 2016]; Available from: http://www.sens.org/research/introduction-to-sens-research.
6. Harley, C.B., et al., *The telomere hypothesis of cellular aging.* Exp. Gerontol., 1992. **27**(4): p. 375-82.

7. West, M.D., *The Immortal Cell*. 2003, New York: Doubleday. 244 p.

8. Fossel, M., *Cells, Aging and Human Disease*. 2004, New York: Oxford University Press. 489 p.

9. Fossel, M., *Use of telomere length as a biomarker for aging and age-related disease.* Current Translational Geriatrics and Experimental Gerontology Reports, 2012. **1**(2): p. 121-127.

10. Fossel, M., *The Telomerase Revolution: The Enzyme That Holds the Key to Human Aging... and Will Soon Lead to Longer, Healthier Lives*. 2015, New York: Ben Bella Books.

11. Cawthon, R.M., et al., *Association between telomere length in blood and mortality in people aged 60 years or older.* Lancet, 2003. **361**(9355): p. 393-5.

12. Rode, L., B.G. Nordestgaard and S.E. Bojesen, *Peripheral blood leukocyte telomere length and mortality among 64 637 individuals from the general population.* J. Nat. Cancer Inst., 2015. **107**(6): p. djv074.

13. Haussmann, M.F., D.W. Winkler and C.M. Vleck, *Longer telomeres associated with higher survival in birds.* Biol. Lett., 2005. **1**(2): p. 212-4.

14. Pauliny, A., et al., *Age-independent telomere length predicts fitness in two bird species.* Mol. Ecol., 2006. **15**(6): p. 1681-7.

15. Herbig, U., et al., *Cellular senescence in aging primates.* Science, 2006. **311**(5765): p. 1257.

16. Argyle, D., et al., *Equine telomeres and telomerase in cellular immortalisation and ageing.* Mech. Ageing Dev., 2003. **124**(6): p. 759-764.

17. McKevitt, T.P., et al., *Telomere lengths in dogs decrease with increasing donor age.* J. Nutr., 2002. **132**(6): p. 1604S-1606S.

18. Brümmendorf, T.H., et al., *Longitudinal studies of telomere length in feline blood cells: implications for hematopoietic stem cell turnover in vivo.* Exp. Hematol., 2002. **30**(10): p. 1147-1152.

19. Vera, E., et al., *The rate of decrease of short telomeres predicts longevity in mammals.* Cell Reports, 2012. **2**(4): p. 732-737.

20. Administration, S.S., *Acuarial Life Table*. 2010: Washington, DC.

21. Krtolica, A., et al., *Senescent fibroblasts promote epithelial cell growth and tumorigenesis: a link between cancer and aging.* Proc. Natl. Acad. Sci., 2001. **98**(21): p. 12072-12077.

22. Campisi, J. and F.d.A. di Fagagna, *Cellular senescence: when bad things happen to good cells.* Nat. Rev. Mol. Cell Bio., 2007. **8**(9): p. 729-740.

23. Kuilman, T. and D.S. Peeper, *Senescence-messaging secretome: SMS-ing cellular stress.* Nature Reviews Cancer, 2009. **9**(2): p. 81-94.

24. Baker, D.J., et al., *Clearance of p16Ink4a-positive senescent cells delays ageing-associated disorders.* Nature, 2011. **479**(7372): p. 232-236.

25. Bernardes de Jesus, B., et al., *Telomerase gene therapy in adult and old mice delays aging and increases longevity without increasing cancer.* EMBO Mol. Med., 2012: p. 691-704.

26. Jaskelioff, M., et al., *Telomerase reactivation reverses tissue degeneration in aged telomerase-deficient mice.* Nature, 2011. **469**(7328): p. 102-106.

27. Mitteldorf, J., *Telomere biology: cancer firewall or aging clock?* Biochemistry (Moscow), 2013. **78**(9): p. 1054-1060.

28. Reiss, A.B. and A.D. Glass, *Atherosclerosis: immune and inflammatory aspects.* J. Investig. Med., 2006. **54**(3): p. 123-31.

29. Marx, J., *Inflammation and cancer: the link grows stronger.* Science, 2004. **306**(5698): p. 966-968.
30. Andersen, K., et al., *Do nonsteroidal anti-inflammatory drugs decrease the risk for Alzheimer's disease?* Neurology, 1995. **45**(8): p. 1441-1445.
31. Sven, E.N., et al., *Does aspirin protect against Alzheimer's dementia? A study in a Swedish population-based sample aged = 80Å years.* Eur. J. Clin. Pharmacol., 2003. **V59**(4): p. 313-319.
32. Pelletier, J.-P., J. Martel-Pelletier and S.B. Abramson, *Osteoarthritis, an inflammatory disease: potential implication for the selection of new therapeutic targets.* Arthritis Rheum., 2001. **44**(6): p. 1237-1247.
33. Fagiolo, U., et al., *Increased cytokine production in mononuclear cells of healthy elderly people.* Eur. J. Immunol., 1993. **23**(9): p. 2375-2378.
34. Chung, H.Y., et al., *Molecular inflammation: underpinnings of aging and age-related diseases.* Ageing research reviews, 2009. **8**(1): p. 18-30.
35. Kaiser, J., *Will an aspirin a day keep cancer away?* Science, 2012. **337**(6101): p. 1471-1473.
36. Salem, M., F. Alenzi and W. Attia, *Thymoquinone, the active ingredient of Nigella sativa seeds, enhances survival and activity of antigen-specific CD8-positive T cells in vitro.* Br. J. Biomed. Sci., 2011. **68**(3): p. 131.
37. George, A.J. and M.A. Ritter, *Thymic involution with ageing: obsolescence or good housekeeping?* Immunol. Today, 1996. **17**(6): p. 267-272.
38. Hosaka, N., et al., *Thymus transplantation, a critical factor for correction of autoimmune disease in aging MRL/+mice.* Proc. Natl. Acad. Sci., 1996. **93**(16): p. 8558-8562.
39. Anisimov, V.N. and V.K. Khavinson, *Peptide bioregulation of aging: results and prospects.* Biogerontology, 2010. **11**(2): p. 139-149.
40. Fahy, G., *Precedents for the biological control of aging: postponement, prevention and reversal of aging processes, In: Approaches to the Control of Aging: Building a Pathway to Human Life Extension,* G.M. Fahy, et al., Editors. 2010, Springer: New York.
41. Bredenkamp, N., C.S. Nowell and C.C. Blackburn, *Regeneration of the aged thymus by a single transcription factor.* Development, 2014. **141**(8): p. 1627-1637.
42. Harrison, D.E., et al., *Rapamycin fed late in life extends life span in genetically heterogeneous mice.* Nature, 2009. **460**(7253): p. 392-5.
43. Wilkinson, J.E., et al., *Rapamycin slows aging in mice.* Aging Cell, 2012: pp. 127-223.
44. Blagosklonny, M.V., *Prospective treatment of age-related diseases by slowing down aging.* Am. J. Pathol., 2012. **181**(4): p. 1142-1146.
45. Marzetti, E. and C. Leeuwenburgh, *Skeletal muscle apoptosis, sarcopenia and frailty at old age.* Exp. Gerontol., 2006. **41**(12): p. 1234-8.
46. Pistilli, E.E., J.R. Jackson and S.E. Alway, *Death receptor-associated pro-apoptotic signaling in aged skeletal muscle.* Apoptosis, 2006. **11**(12): p. 2115-26.
47. Behl, C., *Apoptosis and Alzheimer's disease.* J. Neur. Trans., 2000. **107**(11): p. 1325-1344.
48. Migliaccio, E., et al., *The p66shc adaptor protein controls oxidative stress response and life span in mammals.* Nature, 1999. **402**(6759): p. 309-13.
49. Williams, G., *Pleiotropy, natural selection and the evolution of senescence.* Evolution, 1957. **11**: p. 398-411.
50. Ebling, F.J., *The neuroendocrine timing of puberty.* Reproduction, 2005. **129**(6): p. 675-683.
51. de Magalhães, J.P., J. Curado and G.M. Church, *Meta-analysis of age-related gene expression profiles identifies common signatures of aging.* Bioinformatics, 2009. **25**(7): p. 875-881.

52. Zykovich, A., et al., *Genome-wide DNA methylation changes with age in disease-free human skeletal muscle.* Aging cell, 2014. **13**(2): p. 360-366.
53. Rando, T.A. and H.Y. Chang, *Aging, rejuvenation and epigenetic reprogramming: resetting the aging clock.* Cell, 2012. **148**(1): p. 46-57.
54. Johnson, A.A., et al., *The role of DNA methylation in aging, rejuvenation and age-related disease.* Rejuvenation Research, 2012. **15**(5): p. 483-494.
55. McCay, C.M., et al., *Parabiosis between old and young rats.* Gerontology, 1957. **1**(1): p. 7-17.
56. Conboy, I.M., et al., *Rejuvenation of aged progenitor cells by exposure to a young systemic environment.* Nature, 2005. **433**(7027): p. 760-764.
57. Mayack, S.R., et al., *Systemic signals regulate ageing and rejuvenation of blood stem cell niches.* Nature, 2010. **463**(7280): p. 495-500.
58. Bouchard, J. and S.A. Villeda, *Aging and brain rejuvenation as systemic events.* J. Neurochem., 2014.
59. Egerman, Marc A., et al., *GDF11 increases with age and inhibits skeletal muscle regeneration.* Cell Metabolism, 2015. **22**(1): p. 164-174.
60. Katsimpardi, L., et al., *Vascular and neurogenic rejuvenation of the aging mouse brain by young systemic factors.* Science, 2014. **344**(6184): p. 630-634.
61. Elabd, C., et al., *Oxytocin is an age-specific circulating hormone that is necessary for muscle maintenance and regeneration.* Nature communications, 2014. **5**: pp. 1-11.
62. Conboy, I.M., M.J. Conboy and J. Rebo, *Systemic problems: a perspective on stem cell aging and rejuvenation.* Aging (Albany NY), 2015. **7**(10): p. 754.
63. Merry, B.J. and A.M. Holehan, *Serum profiles of LH, FSH, testosterone and 5 alpha-DHT from 21 to 1000 days of age in ad libitum fed and dietary restricted rats.* Exp. Gerontol., 1981. **16**(6): p. 431-44.
64. Bowles, J.T., *The evolution of aging: a new approach to an old problem of biology.* Med. Hypotheses, 1998. **51**(3): p. 179-221.
65. Mazin, A., *Genome loses all 5-methylcytosine a life span. How is this connected with accumulation of mutations during aging?.* Mol. Biol. (Mosk.), 1993. **27**(1): p. 160.
66. Mazin, A., *Loss of total 5-methylcytosine from the genome during cell culture aging coincides with the Hayflick limit.* Mol. Biol. (Mosk.), 1993. **27**(4): p. 895.
67. Horvath, S., *DNA methylation age of human tissues and cell types.* Genome Biol., 2013. **14**(10): p. R115.
68. Zhang, W., et al., *A Werner syndrome stem cell model unveils heterochromatin alterations as a driver of human aging.* Science, 2015. **348**(6239): p. 1160-1163. DOI: 10.1126/science.aaa1356.
69. Guarente, L., *Sirtuins, aging and medicine.* New Engl. J. Med., 2011. **364**(23): p. 2235-2244.
70. Chavous, D.A., F.R. Jackson and C.M. O'Connor, *Extension of the Drosophila life span by overexpression of a protein repair methyltransferase.* Proc. Nat. Acad. Sci., 2001. **98**(26): p. 14814-14818.
71. Han, S. and A. Brunet, *Histone methylation makes its mark on longevity.* Trends Cell Biol., 2012. **22**(1): p. 42-49.
72. Brunet, A. and S.L. Berger, *Epigenetics of aging and aging-related disease.* J. Gerontol. A Biol., 2014. **69**(Suppl 1): p. S17-S20.
73. Studer, L., E. Vera and D. Cornacchia, *Programming and reprogramming cellular age in the era of induced pluripotency.* Cell Stem Cell, 2015. **16**(6): p. 591-600.
74. Moore, R.Y., *Suprachiasmatic nucleus in sleep–wake regulation.* Sleep Med., 2007. **8**: p. 27-33.

75. Silva, A.P., C. Cavadas and E. Grouzmann, *Neuropeptide Y and its receptors as potential therapeutic drug targets.* Clin. Chim. Acta, 2002. **326**(1): p. 3-25.

76. Aveleira, C.A., M. Botelho and C. Cavadas, *NPY/neuropeptide Y enhances autophagy in the hypothalamus: a mechanism to delay aging?* Autophagy, 2015. **11**(8): p. 1431-1433.

77. Botelho, M. and C. Cavadas, *Neuropeptide Y: an anti-aging player?* Trends Neurosci., 2015. **38**(11): p. 701-711.

78. Chiba, T., et al., *A key role for neuropeptide Y in life span extension and cancer suppression via dietary restriction.* Sci. Rep., 2014. **4**: p. 1-10.

79. Bakos, J., et al., *The role of hypothalamic neuropeptides in neurogenesis and neuritogenesis.* Neural Plast., 2016.

80. Zhang, G., et al., *Hypothalamic programming of systemic ageing involving IKK-[bgr], NF-[kgr]B and GnRH.* Nature, 2013. **advance online publication**.

81. Oeppen, J. and J.W. Vaupel, *Demography. Broken limits to life expectancy.* Science, 2002. **296**(5570): p. 1029-31.

82. Kolbert, E., *The Sixth Extinction: An Unnatural History.* 2014: A&C Black.

83. Pimm, S., et al., *The biodiversity of species and their rates of extinction, distribution and protection.* Science, 2014. **344**(6187): p. 1246752.

84. Pereira, H.M., et al., *Scenarios for global biodiversity in the 21st century.* Science, 2010. **330**(6010): p. 1496-1501.

85. Cox, R., *Environmental Communication and the Public Sphere.* 2015, Washington DC: Sage Publications.

86. Sagan, C. and R. Turco, *A Path Where No Man Thought: Nuclear Winter and the End of the Arms Race.* 1990, New York: Random House.

87. Hooke, R.L., J.F. Martín-Duque and J. Pedraza, *Land transformation by humans: a review.* GSA Today, 2012. **22**(12): p. 4-10.

88. Nelson, M., et al., *Using a closed ecological system to study Earth's biosphere.* Bioscience, 1993. **43**(4): p. 225-236.

89. Singh, H., *Green revolutions reconsidered.* 2001: Oxford University Press.

90. Evenson, R.E. and D. Gollin, *Assessing the impact of the Green Revolution, 1960 to 2000.* Science, 2003. **300**(5620): p. 758-762.

91. Laxminarayan, R., et al., *Antibiotic resistance—the need for global solutions.* The Lancet Infectious Diseases, 2013. **13**(12): p. 1057-1098.

92. Reisner, M., *Cadillac desert: The American West and its disappearing water.* 1993, New York: Penguin.

93. Savas, H.B., et al., *Medical doctors' perceptions of genetically modified foods.* J. Clin. Anal. Med., 2016. **7**(2): p. 172-175.

94. Rissler, J. and M.G. Mellon, *The Ecological Risks of Engineered Crops.* 1996, Cambridge, MA: MIT Press.

Index